THE FLOWERING OF A WARATAH

NEUROLOGY IN AUSTRALIA

A HISTORY

THE FLOWERING
OF A WARATAH

NEUROLOGY
IN AUSTRALIA
A HISTORY

MERVYN J EADIE

Australian Scholarly Publishing

First published 2000. Second edition 2024 by:
Australian Scholarly Publishing Pty Ltd
7 Lt Lothian St North, North Melbourne, Victoria 3051
www.scholarly.info / enquiry@scholarly.info / 06 3 93239 6963

ISBN 978-1-923068-74-2

Cover design Amelia Walker

CONTENTS

Illustrations

Figures

FOREWORD

It is a pleasure to write the foreword to the second edition of *The Flowering of a Waratah* whose lyrical name invokes the symbol of the Australian Association of Neurologists. The subsidiary title, 'A history of Australian Neurology and the Australian Association of Neurologists', conveys the scope of the book, and readers will that find both these topics are covered fully and carefully.

I have known Mervyn Eadie for almost 40 years, first as a medical student at the University of Queensland, later as a junior researcher in its Department of Medicine, and later as a colleague in the Department of Neurology at Royal Brisbane and Women's Hospital. Mervyn is softly spoken and hugely knowledgeable, with a tendency to reflection and is noted for his wise analysis of situations and quiet sense of humour. He is also well-known as a man of letters.

Mervyn is a pre-eminent Australian neurologist. For more than 60 years he has been a member of the Australian Association of Neurologists, which recognized his contribution by establishing the annual MJ Eadie award for Neuroscience. His medical research was focussed on epilepsy and pharmacology, but, fortunately for us, his other field of scholarship is medical history. In this volume, he has written the history of Australian neurology and the history of the Association of Neurologists. For many of these events, he was an eye-witness. He was personally acquainted with some of the Originators of the Association and in other cases was able to speak directly to neurologists who were colleagues of early Australian neurologists. This close relationship with the subjects is apparent throughout.

The first edition was written for the 50th anniversary of the founding of the Association. This new edition has been written as we anticipate the 75th anniversary in 2025. The Council of the Association formed the opinion that as the events relating to the founding of the Association become more remote, it is important that we have a record of our past, to provide perspective for the journey forward. The book has been thoroughly revised, with comments that reflect the passage of essentially another generation. For example, in reflecting on the Originators of the Association Mervyn has sought to emphasize the role of Leonard Cox, whose influence had possibly been under-rated recently.

The history of Australian neurology has been divided into three epochs-the early years when neurology did not exist as a speciality in Australia, the 20 year period around Word War 2, and the years since the 1960s. The history tells of the diseases and the doctors of those times, and the struggle to have neurology accepted as a stand-alone speciality. This is set against a wider discussion of the evolution of neurology as a speciality in Europe, the gradual divorce of psychiatry from neurology and the establishment of the 'canon' of neurology. These accounts are documented in detail, with reference to the early Australian medical literature. The book includes biographies, both of academics and those who were primarily clinicians, of interest to those of who like their history to be stories of people. Mervyn has some favourites such as AW Campbell, a renowned neurologist and neuro-anatomist, whose story is told in detail, and Hunter and Royle, who studied spasticity and whose lives ended in tragic ill-health.

The diseases mentioned in the book are diverse and fascinating, including such titbits as the story of the discovery of kuru and Murray Valley encephalitis. The book also benefits from Mervyn's longevity; writing one hundred years later about encephalitis lethargica in the 1920s, Mervyn is able to recount that 60 years ago he saw a patient with Parkinsons disease as a consequence of this dreadful disease. Such telescoping of history is impressive.

This establishment and subsequent doings of the Association seem to have been calm and uncontroversial. Mervyn emphasizes the intention of the originators that the group should be an Association of neurologists, with high standards required for membership. From the outset of the Association, when there were few members, there has been an emphasis on publication of its proceedings, and the ups and downs of the journals is described first-hand by Mervyn who was the long -serving editor.

The final chapter is a reflection on the development of neurology in Australia, considering how neurology came to be developed despite our small population spread over a large area, and our distance from Europe where neurology was developed much earlier, and benefits from Mervyn's experience and observations over many years.

As well as being a book to read, this volume is also a permanent record. There is an extensive list of references to the history of neurology, that will be of use to future scholars, and the Appendices include the names of office bearers, lists of Scientific meetings and contents of early Proceedings. It is of comfort to know that these are now preserved in a safe, publicly accessible book.

I am sure that members of the Association will find this to be a valuable volume. It is likely that future historians of neurology will find this to be an important record. ANZAN is pleased and thankful Mervyn has undertaken this task.

Pamela McCombe
Immediate Past President
Australian and New Zealand Association of Neurologists

FOREWORD
to the First Edition

The history of a group, an organisation or an association and even a nation confers both a sense of identity and of direction with which to meet and overcome future challenges. In May 1999 at the 90th meeting of the Council of the Australian Association of Neurologists it was determined that an important part of the celebrations to mark the first 50 years of the Association should be a compilation of its history, and that of neurology in Australia. It was also resolved to ask Professor Mervyn Eadie to undertake this task, a request that he accepted with gracious celerity. *The Flowering of a Waratah – A History of Australian Neurology and of the Australian Association of Neurologists* is the agreeable consequence. It comes at an important time in the history of our Association. Not only is original material still accessible, as are most of those members of the Association responsible for its nurture during its first decade and a half and for the seeding of neurologists around Australia, but the practice of neurology is changing fundamentally. Advances in imaging technology and molecular biology are expanding the therapeutic horizons rapidly to levels which would have been almost incomprehensible to the originators of our Association 50 years ago, and yet economic and litigious imperatives and a trend to dependence on so-called evidence-based clinical pathways threaten to constrain the present-day practice of neurology.

The Flowering of a Waratah is as much a testament to the author's own contribution to Australian neurology as it is a history of neurology in Australia. Mervyn Eadie's modest description of his first appointment to the position of 'junior' to John Sutherland, Senior Visiting Neurologist at the Brisbane General Hospital, and his subsequent academic position at the University of Queensland personifies his humble, self-effacing character that has endeared him to so many students and contemporaries. Graduating with honours from the University of Queensland in 1955 he became a member of the Australian Association of Neurologists in 1961 and since then has contributed significantly to Australian neurology at every level he has engaged. Aided by Professor John Morris from Westmead Hospital and Alice Boyce (from the Australian Association of Neurologists' Secretariat),

Mervyn Eadie has combined his natural percipience, ironic humour and immense experience gained over 40 years in active practice in neurology and neuropharmacology with his love of history to produce a wonderful account of the development of neurology in Australia. In doing so he has imbued it with that same crisp exciting readability which is born of an intimate and reverent knowledge of the topic and that mirrors the works of historians such as Sir Arthur Bryant.

Commencing with European settlement in Australia and the medical practitioners of that time, *The Flowering of a Waratah* traces the development of our specialty in Australia from its dependence on medical advances in Britain, Europe and North America to the present day where the high standards of clinical neurology and research are acknowledged internationally. The history not only expands on some of the personalities who have contributed to the present high international standing enjoyed by Australian neurology and some of the reasons for this reputation, including the Australian Association of Neurologists itself, but it also contains the records of membership and financial accounts and of papers presented to early scientific meetings of the Association. Important decisions and considerations of Council meetings, among which are the intriguing and recurring proposition of an independent College of Neurologists and the adoption of the Waratah insigne, are laced with personal and communicated insights into the reasoning of a particular decision or course of action.

The Flowering of a Waratah is a superbly detailed account of the history of neurology in Australia which will enrich the professional lives of future generations of Australian neurologists with a sense of `being', as they and the Australian Association of Neurologists continue to flourish.

W M Carroll
President
Australian Association of Neurologists
December 1999

PREFACE

In Melbourne, on a Saturday morning almost three-quarters of a century ago, four men sat down and resolved that a society should be set up to facilitate the development of the area of medicine in which each of them had a particular and continuing interest, viz. clinical neurology. The society that resulted came to be named the Australian Association of Neurologists, and its existence was formally inaugurated in 1950. To commemorate the 50th anniversary of its foundation, the Association decided that its own story should be recorded and set down in relation to the history of the overall development of neurology in Australia. The outcome was the first edition of this book. A little over two decades later, the Council of the Association, by now the Australian and New Zealand Association of Neurologists, considered that the time had come for the story of Australian neurology and its professional association to be brought up to date, taking in new material that had become available in the interval, and including some additional earlier historical information that had not been available at the time of the previous edition.

The *Shorter Oxford Dictionary* (1973) defined neurology as 'the scientific study or knowledge of the anatomy, function and disease of the nerves and nervous system'. However, in every-day contemporary medical usage, the word 'neurology' seems largely confined to the scientific study, management and understanding of *disease* of the central and peripheral nervous systems. In what follows, the word will be taken in this latter more limited sense, though Australian work in the basic neurosciences which has obvious bearings on such clinical neurology will be touched on.

The recorded history of neurology in Australia extends only over the little more than two centuries since 1788 during which Europeans have dwelt in the country. There seems to be no certain earlier information as to whether neurological illness existed among the indigenous inhabitants prior to then. Perusing the available records since European settlement suggests that the development of neurology in the country can be regarded as having fallen into three overlapping stages.

The first of these three stages spanned a potential maximum of some 150 years, extending almost to the eve of the 1939–1945 World War. During that first stage, with a single most notable exception, what scientific study there was of nervous system disease was carried out by medical practitioners who did not practise exclusively, or often even predominantly, in neurology. Such practitioners first became interested in, or found themselves by circumstances involved in, neurological problems, and were then able to contribute to knowledge concerning these problems before returning to the courses of their more usual professional activities. The solitary exception to this pattern might have been passed over swiftly, being regarded almost as an aberration, had it not been that the man who constituted that exception made a number of very significant scientific contributions to neurological knowledge during his long period of clinical neurological practice in Australia. Moreover, before that time, whilst working overseas, he had established for himself a formidable and enduring international reputation in the neuroscience of his day. Seen in relation to the state of the nervous system knowledge of his day, Alfred Walter Campbell was arguably the greatest neuroscientist his homeland has ever produced. His career, coming near the end of the first (i.e. the pre-neurologist) stage of Australian neurology, warrants separate and detailed consideration.

In the second comparatively short stage of the development of Australian neurology, beginning just before World War II, a generation of full-time practising clinical neurologists emerged. As mentioned, in 1950 they founded a professional association which has endured. In doing this, and by their other endeavours including, in the cases of some founding members, their research, they established the specialty of clinical neurology in the country.

The third stage of the development of Australian neurology began about 1960, and still continues. It has seen neurology grow in numerical strength and maturity of practice while achieving academic recognition in the Australian university system. Over the same period, medicine internationally has become increasingly aware of the general calibre of contemporary Australian neurology, as distinct from the achievements of one or two exceptional talents among its practitioners, which had been the case in the earlier stages of Australian neurological development.

The founding generation of neurologists had constituted the Australian Association of Neurologists in such a way that its members have been involved, at least to some extent, in nearly all the events that have involved neurological medicine in the country since the Association's inception. As a result, the history of the Association largely coincides, not only temporally but in substance, with the second and third phases of the evolution of Australian neurology. Further, the Association in its own right has undertaken a significant additional and continuously growing educational role. However, advances in neurological knowledge are not the exclusive prerogative of clinical neurologists, and discoveries about nervous system disease have continued to be made in Australia, as in earlier times, by those who were neither by training nor by mode of practice, neurologists, though some of them became Associate Members of the Australian Association of Neurologists.

The account that follows is largely arranged chronologically, in terms of the three phases of development mentioned above, though with further subdivision in places. At the time of writing of the present edition of this book, no member of the founding generation of Australian neurologists was still living. Some members of the succeeding generations have also died. The professional lives of these people, and their achievements, can be seen more or less as a whole, and appreciated in the context of their times and circumstances, as far as these can be known. Some of them had played obviously significant parts in the development of Australian neurology. Others, through professional careers of various lengths, had been diligent servants in caring for those whose illnesses they had been called to manage. However, throughout their years in practice they remained relatively inconspicuous outside professional circles and left behind few, or no, enduring and accessible records to facilitate any substantial account of their careers being provided. I can only apologise if details of the careers of such worthy men and women who others may have thought deserved recording have not been included in the present text.

When one turns to the lives and activities of those neurologists still living, whether they continue to play, or have finished playing, significant parts in Australian neurology, it becomes more difficult, and potentially more invidious, to try to form definitive assessments and then commit them to paper. Their stories may well still be quite incomplete. In some ways it would have been easier not to attempt to deal at all with those still living, but to do this would have resulted in substantial gaps in the account of the past three decades. The more recent record would then have been left so unbalanced that the whole account might have been better ended when the founding generation of Australian neurologists left the scene. On the whole, it has seemed best to try to deal with the achievements of living persons to the time of writing, but to set these achievements only in a contemporary and not in a more definitive overall perspective, and not to touch on the personal qualities of such people.

There is also a difficulty in referring to Australian neurology's professional association after 2006, when the Australian Association of Neurologists became the Australian and New Zealand Association. While the merging of the two associations largely formalised an already long-standing *de facto* situation, the expanded title of the Association might have created an expectation that this new edition should deal with the histories of both Australian and New Zealand neurology, but it does not attempt to deal with the latter. To try to avoid possible consequences of the expanded affiliation of the Association, I have tried, wherever possible, not to mention the names of the two countries involved when writing of Australian neurology's professional association as it existed after 2006.

The various difficulties referred to immediately above prompt confession to another limitation of this book – that it is written from within the Australian neurological community by one who has had immediate personal involvement in some of the events and knowledge of some of the people mentioned. Indeed, a number have been close and often long-standing friends. Consequently, there is a possibility that objectivity may at times have unwittingly been sacrificed to the influences of sentiment and emotion. However, attempting to totally eradicate the personal element would very probably remove some sense of immediacy from parts of the text and some details of significance might have been omitted. Hopefully, the reader will be conscious of such considerations and recognise that the book has been written very much from the perspective of one who is grateful to have lived out his professional life amid some of the matters recounted, and amongst some of the people involved in them.

I am very grateful to the Council of the Australian and New Zealand Association of Neurologists for inviting me to undertake both editions of this book, and for making the Association's records available to me. Mrs Alice Boyce, in the Association's office in Sydney, was unfailingly helpful in finding documents and seeking out information required for the first edition of the book. Her successor, Mrs Mandy Jones, with her long experience of the Association's affairs and activities, and her staff members, have been equally helpful, and receptive to requests for information that has facilitated the writing of this extended version of the story. Professional colleagues have been generous in answering queries and providing information, particularly John Morris in relation to the first edition, and those who provided him with the photographs of various Australian neurologists included in that edition. For the first edition of the book, I was also indebted to the late Dr Humphrey Cramond, at the time Honorary Curator of the Library of the Queensland Branch of the Australian Medical Association, for access to that Library's collection of early Australian medical journals, and to Brenda Heagney, then Librarian to the History of Medicine Library of the Royal Australasian College of Physicians in Sydney and to her successors for providing information and photographs. I am also indebted to neurological colleagues for photographs of some of their neurological predecessors who are no longer living and whose activities and achievements are mentioned in the present account.

In particular, I am grateful to my Melbourne based neurological colleague Richard Gerraty who undertook, on behalf of the Council of the Australian and New Zealand Association of Neurologists, the task of arranging the printing and other aspects of the publication of this book, and to Nick Walker and his staff at Australian Scholarly Publishing for their skilled transformation of an untidy and disorganised typescript into a handsome final product.

For the errors in the book, and for its infelicities, the blame is mine. In private compensation for exposing myself to the odium of being responsible for such shortcomings, I have had the quiet pleasure of experiencing a growing empathy with the past events and life of Australian neurology, in resurrecting memories of old friendships, and in possessing a confident hope for the future of Australasian neurological medicine.

MJE
November 2023

Chapter 1

PRE-NEUROLOGIST AUSTRALIAN NEUROLOGY

Neurological disease almost certainly existed in Australia well before European settlement of the country began in 1788. The earlier inhabitants left behind no enduring accounts of their illnesses, and the earliest surviving records come from a time when the notion of nervous system disease covered a somewhat different range of entities from that embraced by the current concept of neurology. Consequently, one can provide only a very inadequate and inevitably incomplete account of the earlier stages of neurology and neurological illness in Australia, though it is one that becomes more detailed as it approaches the time when the founding generation of professional clinical neurologists began to appear in the country in the 1930s and 1940s.

In possibly the first surviving record of neurological illness that had occurred in the country, Gandevia and Cobley (1974) described a death from probable neurological disease that occurred in 1791, only three years after the founding of the original Sydney Cove settlement, viz.

> *Case 5*. Probably either Robert Hogg or Peter Hubbert, a convict attending on Mr White [the Principal Surgeon], in passing from his house to the kitchen, without any covering upon his head, received a stroke from a ray of the sun, which at the time deprived him of speech and motion, and in less than twenty-and-four hours, of his life. The thermometer on that day [4 November 1791] stood at twelve o'clock at 94°...

Neither the ambient temperature, nor the duration of sunlight exposure, appears adequate to explain the event. A cerebral haemorrhage or, possibly, a massive cerebral infarction, seems more probable.

Epilepsy, lues and `locked jaw' were neurological illnesses that were mentioned in at least one `return' setting out the assigned causes of death in Sydney prior to 1800 (Watson 1911). In the more northerly convict settlement of Brisbane (founded in 1823), the Brisbane Hospital records of 1828 listed two admissions for paralysis and, in 1831, one instance of paralysis and another of hemiplegia (Jackson 1924). Among 170 admissions to that hospital in the two-year period 1840–1842 there were 5 diagnoses of epilepsy (Tyrer 1993).

The few early reports mentioned immediately above should be appreciated in the light of the state of then contemporary medical knowledge and medical practice. As mentioned earlier, when the original European settlement of the country began, the idea of `neurology' as a particular area of medical knowledge and practice had not yet appeared. The spectrum of organic disease of the nervous system, i.e. what was later to be considered the content of neurology, was in those days substantially different from what it subsequently became. In 1778, the first of the numerous editions of Samuel-Auguste Tissot's classic *Traité des nerfs et de leurs maladies* appeared. His account was based on a mixed classificational basis that involved both anatomy and concepts of pathogenesis. The text included, as well as chapters on epilepsy and migraine, a consideration of various disorders of `moral' causation, which today would be regarded as within the territory of psychiatry. In 1789, one year after the first European settlement of Australia, William Cullen brought out his *First Lines of the Practice of Physick,* a text that played a major part in the education of several future generations of English-speaking medical students. Cullen's classification of nervous system diseases, for which he coined the collective term `neuroses', was based on clinical phenomenology rather than on pathology or aetiology. Within his rubric of neuroses Cullen included entities such as palpitations, dyspnoea, asthma, whooping cough, pyrosis, colic, diarrhoea, diabetes, mania, melancholia and other insanities, but also disorders which would now be regarded as neurological. It was almost as if Cullen considered that nervous system disease involved the whole range of convulsive disorders that Thomas Willis in 1684 wrote about in his *Pathology of the Brain and Nervous Stock*, many of the neurological disorders Willis dealt with in his *De Anima Brutorum* (1683), and as well almost every conceivable disorder in which visceral motor overactivity occurred in the absence of detected macroscopic pathology. To this array of illness Cullen threw in, for good measure, much of the content of present-day psychiatry as well as some general medicine.

THE 19ᵀᴴ CENTURY

Present-day neurology internationally began to gradually take on something approaching its current shape during the latter half of the 19th century. In what is generally considered the first neurology textbook of modern times, Romberg's *Manual of the Nervous Diseases of Man* (1851), a symptomatic approach to classification similar to that employed by Cullen was used. Consequently, the disorders described included a number of what would now be regarded as non-neurological conditions. However, Abercrombie (1828) had earlier in the 19th century provided a reasonable and logically more satisfactory account of many neurological disorders classified on a basis of demonstrated pathology. In contrast to Romberg's text, by 1871 Hammond in the United States, when writing on nervous system disease, employed a classificational schema largely based on pathology. The text of Hammond's monograph is relatively easily related to the content of present-day neurology. Similarly, Gowers in the first edition of his great two-volume *Manual of Diseases of the Nervous System* (1886 and 1888) employed a classificational approach not unlike that in use today, one based mainly on a mix of aetiology and pathology. The disorders discussed in Gowers' text are reasonably similar to those to be found in many modern-day textbooks of neurology. The psychiatry, and the visceral functional disorders included by the earlier authors, had all but disappeared. Somewhere between 1850 and 1870 the issue of what disorders were to be regarded as neurological and what were not, seems to have been mostly settled, probably largely by informal and mainly unvoiced consensus. The present-day canon of neurology thus became determined at about the time when the present-day specialty of neurology began to emerge in Britain and Western Europe and, around 1860, began to assume the status of a recognisable area of specialised medical practice. What later became the National Hospital for Nervous Diseases in Queen Square, London, was founded in 1860 (Holmes 1954; Anonymous 1960), while J-M Charcot was appointed to the world's first Chair in Neurology in Paris in 1882, at the Salpêtrière, where he had commenced the teaching of neurology 20 years before (Guillain 1959). Despite these events in Europe and Britain, there was to be a delay of another six or seven decades before clinical neurology came to be generally recognised as a medical discipline in Australia.

Nonetheless, in the 19th century, some contributions to neurological knowledge were made on Australian soil. The contributors were not acknowledged neurologists, and for the most part practised mainly in other areas of medicine, or in medicine more generally. Many of their neurological contributions were essentially opportunistic, and occurred when neurological illness manifested itself in ways which were peculiar to Australian conditions. There were also a few contributions that were deliberate attempts to grapple with neurological problems that had more global impacts. Relative to the situation in the northern hemisphere, the delay in the emergence of neurology as such in Australia was probably largely determined by the comparatively short existence of European culture in the country, and by geographical and economic factors. Communications between distant places in those times were relatively slow and difficult, and Australia was a long way from the large European centres where neurology had begun to declare its existence. As well, the substantial distances between major population centres within Australia, and its relatively small though growing total population, resulted in considerable delay before any given locality could accumulate the critical mass of patients capable of supporting the specialised activities of even a single neurologist.

From here on, the present chapter attempts to deal with the neurological work that went on, and the neurological discoveries of some significance that were made between 1880 and the eve of World War II by those who were not self-declared neurologists. It also touches on the few men in the Australia of those times who, at least for a period in their professional lives, seem to have had a major interest in neurological disease, However, it excludes Alfred Walter Campbell, who was a very great neuroscientist relative to the standards and expectations of his times, and who is dealt with separately in the next chapter.

During the years prior to World War II, when communication between Australia and Europe or North America was relatively protracted and could be rather uncertain, Australian medicine maintained an awareness of overseas knowledge, trends and advances, though its own research tended to be published in its local medical journals. This was probably largely due to publication delays if papers were submitted to overseas journals and to the potential uncertainties in maintaining communication with overseas-based journal editors. The *Medical Journal of Australia*, which first appeared under that designation in 1914, and its predecessors, the Melbourne-based *Australian Medical Journal*, which existed from 1856 to 1895, and reappeared between 1910 and 1914 (seemingly being replaced in the interval by the *Intercolonial Quarterly Journal of Medicine and Surgery*

[1894–1896] and the *Intercolonial Medical Journal of Australasia* [1896–1909]), together with the Sydney-based *Australasian Medical Gazette* (1881–1914), seem to have played a proportionately greater educational and local professional news dissemination role than later became the case for medical journals of Australian origin. Perusal of the contents of the old journals yields something of the flavour of the medicine of the time, with its heavy dependence on British, and to a lesser extent Western European and North American, medical thought. A very significant portion of the papers published in Australia on neurological topics in those times provided thorough and contemporaneous reviews of matters which should have held considerable educational value for the Australian medical community but they made no claim to break new ground based on original Australian research achievements. However, such review-type publications sometimes did happen to contain, almost incidentally, details of their authors' personal experiences, or described small clinical experimental studies that had been carried out or mentioned original ideas relevant to the topics being considered. The latter type of review thus included the sort of material that more-recent writers are likely to have made into the main themes of research-type papers, the educational matter relating to the topic simply providing the background to the new information rather than dominating the publication. As a result, accounts of Australian neurological research are sometimes to be found in the old journal articles that seemingly were intended mainly for educational purposes. Nevertheless, it would seem that, after reading enough of the material published in those now distant times, at least in the inter-war period, one may gain the impression that younger specialists, probably in the process of building up their practices after returning from overseas training, sometimes attempted to enhance their local reputations by publishing ostensibly educational material which, as a side issue, tended to testify to the author's clinical expertise. The old literature sometimes also contained observational-type research regarding new or unusual disease behaviour, itself often the outcome of peculiar local circumstances. Virtually no deliberate programs of experimental studies were reported before Royle and Hunter's investigations in the 1920s that will be considered in some detail later in this Chapter.

The old Australian medical journals also included numerous case reports which fell into two classes. Some were formal accounts of individual unusual cases or of small collections of cases. These accounts sometimes contained some discussion of the topic, but often merely reported the case details only, and read as though the material described had been presented at local medical meetings and almost simultaneously submitted to the journal for publication. Others were brief reports of local medical meetings at which interesting cases had been presented. These reports do provide a precis of the case description and sometimes of the related discussion. This affords the present-day reader some idea of the level of local medical knowledge, even though no formally developed consideration of the topics had appeared in print. Such material, though interesting to read, breaks no new research ground, but it gives some indication of the local pattern of disease as it occurred at various times.

Such material provides the basis of the following account of Australian neurological knowledge, thought and discovery that existed in the period before those dedicated to clinical neurology began to become part of the medical community in the country.

AUSTRALIAN NEUROLOGICAL KNOWLEDGE AND PRACTICE

In the years prior to, and soon after World War I, the authors of neurological articles and reports in the pages of the *Medical Journal of Australia* and its immediate forerunners usually did not quote references at all extensively. If they quoted them, they usually did set not them down in much detail. It was not unusual for a substantial paper to contain no, or almost no, references. When reference to authoritative sources was considered necessary, the works most frequently cited were the contemporary editions of Osler's textbook, or Gowers' *Manual of Diseases of the Nervous System* (the first volume of the earliest edition of which had appeared in 1886, and the second two years later). When any original publications from the literature were cited, they were usually of British or German origin, at least until after World War I. Later, works such as Kinnier Wilson's *Modern Problems in Neurology* (1928) seem to have become influential, and the references cited increasingly suggested a considerable familiarity with the international literature.

The range of neurological conditions discussed in the Australian journals in the latter part of the 19th century and in the earlier part of the 20th differed from that which would be expected in today's journals, mainly in that infectious diseases of the nervous system received substantially more emphasis, cerebral vascular disease, notably stroke, was almost totally ignored, and therapeutic aspects were less often mentioned. In the inter-war period, the types of neurological disorder reported increasingly took on a pattern similar to that of more recent years, with the exception of the late 20th century addition of HIV-related syndromes. Work with greater scientific emphasis increasingly tended to be published internationally rather than locally. The enormous therapeutic progress after World War II resulted in the virtual elimination of neurosyphilis and poliomyelitis, and a great reduction in the menace of bacterial meningitis and other forms of intracranial suppuration, all of which had received frequent mention in the literature of earlier years.

Over the 60 years prior to World War II, as judged from the contents of the local medical publications, one can find trends in matters that the Australian medical community must have regarded as being of interest and importance.

Headache

Until after World War I, in the Australian journals there was very little discussion of the general topic of headache, which subsequently became the bread and butter of clinical neurological practice. The systematic account of headache given by McWhae in 1924 did not involve nearly as much emphasis on migraine as might have been expected, tension headache as such was not mentioned, nor was cluster headache under that name or any of its acknowledged synonyms. There was more attention given to ocular and nasal sinus headache than would now be the case. In 1934 an Adelaide ophthalmic surgeon, Barham Black, published a thoroughly competent account of migraine and discussed the various contemporary theories of its pathogenesis and treatment. The account would not have seemed particularly out of date two decades later, but there have been great changes since that time. There was also some observational research on migraine mechanisms which will be discussed later. Ergotamine was recommended, sometimes in a rather distant manner, for the treatment of attacks of the disorder, but there seemed little awareness of the possibility of employing preventative drug therapy.

Trigeminal neuralgia was well recognised before the turn of the century, though at least one published description of it reads more like an account of cluster headache (Hawkes 1903). By 1910, Campbell (see later) was treating trigeminal neuralgia by the injection of alcohol into the main trigeminal nerve or into one of its branches. Later, Clark (1937) recommended a course of action for the management of the disorder, beginning with the exclusion of any local source of sepsis and the use of simple analgesics in milder cases, then butylchloral hydrate with gelsemium, followed by the inhalation of trichlorethylene for severe paroxysms and finally, if relief had not already been achieved, by injection of the Gasserian ganglion. In his opinion, injection of the trigeminal nerve or of its peripheral branches was to be avoided. As early as 1893, O'Hara had reported surgical curettage of the Gasserian ganglion to relieve the condition.

Epilepsy

The Australian writings on epilepsy from quite early times showed an awareness of the entity of Jacksonian motor seizures. Until much later, on the whole there seemed little appreciation of the implications of Hughlings Jackson's (1870) insights into the nature of epileptic seizures, and into the implications that his concept of localisation of function in the cerebral cortex held for the understanding of the epileptic seizure process. Springthorpe, of Melbourne, was one exception to that generalisation. In 1886 he plainly indicated his acceptance of Jackson's interpretation of the process of epileptogenesis. In the following year he (Springthorpe 1887) put the matter in slightly more forcible terms than Jackson probably would have chosen – the main pathological state in epilepsy was: 'An over-explosability of the cells in the cortical layers of the brain.'

Springthorpe seemed to take a particular interest in epilepsy, and in 1888 referred to his collection of 50 cases of the disorder.

There seemed perhaps less emphasis on the idea that epilepsy was idiopathic, or a disease in its own right, than was the case in contemporary Britain, and more ready acceptance that convulsions were an epileptic phenomenon. Angel Money (1896), in Sydney, argued that all distinctions between epilepsy, convulsions, eclampsia, epileptiform and epileptoid seizures should be subsumed into the general term `cerebral paroxysms'. In his account of epilepsy, Youngman (1942), in Brisbane, quite obviously accepted the local origin of epileptic seizures in the brain but did not seem to think through the further implications of this. He was aware of the electroencephalographic changes reported to exist in different types of epileptic seizure. Later this same author (Youngman 1949) seemed to take the position that there was an intrinsic underlying tendency to experience seizures in those with epilepsy, that this tendency was developed to different degrees in different sufferers, and that there was a great variety of potential seizure-provoking factors. Therefore, in his understanding epilepsy could be a symptom with a number of possible causes. Nevertheless, there was always an underlying intrinsic tendency to have seizures in those who suffered from such epilepsy. Such an interpretation seems to have been the result of deduction or intuition on Youngman's part rather than a product of actual analysis of data.

From at least several years prior to 1873 (Smith 1873), bromide had been the mainstay of antiepileptic therapy, particularly in the case of major rather than minor epilepsy (Hawkes 1905), though the use of chloretone (chlorobutanol) was advocated by Bentley (1911, 1912). Borax was reported to have been successful in an instance where bromide therapy had failed (McAdam 1895), but the agent did not become popular. Bentley (1911) summarised the then contemporary situation regarding the treatment of epilepsy thus: 'The greatest optimist must admit that the treatment of epilepsy is in a thoroughly unsatisfactory condition.'

To some extent the therapeutic situation improved with time. 'Luminal' (phenobarbitone) came into use a little after Bentley's sceptic view was published, and seems to have been regarded as more effective than the various bromide salts. By 1942, Youngman was clearly familiar with the use of phenytoin ('Dilantin'), which had become available overseas only two or three years previously. By 1947 troxidone ('Tridione'), now long superseded, was used for the treatment of *petit mal.*

Trepanning of the skull was carried out in quite early times in Australia for epilepsy associated with depressed fractures of the skull (Maund 1856; Whitcomb 1862), in the latter case successfully, at least in the short term.

Cerebral Vascular Disease

Stroke and other cerebral vascular disorders were relatively neglected matters in the Australian literature until after World War I. This apparent neglect probably did not arise from ignorance, but because such disorders were already well enough known and there had been no diagnostic or therapeutic advances in relation to them over many years. Reeves (1861) had written on 14 cases of corpus striatum softening encountered amongst 113 instances of brain softening, and expressed the view that such softening was not always due to ischaemia. Robertson (1881) described two instances of stroke, simply from the point of view of their phenomenology. Interestingly, as early as 1906, Mc Donald had adduced physiologically-based arguments against attempting to reduce the arterial blood pressure after cerebral haemorrhage. Dawson's (1937) discussion of cerebral arteriosclerosis tended to be orientated towards its role in producing higher level cerebral function disorder rather than stroke. By 1938, de Crespigny's account of cerebral vascular disease read much as a latter-day one might, except that syphilitic vascular disease would no longer merit mention, there would be more emphasis on disease of the posterior circulation, and there would not be such paucity of therapeutic options.

Cerebral aneurysm and subarachnoid haemorrhage received little attention until the inter-war years, though Williams (1881) had briefly described the autopsy features of a ruptured posterior inferior cerebellar artery aneurysm. Before the introduction of lumbar puncture, it was difficult to diagnose the occurrence of subarachnoid bleeding during life, and recognition of cerebral aneurysm in the living had to await the advent of angiography, shortly before World War II. When Graeme Robertson (1936) described his case series of intracranial aneurysms, he stated that no diagnosis of cerebral aneurysm had been made at the Melbourne Hospital prior to 1929, but that he was aware of 31 instances of ruptured cerebral aneurysms at the Hospital subsequent to that date. Cleland, a year later (1937), reported 19 instances of small aneurysms on the circle of Willis or its branches that had been encountered in 3670 autopsies carried out in Adelaide. All but two of these aneurysms were not associated with the occurrence of subarachnoid haemorrhage.

INFECTIONS

Syphilis

From quite early times a good deal was written concerning syphilis as it affected the nervous system (e.g. Jamieson 1895-6; Morgan 1920; Minogue 1926), particularly general paresis of the insane, and tabes dorsalis. Stoller and Emmerson (1969) published a description of the history of general paresis of the insane in Victoria, based on their survey of mental hospital records. The first possible instance they traced dated back to 1859, more than a decade before the designation 'general paresis' came into use. They noted that this particular diagnosis had first been recorded in 1867 and was made frequently after 1872.

There was a good deal of interest in the malarial treatment of general paresis in the 1920s and 1930s (Ellery 1926; Dawson 1928) and soon afterwards in its treatment by electrically-induced fever (Prior 1937). In reviewing the treatment of neurosyphilis, Cox (1949b) indicated that penicillin was beginning to supplant the older agents (mercury, arsenic, bismuth and potassium iodide). In that same year, Susman (1949) vigorously extolled the virtues of penicillin in treating neurosyphilis, and expressed the opinion that arsenic and bismuth therapy had become obsolescent.

Meningitis

Bacterial, mainly meningococcal, meningitis (often called 'cerebro-spinal fever') occurred sporadically (Hood 1902), and also in epidemics in Australia (Fairley & Guest 1915; Cleland 1916; Calov 1940), while instances of tuberculous meningitis were reported. In the period 1938–1940 there was a small flurry of publications attesting to the efficacy of the newly available sulphonamides in treating various forms of bacterial meningitis (Anderson and English 1938; Robinson 1939; Hamilton 1940a; Lowe 1940). Soon after that, Milroy and Hughes (1945) reported on the cure of pneumococcal meningitis by injected penicillin, and in the next year Turner (1946) described that antibiotic's effectiveness in childhood purulent meningitis.

Sawers and Thomson (1935) reviewed four previous Australian reports of torula (cryptococcal) meningitis, the first dating back to Swift and Bull (1917), while adding a fifth instance of the disorder. Soon after, de Crespigny (1944) devoted a Rennie Memorial Lecture to the topic of torula meningitis and two years later Cox and Tolhurst (1946) published a monograph dealing with the subject.

Encephalitis and Myelitis

There were also outbreaks of viral encephalitis at times in Australia. These will be discussed separately later in this chapter, because of their particular local interest. Aseptic meningitis did not seem to be diagnosed as such during the times under consideration, possibly because any instances that were recognised were categorised as non-paralytic poliomyelitis. The latter disorder had occurred in epidemic form in some of the years under consideration and will also be discussed below.

Rabies

Rabies has never been an appreciable problem in Australia, because of the effective quarantine practices that have operated. However, Crowther (1946) described a set of events which had occurred in Hobart long before his time, and which raised the spectre of the dreaded disease. Crowther's account, based on reports in the local newspapers, deserves to be read in its entirety, partly for its discursive charm. In January 1867, a boy in Hobart was bitten on the lip by a half-bred spaniel. One month later, the boy became ill with symptoms suggestive of rabies, and died within a few days. The dog, which also died soon afterwards following further wayward behaviour, had in the interval bitten two other citizens. There was consternation, and a period of anxious waiting for the whole local community, to say nothing of those bitten, until it became apparent that neither of the bitten persons had become ill. In retrospect, Crowther thought the boy had died of tetanus, but the majority of the local medical profession at the time of the events was convinced that he had suffered from rabies.

BRAIN TUMOURS

Cerebral tumour was not a prominent topic in the old Australian medical literature, though there were isolated reports of interesting cases, suggesting that the disorder did not go unrecognised, e.g. Robertson (1860). Quite soon after the initial overseas reports of the successful surgery of cerebral tumour, beginning with Macewen in Glasgow in 1879, there appeared accounts of isolated craniotomies carried out for cerebral tumours in various parts of Australia, sometimes even in rural areas. For instance, in 1892, Parry in rural New South Wales had operated unsuccessfully on a cerebral hydatid cyst in a 9-year-old boy. Rudall (1859) had earlier demonstrated the presence of such a cyst at autopsy. Syme (1895), in Melbourne, reported the successful removal of what almost certainly was a meningioma. Harold Dew, later Professor of Surgery in the University of Sydney, in 1922 reported an operative series of 85 cerebral tumour cases, 55% of them gliomas. In the 1930s, there was a considerable increase in the amount written about cerebral tumour in Australia, much of it from the pens of Leonard Cox (see Chapter 3) and the initial generation of Australian neurosurgeons, e.g. Gilbert Phillips, Rex Money and Douglas Miller, whilst Dew (1936) returned to the topic and reviewed the biology of the meningiomas in a Bancroft Oration.

INVOLUNTARY MOVEMENT DISORDERS

Parkinsonism

Curiously little was written of Parkinson's disease during the earlier part of the period under consideration, though the disorder was recognised (Huxtable 1892a). Parkinsonism followed in the wake of the Australian epidemic of encephalitis lethargica (see later) but seemed to arouse no especial local interest. The treatment of Parkinson's disease in those times comprised various agents with anticholinergic properties (Hughes 1940). Interestingly, in 1948 the Sydney neurosurgeon W Lister Reid reported favourable results in 15 patients from what was considered an experimental procedure, the surgical excision of Brodman's cerebral cortical area 6.

Chorea

When Stawell (1915), at a medical meeting in Melbourne, expressed the belief that he had provided his hearers with the first description of Huntington's disease occurring in a patient in Victoria, psychiatrists in his audience promptly announced that there were other cases to be found in Victorian mental institutions. Jones (1917) described a Tasmanian family affected with the disorder. Brothers (1964) traced the history of the disease in Tasmania and Victoria to a family of Huguenot origin which had emigrated to Tasmania from Somerset in the west country of England as long before as 1842 (Brothers gave the date as 1848, but it was subsequently corrected by Pridmore in 1990). Brothers did not make it clear whether this was the same Tasmanian family reported earlier by Jones (1917). The first instance of the disease in the family had been recognised in 1878. It is perhaps of some interest that there was no record of Huntington's disease in the convicts shipped to Australia in earlier times.

Sydenham's chorea was known in Australia in the latter half of the 19th century (Jamieson 1873), and its relationship to rheumatic fever recognised

(Williams 1937). Fulton (1879) had used injections of curare to try to relieve choreic movements.

Wilson's Disease

There were a few reports of clinically recognised progressive lenticular degeneration (Swift 1917; Macdonald 1927; Minogue 1927). Most of these lacked any indication of the presence of a similar disorder in the affected person's family. Often the clinical details appeared insufficient to sustain the diagnosis that had been made.

DEMYELINATING DISEASE

Frith (1988) has provided a careful account of the history of multiple sclerosis in Australia up to her time of writing . As long ago as 1875, Newman had discussed the disorder of multiple sclerosis in the pages of the *Australian Medical Journal* under its no longer used designation of `insular sclerosis`. However, he described no Australian case. In retrospect, on the basis of the details published, the clinical diagnoses of the earlier reported Australian instances of what was then termed insular or disseminated sclerosis often appear quite uncertain (e.g. Huxtable 1892b; Officer 1903). Nevertheless, a pathologically-confirmed instance of the disorder was described by Flashman and Latham in 1915. As early as 1886 James Jamieson, of Melbourne, had reported two instances of unusual peripheral neuritis, in the second of which he had initially thought the diagnosis was that of disseminated sclerosis. Frith, with some justification, pointed out that his initial diagnosis appeared a great deal more probable than the designation under which the case was published. Until the mid-1920s, reports such as those of Griffiths (1922) and Maudsley (1925) seemed not to reveal any appreciation that the clinical diagnosis of the common relapsing-remitting form of the disorder depended heavily on evidence that the disease that was present had affected multiple different areas of the central nervous system at different times as it ran its course. By 1926, that insight seemed to result in increased numbers of the clinically probable disease being described (Hurley 1926; Maudsley 1926; Sewell 1926; Johnston 1927). However, the formal clinical diagnostic essentials were not acknowledged as such at the time.

Cox *et al.* (1949) carried out a therapeutic trial of anticoagulation in an attempt to prevent worsening of disability in multiple sclerosis. The rationale for the treatment lay in the idea that intracranial venous thrombosis was causally related to the demyelination of the disorder. The investigators concluded that the treatment was ineffective. By present-day standards, their trial design was deficient, and no proper statistical analysis of the results was carried out.

Pathologically proven diffuse sclerosis was reported in Australia by De Crespigny and Woollard (1929) and by Holmes à Court and Latham (1935), and there was a clinically diagnosed instance reported by Flynn and Greenaway (1935). Just prior to, and during World War II, E Weston Hurst, in Adelaide, with various co-workers, described instances of various types of demyelinating disease, whilst Hurst himself described the new entity of acute haemorrhagic leucoencephalitis (Hurst 1941a, b). Hurst's experimental work is discussed later in this chapter.

TROPICAL NEUROLOGICAL DISORDERS

There were Australian reports of uncommon neurological disorders that are not often encountered in more temperate climates, e.g. tick-bite paralysis (Cleland 1912; Eaton 1913), to be discussed further a little later in this book. In the earlier part of the period under consideration, certain common tropical diseases tended to go unrecognised in Australia. Those who practised medicine in the country in those days often had been trained in Europe or in Britain, or later in Melbourne (which produced the first Australian medical graduates). In these places, medical students were unlikely to gain much experience of tropical diseases. When graduates from these overseas and temperate zone climates began to practise in Australia and first came across instances of certain tropical diseases, they were not familiar with the disorders and therefore failed to diagnose them. This was particularly so in the case of leprosy.

Leprosy

In Australia, leprosy appears to have first been encountered in Chinese seamen in the country's seaports, and in Chinese and Polynesian immigrants. After a time, it was also recognised among Aboriginal people in northern Australia. Thompson (1898), in his review of the history of the disorder in Australia, stated that it had not occurred in Aboriginals until 1892, when an instance was noted at Maryborough, in Queensland. Possibly leprosy-affected persons from tropical countries to the north of Australia had made their way into the country other than through the seaports and had then come in contact with Aboriginals and transmitted the infection to some of them. Creed (1889) stated that there were no known lepers in Australia in 1856, apart from 13 in Victoria. By his time of writing there were still 5 in Victoria, and 10 in New South Wales, but none in South Australia or Tasmania. He could not obtain figures for Queensland. Creed also stated that there was only one European among the leprosy sufferers, in keeping with what Shields (1889) wrote:

> In reference to the prevalence of leprosy in Australia, the disease is, with few exceptions, confined to the Chinese. It is known in one case only, and that in New South Wales, to infect a European. In Victoria there are five lepers (all Chinese) in the leper camp at Point Nepean.

However, Joseph Bancroft, of fame for his discoveries in relation to filariasis, wrote in 1892 of how, when he had first taken up duty in the old Brisbane Hospital in 1868, he had failed to recognise leprosy in a patient of German origin. Bancroft indicated that information in earlier Brisbane Hospital records suggested that there had been an even earlier, but unrecognised, instance of the disease in a patient of Chinese origin who had been admitted to the Hospital as early as 1855. Somewhat in contrast to these figures concerning the rarity of leprosy in persons of European origin, an Editorial in the *Australasian Medical Gazette,* in 1892, stated that there were 8 affected white persons in New South Wales, all of whom were detained in lazarets.

Because in earlier years, it had been widely and reassuringly accepted that leprosy in Australia was to be found only in Asian immigrants and in persons of South Sea island origin, there was some consternation when the first instance of the disorder occurred in an Australian-born citizen of European descent. By 1926 there were 16 persons in the lazaret of the Coast Hospital in Sydney, and a total of 13 white lepers in New South Wales, 51 in Queensland, and two in Western Australia, but none in the remaining three States (Molesworth 1926). Sufferers from leprosy were quarantined in lazarets situated well away from the unaffected general community and kept there for the remainder of their lives unless, as occasionally appeared to happen, spontaneous cure occurred. That situation continued until the advent of sulphone therapy after the end of World War II.

Beri beri

Instances of beri beri neuritis were reported in Asian seamen, and in Chinese immigrants in Melbourne in 1888, and in Sydney from 1890 onwards (Graham 1893; Paton 1894). As was the case for leprosy, the nature and cause of the polyneuritic disorder was not recognised for a time.

MISCELLANEOUS NEUROLOGICAL DISORDERS

In the later part of the 19th century and the decades around the turn of the century the case reports which appeared in the pages of the *Medical Journal of Australia* and its precursors the *Australian Medical Journal,* the *Australasian Medical Gazette* and the *Intercolonial Medical Journal* included instances of many neurological conditions which would even today be regarded as uncommon, thought of interest to the general medical readership. Further, the clinical details of the descriptions as published suggest that the diagnoses made usually would withstand the scrutiny of modern knowledge. There were, for instance, reports of myasthenia gravis (Hogg 1906), polyneuritis, which often probably was the Guillain-Barré syndrome, which was not well recognised until after the end of World War I (Crago 1890; Thomson 1898; Mills 1919), Duchenne muscular dystrophy (Smith 1871; Jamieson 1894), myotonia congenita (Fleetwood 1889; Campbell 1919), epiloia, i.e tuberose sclerosis (Lind 1924), paramyoclonus multiplex (possibly simply a severe Janz syndrome – Verco 1912), Leber's optic atrophy (Pockley 1915; Hogg 1915, 1928; Moriet 1921), carotido-cavernous fistula (Gibson 1896, 1905), Friedreich's ataxia (Stawell 1895; Spark 1897; Litchfield *et al.* 1917), Marie's cerebellar ataxia (largely equivalent to what was later termed olivo-ponto-cerebellar atrophy – Morris 1908), amyotrophic lateral sclerosis (Howson 1918; Murphy 1924), geniculate zoster (Findlay 1933), post-herpetic neuralgia (Marten 1897), subacute combined degeneration (Evans 1925), diabetic pseudo-tabes (Bostock 1926), diptheritic paralysis (Jamieson 1883), arsenical neuritis (Hughes 1927), meralgia paraesthetica (Rennie 1902) and congenital word blindness (Macleod 1920).

There was no record of botulism in the country until 1942, when two outbreaks occurred, both associated with eating canned beetroot (Gray 1948).

As well as the reports of unusual and interesting disorders, new treatments of real value came into use at times. Thus Leonard Cox (1938a) wrote on the effectiveness of injected neostigmine in relieving the manifestations of myasthenia gravis. At an earlier stage, ephedrine and potassium chloride had been used to manage the disorder. At much the same time, neostigmine was also tried, and allegedly provided benefit, in certain forms of myopathy (Taylor 1938).

NEUROLOGICAL INVESTIGATIONS

Over the period under consideration, various ancillary investigations became available to assist in the diagnosis of neurological disorders, and the recognition of certain conditions during life became possible by virtue of these investigations.

Radiology was available in Australia from quite early times. Within a few months of the announcement of Rontgen's discovery in 1895, Balls-Headley (1896) in Melbourne described the use of X-rays to demonstrate a needle buried in a girl's foot. Clendinnen (1897) reported the use of the technique to display the cranial blood vessels at post mortem. In the following year Hopkins (1898) gave an account of Clendinnen's use of the technique to locate a bullet within a living patient's brain.

Whilst it was not necessarily for the first time in Australia, a lumbar puncture for cerebro-spinal fluid examination had been carried out in Victoria in 1907 (Stoller and Emmerson 1969), more than a decade after the procedure was first described by Quinke (in 1891). Later, an interest was taken in the chemical composition of the cerebro-spinal fluid, notably its protein content (Phillips 1937) and in its Lange colloidal gold reaction (Buchanan 1937), which in those times was considered important in the diagnosis of neurosyphilis. John Fullarton Mackeddie (1868–1944), Physician to In-Patients at the Alfred Hospital in Melbourne, who played a very influential part in the foundation of the Baker Institute (Kennedy 1944), wrote of the technique of cisternal puncture in 1926, and of myelography (using `lipiodol') injected via the cisternal and the lumbar routes in 1927, 1929 and 1931. Edye (1926) of Sydney, independently described the technique of cisternal puncture. Ventriculography, originally described by Dandy in 1918, was the subject of reports by Noble and by Monson, both of whom described the same patient from Sydney, in 1926. Pneumoencephalography was described by Buchanan, of Sydney, in 1929, though there are intimations that Leonard Cox, in Melbourne, had used the technique earlier. The Adelaide neurosurgeon, Leonard Lindon, in 1936 published an account of cerebral arteriography using `Thorotrast' as the contrast medium This was some 6 years after Moniz had first described his work with the investigational technique.

In 1939, almost a decade after Berger had described the possibility of recording the electrical activity of the human brain, the Sydney neurosurgeon Gilbert Phillips wrote of the electroencephalographic abnormalities found in epileptic seizure sufferers, and the psychiatrist N V Youngman did likewise soon afterwards (1942). On the basis of their accounts, it is difficult to know whether they were already using the technique in Australia when their papers appeared. Geoffrey Trahair (1910–1950) a psychiatrist who died young and who was the first acknowledged electroencephalographer in Australia (Phillips 1951), made it clear that an electroencephalograph had been in use in Sydney in the hands of Phillips and A K McIntyre (Trahair 1950) as early as 1941 or 1942 (Trahair and Garvan 1948), and that no similar apparatus was available elsewhere in Australia at the time.

In general, in the years before World War II there appears to have been a lag of some 5 to 10 years between the time when a new neurological investigational technique was reported overseas, and when the first accounts of its use in Australia appeared. Of course, it is possible that the method in question may have been employed earlier somewhere in the country, but that use is not recorded in a present-day accessible source.

RESEARCH INTO TOPICS OF GLOBAL RELEVANCE

Spasticity and its Attempted Surgical Relief

The first deliberate and sustained effort in Australia to investigate a neuroscience question of international significance, and at the same time provide a therapeutic benefit for patients, occurred in the Department of Anatomy of the University of Sydney in the third decade of the 20th century.

The attempt originated from a finding in a serpent and, like a much earlier biblical event which was reportedly instigated by a serpent, produced enticing prospects which culminated in disaster. The more recent story can be pieced together from a series of papers which began to appear in the *Medical Journal of Australia* in 1924 and 1925, and later in two obituaries published in the same journal, and in a formal biography of one of the participants, John Irvine Hunter (Blunt 1985).

In 1879 Tchiriew had discovered two types of nerve ending in snake muscle, the familiar motor end plates in which myelinated fibres from anterior horn cells terminated, and a new type of ending, *terminations en grappes* (Hunter and Latham 1925). The nature of the latter endings, and their functional significance and relation to the sympathetic nervous system, became a controversial matter, particularly as knowledge of nerve and muscle physiology accumulated, largely stimulated by Sherrington's work in Britain. In a series of papers from 1909 onwards, the Dutch histologist Boeke produced evidence that skeletal muscle possessed a double innervation comprising both myelinated and unmyelinated fibres. The unmyelinated fibres ended in the *terminations en grappes* and were of sympathetic origin. Others disagreed with this interpretation. The members of the Department of Anatomy at Sydney University became interested in the matter and J T Wilson, who had held the Challis Chair of Anatomy at that institution for some 30 years, subsequently published a major review dealing with the question. A Sydney orthopaedic surgeon, Norman Royle (Birkett 1944), who had previously been a Demonstrator in Anatomy in Wilson's department, took up the problem of spasticity and its possible treatment. Royle began to do experimental work on spasticity in the Department of Anatomy. Around 1920, a young medical student of exceptional ability and energy, John Irvine Hunter (Anonymous 1924), born in 1898, was also working in the Department as a Prosector in Anatomy whilst completing his medical course. Hunter almost certainly became aware of Royle's work on the anatomical background to spasticity somewhere around this time. Hunter, patently possessed of some considerable measure of genius, although still a medical undergraduate, had already carried out a number of experimental anatomical studies. After he graduated in Medicine from the University of Sydney (in March 1920), he was almost immediately appointed Demonstrator in Anatomy. Shortly afterwards he became Associate Professor of Anatomy in the University.

In 1920 Wilson was appointed to the Chair of Anatomy at the University of Cambridge and resigned his post in Sydney. The University of Sydney did not replace him immediately, but arranged for Hunter to spend time overseas, parts of it in Wilson's department in Cambridge, parts with Grafton Elliott Smith, a Sydney graduate of an earlier day who was by then Professor of Anatomy at University College, London, and additional time with Ariens Kappers at Amsterdam. In these places Hunter carried out further anatomical research, including a study of the fore-brain of a kiwi which earned him a Doctorate of Medicine from Sydney. He then returned to Sydney in 1923, and at the early age of 25 became Wilson's successor in the Challis Chair of Anatomy. He brought back with him to Sydney a slide that Kuchinsky in London gave him. This slide demonstrated the dual innervation of python muscle. Hunter also brought back the knowledge that Kuchinsky had concluded that the myelinated and unmyelinated nerves in muscle never ended on the same muscle fibre. Hunter seems to have seen a possible application for Kuchinsky's conclusion in the investigation that Royle continued to pursue in relation to the basis of spasticity in what had now become Hunter's department.

At that time there was a school of thought which considered that muscle tone involved two elements, contractile tone and plastic tone. If there was a double innervation of skeletal muscle, and two different types of nerve fibre termination (one originating from anterior horn cells, the other part of the sympathetic nervous system) and two separate classes of muscle fibre, it was not unreasonable to hypothesise that the anatomical background to the two types of tone might lie in this double innervation. It was already well established that division of the fibres emanating from anterior horn cells would produce paralysis, but would section of the sympathetic fibres alter tone in a clinically useful way? Hunter and Royle began to collaborate. Royle produced spasticity in experimental animals by spinal cord section, and later by decerebration, and then studied the effects of previous or subsequent sympathectomy on the spasticity produced by the earlier surgery. Royle became convinced that the surgery did reduce the spasticity in his experimental animals. Meanwhile Hunter apparently carried out some experimental studies of his own on fowls and embarked on a program of histological studies on the innervation of muscle in conjunction with Oliver Latham (whose career is discussed later).

Royle reached a stage in his research where he felt justified in carrying out sympathectomies on two patients with spasticity. He convinced himself, and provided cinematographic evidence sufficient to satisfy others, that their disability from spasticity was reduced by the surgery. The work was presented at a meeting of the New South Wales branch of the British Medical Association held in the Anatomy Department of Sydney University on 23 October 1923, and subsequently was published (Hunter 1924a; Royle 1924a). A very distinguished visitor was present in the audience – Sir William Macewen, Regius Professor of Surgery in the University of Glasgow, perhaps the greatest innovator in all the history of surgery, the founding father of neurosurgery and the first man to ever successfully remove a diseased whole human lung. Macewen, a shrewd old man, as judged from the precis of his comments reported after the presentation, was a little hesitant to commit himself too enthusiastically about the discoveries and seemed rather to try to skirt around the issue. However, Hunter's youth and transparent genius, the obvious practical implication of Royle's surgery and its potential benefits for neurological patients, and the fact that, for the first time, Australian research appeared to have produced an outcome of international significance, combined to have a major impact in local medical circles. The printed report of the meeting seemed to catch the spirit in which the research appears to have been appreciated in its home environment (*Medical Journal of Australia* 1924, p 98):

> Dr R Gordon Craig, in thanking Dr Royle and Professor Hunter for their splendid demonstration, said that the Medical School at their University was emerging from its infant into its adult life. ... Formerly they had been content to depend for their scientific information on the researches conducted in the old world. Now they had among them men who were able to contribute to knowledge.

A little later the results of Royle's surgery also produced a very considerable impression on a delegation of visiting American surgeons, including William Mayo. This resulted in Hunter and Royle being invited to travel to New York in October 1924 to deliver the J B Murphy Lecture to the American College of Surgeons and thus provide a vehicle for making their findings more widely available. Before they did this, they had presented further relevant material at a regional meeting of the British Medical Association at Lismore in northern New South Wales (on 12 April 1924). There Royle (1924b) largely confined himself to extensive details of the surgical operations he was carrying out to divide the grey rami of the sympathetic trunk. However, he mentioned that he had performed additional successful operations since the two described in his initial communication some months previously. Hunter (1924b) gave a very long and competent account of the relevant background literature concerning the procedure and briefly described some experimental observations of his own concerning the effect of sympathectomy on the wing posture of the fowl. In the same issue of the *Medical Journal of Australia* in which the meeting details were reported, he also provided comments on the anatomy relevant to Royle's operative procedure (Hunter 1924c). One cannot but wonder whether an audience which presumably comprised mainly local general practitioners may have been rather overwhelmed by the amount and depth of the scientific data provided for their edification. From the material published to this point, one might have gained the impression that Hunter's role had been largely to stimulate and facilitate Royle's work and to explain its theoretical background in anatomy and neurophysiology with great lucidity. But in the meantime, Hunter had been carrying out histological research in conjunction with Oliver Latham, as mentioned above (Hunter and Latham 1925), though this work did not appear in print until after the events to be recounted below. The conclusion to Hunter and Latham's paper summarised their findings:

> As far as our work goes these two types of nerve terminations *en grappes* and *en plaques* do not exist in the same muscle fibres but each supply separate groups and we have found little evidence incompatible with the theory that these striped musculatures are divided into alternate groups of muscle fibres served respectively by branches from the somatic and sympathetic nervous systems...

Thus they considered they had established the microscopic evidence which provided the rationale for the procedure of sympathectomy in the treatment of spasticity.

After their presentation to the American College of Surgeons in New York, Hunter (not long married) and Royle travelled to Britain. There the lecture Hunter had been invited to give in London had to be cancelled because the young man had become ill. He died in University College Hospital on 10 November 1924, just before the lecture had been due to be delivered. At the time, it was believed he had contacted enteric fever and had died from it. However, in Boston, Royle also became ill and remained so for long enough to prevent his contributing to the tributes to Hunter which were paid by his senior colleagues at the University of Sydney during the ensuing weeks (*Medical Journal of Australia,* 10 January 1925). Royle was later able to return to work, remained productive and carried out further sympathectomies for spasticity and other disorders, e.g. retinitis pigmentosa (Royle 1930, 1932), and for what he had diagnosed as disseminated sclerosis (Royle 1933). He also carried out some experimental neuropharmacological work, using ephedrine to reduce spinal cord oedema which he postulated caused anterior horn cell injury in acute poliomyelitis (Royle 1935), and engaged in various experimental physiology studies (Royle 1937). Sadly, Royle's career came to a premature termination for, from 1930 onwards, he began to develop manifestations of post-encephalitic Parkinsonism. When this became known, speculation arose, at least among the members of Hunter's former Department in Sydney, that both Hunter and Royle had contacted encephalitis lethargica whilst in America, where the disorder was then still occurring. It was suggested that Hunter had died in the acute phase of the illness, whereas Royle had experienced a mild initial illness, but later developed its delayed, progressive and debilitating extrapyramidal consequences.

Thus the whole splendid endeavour to relieve spasticity ended in disaster for those intimately involved in it. For Hunter, the disaster was immediate, but spared him the realisation that his work was invalid and his conclusions incorrect. For Royle, the disaster was more delayed and protracted, and possibly compounded by the realisation that he had survived long enough to become aware that neither aspect of the work for which such high hopes had been held, the neuro-anatomical findings on which it had been based, and the surgical treatment, had proved sustainable or consistently reproducible in the hands of others. As early as 1926, in the face of criticism of Hunter and Royle's work, Editorial comment in the *Medical Journal of Australia* (1926) found it desirable to mount the argument that failure of a surgical procedure to provide an expected benefit did not necessarily prove that the rationale for the procedure was invalid. Royle (1927), seemingly wounded by criticism of his results and of their theoretical basis, including that from the neurophysiologist E D Adrian (subsequently Lord Adrian, and a Nobel Laureate), threw down the challenge that no one else had done sympathectomies in goats, the species in which he had obtained his experimental relief of spasticity. In Melbourne, Tiegs and Coates (1928) rejected that defence by their failure to show that sympathetic ramisection in goats altered limb posture, the knee jerk or the tension in the tendo archilles. Their report triggered correspondence from Royle (1928), supported by A W Campbell (1928a), which tried to explain the discrepancies in the findings of the two groups of workers. Gradually, it became established that, although unmyelinated sympathetic nervous system fibres went to skeletal muscle, they there innervated blood vessels and not skeletal muscle fibres. In addition, the future Sydney neurosurgeon Gilbert Phillips (1931), working in the Anatomy Department of Sydney University, established that the sympathetic nervous system was not the source of the efferent limb of the reflex subserving posture maintenance.

Why Royle's operations should have appeared to relieve spasticity is unclear. It was suggested that it was the post-operative physiotherapy rather than the surgery which produced the benefit, for Royle had been a physical education teacher before he studied medicine and was interested in the application of physiotherapy. However, Royle countered by pointing out that the benefit from the operation was present even on the first post-operative day. Only some years after his original work with Hunter, did Royle (1933) finally acknowledge the correctness of the investigation to be described immediately below. This showed that there was no sympathetic innervation of voluntary muscle. However, Royle (1937) then took recourse in ascribing the relief of spasticity produced by sympathetic ramisection to the improved spinal cord circulation which the procedure produced, mounting an argument that the faster local circulation gave oxygen less time to act in the spinal cord so that neuronal function tended to be suppressed. His was obviously a physiologically untenable explanation. Perhaps Royle's surgery, in avulsing the grey rami communicantes of the sympathetic trunk (for he avulsed the rami rather than simply dividing them), disturbed the function of gamma efferent fibres or even those arising from alpha motor neurons. Interestingly, Royle's early account of the surgery (Royle 1924a) mentioned muscle twitchings in the leg on the sympathetomised side after the operations, suggesting that motor nerve fibres had been affected by his procedure. The long-term outcomes of Royle's own surgery do not appear to have ever been reported in detail. Unfortunately, before making their results public, neither Hunter nor Royle appears to have examined Royle's experimental animals to see what damage to neural structures had been produced by the surgery. Underlying their concept seems to have been the assumption that, because there were unmyelinated nerve fibres in muscle, and unmyelinated fibres in the sympathetic nerves which went to muscle, the two sets of unmyelinated fibres were the same fibres.

Despite its imperfections and its ultimate abandonment, the work of Hunter and Royle was a courageous and imaginative attempt to deal with a very significant global medical problem. Hunter, who was widely admired for his personal qualities and became something of a contemporary local idol because of his enormous talents and already considerable scientific attainments, was to be transformed into a figure of almost legendary statue in the memory of the Sydney School of Medicine. The fact that he and Royle were ultimately proven incorrect was largely lost sight of in the regret evoked by awareness of the unfulfilled promise of a life of genius so prematurely and abruptly cut off. Herbert John Wilkinson (1891–1963), the foundation Professor of Anatomy in the University of Queensland (Hickey 1963), had been a medical student in Hunter's Department during the latter's brief period in the Challis Chair of Anatomy. After his own graduation, Wilkinson became a member of the academic staff of that Department. In later life, Wilkinson spoke of Hunter to his own students and conveyed almost a sense of reverence and hero worship. Yet long afterwards, one of Wilkinson's own former junior colleagues in the Queensland Department of Anatomy, Geoffrey Kenny (1988) published information which he must have received through his contacts with Wilkinson. This information produced the insight that a third, though much lesser, calamity emanated from the Sydney work on the dual innervation of muscle, and that the victim of that latter calamity was Wilkinson himself.

After Hunter's death Wilkinson, as a young academic in the Sydney Department of Anatomy, had taken up, almost by inheritance, the question of the double innervation of skeletal muscle. After very careful and detailed investigation in Sydney and overseas he came to the definite conclusion that the sympathetic nerves which entered muscle supplied the blood vessels only, and not the muscle fibres themselves (Wilkinson 1929). Thus he found himself in the situation that, in the pursuit of truth, he had come to erode, as it were from within, a major part of the intellectual edifice on which rested the fame of the local hero and idol John Irvine Hunter. It must have been a very difficult realisation for Wilkinson, and also for his colleagues in the Sydney Department of Anatomy, and in the University more largely. Moreover, it involved Wilkinson in an ongoing controversy with Boeke, so that it was quite a number of years before the essential correctness of the former's views became generally accepted. Wilkinson's subsequent academic career was made away from Sydney, first in Adelaide from 1930 as Elder Professor of Anatomy, and then in the University of Queensland from 1936 to 1959, where he seemed to be almost at pains to avoid mentioning to students the major role he had come to play in correcting Hunter's mistake.

Thus, in the end, Sydney men came to correct the earlier error of Sydney men, and the first Australian systematic research into a major neuroscience problem ultimately produced a valid and scientifically sustainable outcome, though one disappointing in terms of the earlier high expectations. However, the man who first obtained the correct answer received (and indeed seemed to expect) far less fame than the earlier investigators who drew mistaken conclusions and yet who, through the intervention of fate, became the heroes of a seeming catastrophe. Yet it was a catastrophe which had the effect of heightening Australian consciousness of, and pride in, the capacity and promise of its medical science. Interestingly, and almost as an accidental by-product of the endeavour, according to Greenwood's (1967) interpretation, Royle's operation had opened up the possibility of sympathetic trunk surgery instead of peri-arterial sympathectomy, for the relief of vasospastic disorders.

Poliomyelitis and Sister Kenny

The occurrence of poliomyelitis in epidemic form was noted in the latter part of the 19th century in the Australian medical literature, and in the first half of the 20th century there were a number of well-documented outbreaks of the disorder during the Australian summers (e.g. Ham 1905). The disease came to be greatly feared in the community. The advent of the injected Salk vaccine in the latter 1950s, and of the oral Sabin vaccine a little later, completely transformed the situation. It is now only the surviving members of an aged generation in the country who can recall the anxieties that their parents experienced each summer, fearing that their children might contract the dreaded `infantile paralysis'.

Australia neurology, and indeed Australian medicine, had little or no notable impact on knowledge of the biology or treatment of poliomyelitis. However, one Australian woman, Elizabeth Kenny, brought about a transformation in the management of the disorder, and in the quality of life of those who were handicapped by it, or were in immediate danger of being so (Macnamara 1953).

Elizabeth Kenny was born in 1880 and lived out much of her life in country towns in south-east Queensland and northern New South Wales. As a young woman she found her way into the nursing profession through rather informal means. After joining the Army Nursing Service during World War I she was ultimately promoted to the level of nursing sister, and thereafter was usually referred to as Sister Kenny. In the post-war years she worked as a nurse in small country towns on the Darling Downs in Queensland. There she found her own way to an original approach to treating the disability of poliomyelitis (and also that of spasticity). From an early stage in the illness, she replaced the conventional initial therapeutic inactivity, or the use of immune serum in the pre-paralytic phase (Macnamara 1929), and the subsequent immobilisation of limbs, and the splinting (Vickers 1921; Clubbe 1925), with massage, the application of heat, and rather intensive passive and active exercises. As time passed, she found increasing support for her methods in the general community. Local people became convinced of their efficacy, and she also received support from some local medical men, though the majority of the medical profession was opposed to her methods which were condemned by a Queensland Royal Commission in the mid-1930s.

Elizabeth Kenny appears to have been a woman of some considerable strength of character and inner conviction, and her attitudes hardened in the face of medical opposition to her approach. The story of the struggle has been told, from the standpoint of one who had access to the Queensland Health Department records, by Ross Patrick (1985). With growing local community and some medical support, and State government backing, clinics utilising Sister Kenny's approach to the management of poliomyelitis were opened in certain cities in Queensland. The State Government gave her an introduction to health authorities in the United States of America and there, after some delay, her methods were taken up on a much larger scale than in her homeland. Gradually she became a famous and revered public figure in the United States, whose President at the time, Franklin Delano Roosevelt, had been partly crippled by poliomyelitis earlier in his life.

By the time of her death in 1952 it seems to have become fairly generally accepted that Sister Kenny's methods were more successful than those which they had displaced. In contrast, her novel ideas of the pathogenesis of poliomyelitis, viz. that the disability in the disorder was due to viral damage to peripheral tissues, were recognised as scientifically unsustainable. Her fame may have rested on a false theoretical premise, but she had empirically, and by the strength of her personality and conviction, very significantly improved the outlook for many afflicted by a crippling neurological disorder. From an international community viewpoint, Elizabeth Kenny would probably appear the most famous figure concerned with neurological disease ever produced by Australia, though from a more scientific standpoint that assessment could scarcely be sustained.

INVESTIGATIONS INTO PECULIARLY AUSTRALIAN DISORDERS

Childhood Lead Poisoning

At the third session of the Intercolonial Medical Congress of Australasia held in Sydney in 1892 one of the papers presented was entitled 'Notes on lead poisoning as observed among children in Brisbane'. There were five authors, of whom the first named was J Lockhart Gibson. The purpose of the presentation was to report an unusual event, the admission to the Hospital for Sick Children in Brisbane in the first seven months of 1892 of ten instances of lead poisoning. The dominant feature of the poisoning was reported to be the gradual onset of a reasonably bilaterally symmetrical paresis of the distal muscles of the limbs with the development of wasting of the affected muscles. The weakness usually began in the lower limbs. In half of the cases, before the development of the paralysis, there were attacks of abdominal pain usually accompanied by vomiting and, in two of the cases, convulsing. Lead was found in the urine of the two children in whom its presence was sought. Such a disorder had not previously been recognised among children in Brisbane, though the authors of the presentation confessed that they might have failed to make the true diagnosis on occasions in the past. Further cases continued to occur in Queensland and additional communications concerning the matter appeared in the local medical literature. It became clear that the clinical spectrum of the disorder was more extensive than the original description had suggested. In particular, an encephalopathic presentation was recognised, dominated by the manifestations of intracranial hypertension. A possible example had been reported in the June 1891 issue of the *Australasian Medical Gazette,* a case of acute ophthalmoplegia with double optic neuritis, the latter term being used for what would later be termed bilateral papilloedema. The author of the report was F Antill Pockley, a Sydney ophthalmic surgeon, and the patient was a six-year-old girl brought to him in 1888 with the rapid onset of total blindness. When living in Brisbane five weeks previously, she had developed sudden abdominal pain and persistent vomiting. Two weeks later a temporary squint appeared, and on the next day she had a convulsion. Further convulsions and screaming fits occurred and it was realised that the child had become blind. When examined in Sydney, she had severe bilateral papilloedema, almost total loss of external eye movements, and was completely blind. Intellectually she was normal and there was no other abnormality on examination. Afterwards there was some return of eye movements and the papilloedema was replaced by bilateral optic atrophy. This was perhaps the first recorded example of a type of case history which became commonplace in Brisbane over the next few years, but in this early instance the possibility of lead poisoning was not considered. Similar events in Brisbane were first reported as instances of `localised basal meningitis' (Gibson *et al.* 1892). By 1897 it had become clear to Turner and Gibson that the entity represented by this diagnosis was an expression of lead poisoning (Turner 1897).

In the *Medical Journal of Australia* for 11 February 1922 the Council of the Queensland Branch of the British Medical Association endorsed a report in which the unnamed authors described in some detail the course of the Queensland outbreak of childhood lead poisoning up to that time (Anonymous 1922). By 1908 some 262 instances of lead poisoning had been admitted to the Hospital for Sick Children in Brisbane (Turner 1908). At this time, 20 new cases a year were appearing, and affected children had been referred from various Queensland towns as well as from Brisbane. Later a series of cases was reported from Townsville in North Queensland

(Breinl and Young 1914). From 1917 to 1926, no fewer than 428 children with lead poisoning were admitted to the Brisbane Hospital for Sick Children, whereas over the same period there were only 4 such admissions to the Royal Alexandra Hospital for Children in more populous Sydney, and 3 to the Melbourne Children's Hospital (Nye 1933). Coincident with these events, there had been no outbreak of lead poisoning in Australian adults, the few instances which occurred being explained by industrial exposure, particularly that occurring at the mining town of Broken Hill. The clinical picture recognised by 1908 involved more than the abdominal symptoms and muscle atrophy which featured prominently in the initial report. There was greater emphasis on convulsions, which were termed eclampsia after the then contemporary use of that word, and on the encephalopathic pattern of presentation of the poisoning mentioned above with its headache, papilloedema, and bilateral abducens palsies, going on to blindness. At lumbar puncture, the intracranial pressure was raised (Gibson 1912). Also, the presence of anaemia and transitory albuminuria was mentioned, with the possibility of chronic interstitial nephritis as a rare complication, though the passage of time proved the latter to be far from rare (Nye 1933).

The interest in this relatively localised outbreak of lead poisoning did not lie so much in the matter of diagnosis, which became clear enough early on, but in why so many cases should occur in Queensland children but not in Queensland adults or in children elsewhere in Australia. Because the symptoms lessened or disappeared when the affected children were hospitalised, and might recur after they returned to their homes, it seemed likely that the lead exposure occurred somewhere in the domestic environment (Turner 1897). Originally it was suggested that the affected children had chewed the tin foil which was used for the wrapping of various sweets and cigarettes (Turner 1897). However, there was never adequate evidence to sustain this hypothesis. The next possibility raised was that the children had drunk water which contained lead. At the time, the roofs of Queensland houses were often made of galvanised iron which was fixed to the underlying roof timbers with lead-headed nails. Rain water from the roof was collected into galvanised iron tanks for domestic use, and it was thought that Queensland children might have been exposed to lead from drinking this water. This might have explained why Queensland children, but not children from more southerly parts of Australia, where iron roofing was less common, developed lead poisoning. It did not explain why their parents and often their siblings escaped. At one stage the Queensland Government Analyst did report the presence of lead in the water from galvanised iron tanks, but this finding was later found to be due to analytical error. What proved to be the probable cause of the lead exposure was first suggested by Turner in 1899, but then forgotten until it was resurrected by Gibson in 1904. The proposed mechanism was as follows, in Turner's (1908) words:

> Nearly all the dwellings in Queensland are built of wood, and in the towns the wood is covered by paint, consisting largely of white-lead. Exposed to our hot summer sun, this paint rapidly weathers, and becomes reduced to a powdery condition. This is particularly noticeable on verandah railings. The verandahs are favourable playgrounds for young children, who clasp the railings with their moist hands, which become covered with poison. Thence it finds its way to the child's mouth, especially in children who suck their fingers or bite their nails.

This putative mechanism was never fully established by rigorous scientific proof and the controlled studies which would satisfy later standards of medical evidence. Nonetheless, the Queensland medical profession was convinced by the circumstantial evidence. The gravity of the situation justified launching a publicity campaign to educate the public, to ban the use of lead paint, particularly on the external surfaces of dwellings, and to have such paint removed if present, or covered over. The pages of the *Medical Journal of Australia* of 11 March and 1 April 1922 contain a deal of rather acrimonious, though courteous, correspondence between Dr S. A. Smith of Sydney and a number of members of the Queensland Branch of the British Medical Association in Australia. The controversy centred on the source of the lead exposure, though it spilled over into other areas. Smith had sought a higher level of scientific proof of lead ingestion than was available. Nevertheless, Queensland Government action and legislation to the desired end followed, later in 1922. Thereafter the incidence of cases of acute lead poisoning gradually diminished and after some years the illness ceased to be a local medical problem. Unfortunately, residual consequences of lead exposure in earlier life continued to account for cases of chronic kidney disease in Queensland until after World War II.

Queensland childhood lead poisoning constituted a unique outbreak of neurotoxicity due to heavy metal exposure, which came about as a consequence of employing a European domestic practice in a tropical environment. The problem was investigated by those on the spot, and in time they came to understand its basis and produced an effective remedy for it.

Pink Disease of Childhood

Australian medicine in its pre-neurologist days made a significant contribution to world knowledge of another childhood disorder with neurological connotations. Unlike the situation with lead poisoning of childhood, where the novel features were the circumstance of occurrence of the phenomenon and the factors responsible for it, pink disease appeared to be a new phenomenon which was first described in Australia, though its true cause was ultimately determined by workers in other lands.

In 1914, Harry Swift, an Adelaide physician and paediatrician (Newland 1937), described a condition which he called 'erythroedema', a name he continued to advocate (Swift 1923) even when others preferred to call the disorder 'pink disease' or 'acrodynia'. Swift (1914) stated that in the previous two years he had seen 14 instances of a disorder in children aged between six and 15 months. The symptoms began with loss of appetite, restlessness, crying, fretting and sleeping poorly. After a few days their hands and feet became swollen and red, though they were cold and clammy to the feel. The skin of the palms of the hands became sodden and tended to desquamate. Swift noticed the resemblance between the appearance of the fingers and hands and that found in patients with peripheral neuritis. The muscles, particularly the larger ones in the limbs, became wasted and hypotonic. Movement became slow and prolonged effort could not be sustained. The prognosis in all cases proved to be favourable. Recovery after hospitalisation occurred slowly over a period of months. Diagnostically, Swift remarked on the affinities between the disorder and peripheral neuritis, but also recognised that there were certain differences. He concluded that the disorder was 'an intestinal toxaemia giving rise to an angio-neurosis', without explaining the basis of his pronouncement.

At the time of Swift's account, the disorder was thought to be a new disease, though Littlejohn (1923) noted that there had been anecdotal reports of the same condition in Australia over the three decades previous to his own time of writing. Clubbe, of Sydney, had coined the name 'pink disease' for it. After Swift's report, there were additional published descriptions of the disorder both from Australia and overseas. In 1931 a monograph by Rocaz appeared and two years later was translated into English by Wood, who had reported further Australian cases from Melbourne in 1921. Rocaz believed that the first description of the disorder had been given by a German physician, Selter, who had named it 'tropho-dermatoneurosis'. However, Rocas acknowledged the important role of the Australian physicians in making the condition known in the world literature, though the subsequent flood of publications concerning the disorder came mainly from Europe and the United States. McDonald (1933) provided a competent account of knowledge of the condition in the *Medical Journal of Australia,* and discussed the postulated aetiologies, indicating that none appeared satisfactory. Penfold *et al.* (1932), at the Baker Institute in Melbourne, had searched unsuccessfully for a bacterial cause of the disorder. Later there were suggestions that a fungus growing on cereals, a virus (whose nature was unspecified), or vitamin B1 deficiency was responsible. However, Southby (1940) reverted to favouring a viral aetiology for the disorder (Clements 1940). A decade later, Cheek (1950) and Cheek and Hicks (1950) in Adelaide found evidence of hyponatraemia in children affected by pink disease. They considered that the disorder was due to adrenal deficiency. A year after that, Williams *et al.* (1951) in Melbourne failed to confirm Cheek's findings. In 1960, Clements published Australian hospital admission data for cases of pink disease and also Australian and British mortality data for the disorder. Both the incidence and the mortality had declined from the early 1950s onwards. For practical purposes the condition disappeared after various lines of evidence established that it was a toxic effect of mercury contained in teething powders given to children. Once the practice of using these powders ceased, and the powders themselves became unavailable, the disorder disappeared from medical notice. Although the laboratory work which established the presence of excessive levels of mercury in affected children was carried out overseas, it is of some interest that Clements (1960) mentioned that Bancroft, of Brisbane, in 1881 had reported to the local Board of Health that he 'sees many children brought to death's door from the parents dosing them with a powerful powder of mercury', whilst Evans (1931) in discussing the differential diagnosis of pink disease, commented 'Lastly, the blame may be laid at the door of the homely old-fashioned tooth in its process of eruption', words more prophetic than was realised at the time.

Thus the Australian role in the understanding of this now extinct peripheral neuropathy of infancy was essentially that of the clinical observation of new phenomena, though it was observation on a comparatively large scale and it brought the disorder to international notice. There was also a continuing, though ultimately unsuccessful, Australian attempt to determine the disorder's cause.

Australian 'X' Disease

In 1917, again in 1918, and also in 1925, outbreaks of what appeared to be a novel viral encephalitis occurred mainly in northern and western Queensland and in western New South Wales. The disorder came to be known as 'X' disease, though it was sometimes referred to in the literature as the 'mysterious' disease. A number of reports of local outbreaks appeared in the *Medical Journal of Australia,* and it was studied in the laboratory first by Breinl in Townsville and later by Cleland and Campbell in Sydney, who after the outbreak published overviews of the events. The disorder occurred at a time when the pandemic of encephalitis lethargica had been occurring in the northern hemisphere (from 1915 to 1926), and this inevitably at first led to suspicion that this disorder had also appeared in Australia (Wilson 1918). However, from the old records, and from subsequent events, it is quite clear that 'X' disease was not encephalitis lethargica, though the latter did occur in Australia, but appeared later than in Europe and North America. There was no significant Australian contribution to research on encephalitis lethargica as such. In contrast, the investigation of 'X' disease, which appears not to have been recognised elsewhere in the world at the time, was entirely in Australian hands throughout. More or less synchronously with 'X' disease, an influenza pandemic (the Spanish or black 'flu') was raging in Australia and elsewhere, but this does not seem to have led to difficulty in recognising the simultaneous presence of an Australian outbreak of encephalitis. It may be easier to deal with Australian 'X' disease after first describing the Australian experience of encephalitis lethargica.

Encephalitis lethargica

The first recorded instance of encephalitis lethargica in Australia, at least along its eastern seaboard, appears to have occurred in Tasmania in May 1919. It involved a soldier who had returned from service overseas in World War I (*Medical Journal of Australia* 1: 204, 1920). Shortly after, in the same year, there was a series of reports of the disease from Victoria (Downing 1919; Stawell 1919, 1920, 1923; Wilkinson 1920). Until 1923, further cases occurred in that State. In New South Wales 35 cases were admitted to Sydney Hospital in 1922 and 1923 (Holmes á Court 1923) and other cases were described (Smith 1920; Mills 1922). Revisiting the situation a little later, Collins (1928) stated that 50 instances of encephalitis lethargica had been admitted to the Royal Prince Alfred Hospital, Sydney, between 1919 and 1927, with 9 deaths occurring. Latham (1934) reported that he had received for examination in his laboratory in Sydney 80 brains from persons with encephalitis lethargica. The earliest reports from Queensland came from the Ipswich area, a little way west of Brisbane, where in May 1922 some 31 cases of an acute encephalitis had been seen in the previous few months (Trumpy 1922). Mathewson (1922) considered that some of these cases resembled clinically the instances of 'X' disease he had seen a few years earlier. However, some of the cases had clinical findings which made encephalitis lethargica more likely, and Cleland (1923) believed that this disorder accounted for the Ipswich outbreak. From personal experience of patients with post-encephalitic Parkinsonism seen more than 60 years ago, it would seem that there were instances of encephalitis lethargica in nearby Brisbane at much the same time as in Ipswich, and for two or three years afterwards. According to Cleland's (1923) evidence, the State of Victoria bore the brunt of the Australian outbreak of encephalitis lethargica. This outbreak did not occur synchronously with 'X' disease, and the geographical distributions of the two disorders differed. Encephalitis lethargica tended to appear mainly in the more populous areas, whereas 'X' disease occurred in more sparsely populated North Queensland and in rural areas along the Darling River basin. Moreover, Parkinsonism tended to develop after a time in those who became ill with what was often regarded as influenza at the time when local cases of encephalitis lethargica were occurring, whereas with one exception Parkinsonism did not occur as a sequel of 'X' disease. The exception was reported by Burnell (1922) in a 7-year-old girl in Broken

Hill in south-western New South Wales, whom he had earlier diagnosed as suffering from 'X' disease in 1918. Much later, serological evidence from patients with post-encephalitic Parkinsonism provided no evidence that the virus believed responsible for `X' disease had played a part in the aetiology of Australian Parkinsonism (Eadie *et al.* 1965).

The 'X' Disease Outbreaks

The first recognised case of 'X' disease was reported from Bourke, in western New South Wales, in 1917 (Litchfield 1917). Breinl, from the Australian Institute of Tropical Medicine in Townsville in North Queensland issued a preliminary report of a local outbreak of acute encephalitis one week later (Breinl 1917). Burnell (1917) reported 16 cases from Broken Hill and Cleland (1917) found a total of 57 (of whom 34 died) in the State of New South Wales in the 1917 outbreak. Breinl (1918) described a further 9 instances in Townsville, Anderson (1917) 14 at Goondiwindi in western Queensland near the New South Wales border which had occurred between February and May 1917, and there were said to be 17 childhood cases in Brisbane, in the extreme south-east corner of Queensland, after the end of March 1917, with a 65% mortality (Matthewson and Latham 1917). The outbreak of acute encephalitis lasted some four months, beginning in midsummer, reaching a peak in February and March, with cases ceasing to appear after May 1917.

In the following summer, the set of events was repeated in western New South Wales with cases being reported again from Broken Hill by Burnell (1918). Although fewer individual reports appeared in the local medical literature, when Cleland and Campbell (1920a) described the epidemiology of the outbreaks they were aware of a total of 134 cases in New South Wales. This suggests that another 77 had occurred in that State in 1918, again in the summer months.

Further cases were described in 1925 in Townsville (Baldwin and Heydon 1925) and in Broken Hill (Kneebone and Cleland 1926). Thereafter, for a generation, the disease in Australia disappeared from medical notice.

The Clinical Features

Clinically, the disorder behaved as a viral polioclastic encephalomyelitis. Cleland and Campbell (1920a) described it as follows:

The disease was abrupt in onset and severe. Children chiefly were affected (ninety-five cases) but adults did not escape (thirty-nine cases). General signs of cerebro-spinal irritation, namely, convulsions, rigidity, increased reflexes, mental obfuscation and loss of consciousness, accompanied by high fever, were the dominant features. Paralysis of voluntary muscles did not occur in more than one out of ten cases. Four and a half days was the average duration of the illness, and it was fatal in no less than 70% of cases, fatality figures which were more than double those of any recorded epidemic of acute poliomyelitis (infantile paralysis).

Breinl (1918) examined the cerebro-spinal fluid in several of his cases of 'X' disease and reported that it always appeared to be under normal pressure though it sometimes contained a mild excess of lymphocytes, or lymphocytes and leucocytes. It was always sterile on culture for the presence of bacteria.

The Pathogenesis

The main initial investigations into the nature of 'X' disease were carried out by Anton Breinl, at the Australian Institute of Tropical Medicine in Townsville, and by J Burton Cleland and Alfred Walter Campbell, in Sydney.

Breinl (died 1944) was an Austrian who had commenced a career in the investigation of tropical diseases whilst based in the School of Tropical Medicine at Liverpool. He came to the Townsville Institute as Director in 1911 and over the next decade carried out a number of studies into local and nearby tropical health problems. His life story, and that of his Institute, were described in some detail by Douglas (1977). Cleland at the time was Principal Microbiologist to the Department of Public Health, New South Wales. Later he had a very distinguished and productive career as Professor of Pathology in the University of Adelaide. Campbell, as mentioned earlier, was a very great neuroscientist whose career is described in the next chapter.

Breinl (1918) carried out autopsies on seven of his cases of 'X' disease and described histological appearances in their brains and spinal cords, mainly comprising perivenous cuffing with round cells, which he interpreted as being consistent with poliomyelitis. However, he recognised that the brain was involved more extensively than was usual in poliomyelitis. The pia mater might show leucocyte and round cell infiltration and the brain substance might contain pinpoint haemorrhages. Cleland and Campbell (1919) generally concurred with these findings but added the observation that changes in anterior horn cells were distinctly less frequent than in poliomyelitis.

Breinl (1918), and also Campbell *et al.* (1918), demonstrated that the causative agent in nervous tissue and cerebrospinal fluid was transmissible to monkeys by intracerebral inoculation, and in these animals produced an encephalitic illness. On this basis, and taken in conjunction with his clinical and histological data, Breinl concluded that the illness was a clinically aberrant form of acute poliomyelitis, though he was careful to point out the unusual severity of the brain involvement. In contrast, as they accumulated further evidence, Cleland and Campbell (1919) increasingly inclined to the view that the disease was a new and discrete entity. Not only was the course of the illness different from that of poliomyelitis, with a greater mortality and less hazard of residual paralysis, but histologically the damage to anterior horn cells was less severe, and the causative agent could be transmitted to species such as a sheep, a calf and a foal (Cleland and Campbell 1920b) to which the virus of poliomyelitis could not be transmitted. Thus the existence of a new viral encephalitis peculiar to parts of Australia was established.

Noting the geographical distribution of the cases in consecutive years, and the seasonal occurrence, Cleland and Campbell (1920a) gave thought to the mode of disease transmission to humans. In this paper they discussed the possibility of there being an animal reservoir of the virus, and of its human dissemination by travel along the Australian railway network. However, no firm conclusion was possible.

There, despite the 1925 cases, and Macfarlane Burnet's (1934) suggestion that the louping ill virus might have been responsible for the outbreaks, the story rested for a little over a quarter of a century, which takes the matter to just beyond the temporal confine imposed on the present chapter. Also, contrary to the notion that the present chapter deals with neurology in the hands of non-neurologists, an Australian neurologist, E Graeme Robertson, was involved in the later stages of the study of the matter, though not in the principal role. Despite these considerations, the events of 1951, and later, will be pursued here, albeit briefly, to complete the account of Australian 'X' disease.

Murray Valley Encephalitis

In 1951 an outbreak of acute encephalitis occurred in the Murray River valley in southern New South Wales and northern Victoria. Clinically and histopathologically, it behaved as an acute viral encephalitis and was recognised to resemble Australian 'X' disease (Anderson 1952; Anderson *et al.* 1952; French 1952; Robertson 1952; Robertson and McLorinan 1952; McLean and Stevenson 1954). By this time, much more sophisticated facilities for virological investigation were available in Australia, and evidence accumulated that this Murray Valley encephalitis was an arthropod-borne viral infection closely allied to Japanese B encephalitis. The latter infection is believed to be endemic in New Guinea and Northern Australia (Anderson *et al.* 1960). It becomes epidemic when seasonal weather conditions cause wild birds carrying the virus to migrate south, which they do principally to the Murray–Darling River basin (Miles and Howes 1953). Under such climatic and geographical conditions, and when the residual level of immunity in the local communities has again become low enough, the clinical disease reappears. Sporadic cases and small outbreaks have continued to be reported since 1951 (Burrow *et al.* 1998). It has become widely accepted the 'X' disease and Murray Valley encephalitis were the one and same illness (Burnet 1952a; 1952b).

OTHER ORIGINAL WORK

Headache

Francis Hare, of Brisbane, in a series of three papers on the paroxysmal neuroses (1903), attempted to forge a unifying concept of a vasospastic pathogenesis for a variety of disorders which embraced epilepsy, migraine and asthma, among other conditions. The word 'neuroses' apparently was employed in Cullen's old general sense of a nervous system disorder, or of a nervous system disorder for which no pathological basis could be detected at the time. With the exception of migraine, the range of disorders Hare considered was more or less the spectrum of illness which Willis long before (1684) had considered to be convulsive in nature. Hare's concept of their pathogenesis really represented a return to ideas in vogue a century previously. These ideas at that earlier time had never had adequate experimental confirmation, and Hare failed to provide one, except in the case of migraine. The observations he made about the effects of temporary occlusion of various scalp arteries by local pressure during migraine attacks proved very reminiscent of those later described by Wolff (1963) in his classic *Headache and Other Head Pain.* Probably, having been published in a colonial medical journal in a country far from the mainstream of medical intellectual activity, Hare's ideas and observations about the mechanism of migraine went largely unnoticed internationally. Possibly they were also to some extent submerged by Hare's other observations and conclusions which must have appeared unsatisfactory even in the state of then contemporary knowledge. Yet, though Hare's observations were uncontrolled, and were not expressed in the quantitative terms that would have been considered desirable, if not essential, to later research standards, they still appear valid and would demand consideration in any adequate explanation of the pathogenesis of migraine.

There were also some small-scale Australian investigations into the treatment of headache. Sippe (1938), a Brisbane physician, believed that migraine had an allergic basis. He therefore tested the efficacies of various diets that were designed to eliminate the intake of specific items of food in preventing attacks of the disorder. In 105 cases managed in this way he reported a 61.9% cure rate, though he seemed aware that he had tended to select the cases in whom he used the treatment. As well, he studied no control group. Lister Reid (1940) described the success of repeated subcutaneous injections of histamine in the prevention of recurrent migraine in five subjects, again without any control observations. Kelly (1942) investigated the effectiveness of injecting local anaesthetic into tender areas in the posterior neck muscles in the relief of what he categorised as chronic traumatic and rheumatic headache in 40 patients. It would be difficult to translate the diagnoses in his subjects into modern-day headache categories, though tension-type headache might be the best approximation.

Epilepsy

Hare (1903) chose to reject the theories of the primary neurogenic origin of epileptic seizures that had come into vogue by his time, mainly as a result of the studies of Hughlings Jackson and Gowers. Hare preferred to return to the earlier vasomotor hypotheses of the origin of the disorder. The ideas he espoused were really variants of Brown-Séquard's (1860) concept of epileptogenesis, rather than an original hypothesis, and by Hare's own admission were based primarily on what he recognised was an assumption that `I shall assume provisionally that in epilepsy, as in most cases of migraine and asthma, there is an initial widespread area of vaso-constriction...'

Hare's ideas attracted some temporary local interest in Australia, but they patently lacked the necessary evidential basis to be developed further in relation to epilepsy, and they led nowhere.

George Rennie (1905a), a man apparently of a more sober cast of mind, addressed the question as to whether epilepsy could be cured. He raised the important issue of what phenomena should be embraced within the rubric of `epilepsy'. Was it to be only those instances in which an underlying pathology could be found to explain epileptic seizures, the view taken by Delaisauve (1854) and Reynolds (1861) some half a century earlier? And what constituted a `cure' for epilepsy? For how long need the sufferer remain seizure free to be considered cured? These were matters which should have been raised sooner and far more often in the international literature than they had been, and Rennie's considering them in 1905 gives some indication of his intellectual qualities.

Within the mental hospital system, some work was also done on metabolic changes, specifically in relation to calcium concentrations in the blood, in relation to epilepsy (Prior & Jones 1916). In this connection `epilepsy' referred to convulsive seizures as they occurred in patients who needed to be confined to such institutions. There seemed little recognition on the part of the authors that their conclusions might not apply to epilepsy as it was present in the wider population. Lalor and Haddow (1920), again working in a mental hospital environment, argued for a toxaemic causation for idiopathic epilepsy on the basis of their measurements of the urinary excretion of urea in epileptic patients.

VARIOUS ENCEPHALITIDES

The Australian outbreaks of 'X' disease and *encephalitis lethargica* seemed to lead to a continuing interest in the topic of the encephalitides over the next decade, or rather longer. From the local varieties of encephalitis, interest first extended to the viral encephalitides in general (Duhig 1922) and then to the various acute disseminated demyelinative encephalomyelitides, whose autoimmune basis was then unknown, e.g. those associated with varicella (Lockwood 1931) and measles (Chinner 1940), and to a localised brain stem variety reported by De Crespigny and Hurst (1942). The neuropathologist Oliver Latham took up the subject from a diagnostic and a pathogenic standpoint on several occasions (1927, 1930, 1931). E

Weston Hurst, in Adelaide at the Institute for Medical and Veterinary Science in the later 1930s, did investigational work on the production of experimental demyelination. He achieved this in experimental animals by means of repeated sublethal exposures to cyanide, or sodium azide. Before Hurst had completed his investigations, he described them (1941 a, b) in his initial Rennie Memorial Lecture given to the Royal Australasian College of Physicians. This lecture contained an admirable and critical account of demyelinating diseases in animals and humans. Incidentally, in this lecture Hurst remarked on the unexpectedly low prevalence of multiple sclerosis in South Australia, as compared with the United Kingdom and other countries, an observation confirmed by epidemiological studies carried out three decades later.

The Argyll-Robertson Pupil

H J Wilkinson was mentioned previously in this chapter for his role in correcting Hunter's misinterpretation of the role of sympathetic nerve fibres in skeletal muscle. Whilst still in the Anatomy School of Sydney University, Wilkinson (1927) carried out a series of physiological and neuroanatomical studies which led him to the conclusion that the afferent pathways from the retina (for light) and the proprioceptive pathway from the extrinsic eye muscles (important for convergence) reached the oculomotor nuclei through different routes in the periaqueductal region of the midbrain. At this site, syphilitic inflammation was therefore able to involve the former pathway selectively to inactivate the pupillary response to light, whilst allowing preservation of the response to accommodation.

CEREBRAL VASCULAR DISEASE

In 1937, A A Abbie, who later became Professor of Anatomy in the University of Adelaide, published detailed studies of the arterial blood supply of the deep central regions of the human cerebral hemispheres which corrected certain errors contained in the earlier accounts of Duret and Heubner (both in 1874). Abbie also showed that the lenticulo-optic artery of Duret did not exist. Abbie's work was significant from the point of view of interpreting the consequences of vascular lesions of the internal capsule and neighbouring brain areas.

Peripheral Nerve Pathology

Goulston (1930) published in the *Medical Journal of Australia* a long and detailed account of the damage caused to peripheral nerves in experimental animals by the effects of radiation from radium needles inserted near the nerves studied.

Myasthenia Gravis

Corkill and Ennor (1937) described their investigation of blood esterase activity in two cases of neostigmine-responsive myasthenia gravis. The esterase activity was not increased. Despite this finding, the researchers were not prepared to discount the possibility that the disorder could be due to increased circulating esterase activity, or decreased acetylcholine production. Competition for post-junctional acetylcholine receptors was not raised as an additional possibility.

Tick-Bite Paralysis

Instances of paralysis associated with tick bites had been reported from eastern Australia as early as 1884 (Bancroft 1884). Of these instances, at least two had been fatal (Bancroft 1884; Ferguson 1924). Probably prompted by this knowledge, Clunies Ross, in the Veterinary Science Department of the University of Sydney, carried out an investigation which led to the recognition of the existence of a tick-derived neurotoxin as the causative agency (Editorial 1927). Later the Sydney paediatrician Donald Hamilton (1940b) reviewed the topic and added further cases of the disorder to the literature.

Myotonia

Covernton and Draper (1947) published a comprehensive clinical and experimental study of myotonia in animals and humans which was extracted from the former's MD thesis (from the University of Adelaide). Some of the pharmacological observations e.g. relating to the effects of neostigmine, adrenaline and carbaminyl chloride, were of theoretical importance.

Finger-cherry Blindness

From 1894 onwards (Flecker 1944), instances were reported of sudden bilateral blindness which affected children a few hours after eating the fruit of the finger-cherry plant *(Rhodomyrtus macrocarpa)* which grew in North Queensland. The toxicity appeared restricted to the optic nerves.

The resultant blindness was permanent and was accompanied by bilateral optic atrophy. The disorder ceased to occur after 1915, when an educational campaign was mounted to alert children and their parents to the dangers of ingesting the fruit of the plant. The nature of the toxin does not appear to have been determined.

Bromide Clinical Pharmacology

The modern medical mind is attuned to the notion that the study of clinical pharmacology is a post-World War II development. It may therefore seem a little surprising to some that, as long ago as 1932, Sippe and Bostock, in Brisbane, carried out what was in essence a clinical neuropharmacological study of the toxicity of bromides, which were at that time still in use in the treatment of epilepsy. Whilst these workers could not establish an optimal bromide concentration in blood which correlated with clinical benefit, they did obtain some evidence of a bromide threshold concentration of 200 mg per 100 mls, above which neurotoxicity was likely.

FORERUNNERS OF THE AUSTRALIAN CLINICAL NEUROLOGISTS

Leaving aside A W Campbell, who will be dealt with in the next chapter, over the period before men began to practise exclusively in clinical neurology in Australia there were certain physicians who achieved local reputations for their interest and skill in neurological matters. These physicians included George Rennie, Sidney Sewell, Henry Maudsley and James Froude Flashman. There was also a neuropathologist Oliver Latham, who was involved in numerous neurological collaborations over the course of half a century. In those times there were also other persons who had been accorded the title of neurologist to various institutions within Australia. Some of these were primarily psychiatrists e.g. Grey Ewan at Newcastle, John Bostock in Brisbane, Reg S Ellery in Melbourne. Some were physicians, such as H K Fry (1886–1959), who between 1920 and 1924 held the appointment of Honorary Assistant Physician in Neurology at the Adelaide Hospital (Rischbieth 1994). When Fry resigned the position, though remaining as a Physician to the Hospital, he was not replaced. This particular neurological appointment was not mentioned in Burston's (1988) obituary of Fry. It has been difficult to trace information about any original contribution to the advancement of neurology that Fry made, locally or more globally. There was also the anatomist John Irvine Hunter, who briefly held the title of Honorary Neurologist to the Lewisham Hospital in Sydney. None of these men was a committed neurologist in the modern sense, Rennie probably being the closest approximation.

George Edward Rennie (1861–1923)

George Rennie appears to have been the first medical man in Australia to have taken a major and sustained interest in organic neurological disease, though he continued to practise as a general physician throughout his career. Details of his life have been obtained from his obituaries (Anonymous 1923; Crago 1923; Clayton 1923) and the introductions to some of the lectures commemorating him which are given at intervals at meetings of the Royal Australasian College of Physicians.

Born in Sydney in 1861, educated at Sydney Grammar School and the University of Sydney, where he received a BA degree in 1882, Rennie went on to University College, London, to take medical qualifications (the University of Sydney at the time had no full medical course). In 1887 he became MB (London) and a Member of the Royal College of Surgeons. In the following year he was awarded a Doctorate of Medicine by the University of London.

After returning to Sydney in 1889 Rennie worked as a pathologist and physician, becoming Honorary Assistant Physician to the Royal Prince Alfred Hospital in 1894, and being appointed Honorary Physician to that institution four years later. However, in that same year, he returned to London to take the Membership of the Royal College of Physicians (of which he later became a Fellow). When he returned to Sydney in 1900, he reverted to being an Honorary Assistant Physician at the Royal Prince Alfred Hospital. In 1906 he again became Honorary Physician to that Hospital and was its Senior Physician from 1912 until 1921, when he retired under the age limit rules.

Throughout his consultant career, Rennie's main professional interest appears to have been in clinical neurology, and he seems to have been regarded as providing the leading neurological opinion in the New South Wales of his time. There is a good deal of testimony concerning his abilities as a clinician and medical teacher. He seems to have been a man of integrity and honour who served his community well. For over a dozen years, as well as conducting his practice and working at his hospital, he edited the

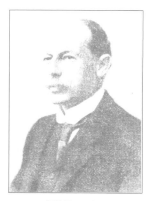

G E Rennie

Australasian Medical Gazette whilst it grew from a monthly to a weekly journal, the major one in the Commonwealth of Australia. When it was subsumed into the *Medical Journal of Australia* in 1914, Rennie relinquished its editorship.

Over the years, Rennie published a significant number of neurological papers. Some were essentially reports of unusual cases, e.g. exophthalmic goitre associated with myasthenia gravis (1919) or of small case series, but several were significant reviews of important topics in the applied physiology of the nervous system. Thus he wrote, for example, on death after apparently minor head injuries (1895), the functional anatomy of the cerebellum (1897), meralgia paraesthetica (1902), the physiology of voluntary movement (1903), the curability of epilepsy (1905a), the treatment of peripheral nerve disease (1905b), the possibility of occupation and peripheral trauma determining the site of syphilitic cerebral pathology (1915), and the effects of spinal cord transection (1921). His discussion (Rennie 1905b) of the possibilities of treating chronic neurological disorders revealed how limited the range of therapeutic options then was, largely comprising mercury and potassium iodide, and massage, exercise and the application of electricity. There were also so-called `nerve-tonics'. Curiously, he did not mention the use of bromide for epilepsy. Rennie's papers showed thorough familiarity with the then contemporary literature, and considerable ability to collate facts and to reason from them. However, the papers contained no indication that Rennie had carried out any original investigative work, or that he had reasoned his way to new insights about the nervous system. There is every reason to infer from his publications that he would have been an excellent teacher of students, but great teachers are seldom remembered beyond the generations that they teach unless their teaching is perpetuated in some durable form and also continues to remain relevant.

Rennie's sustained publication record, and his practice interests, might allow one to argue that he was the first Australian neurologist. He had begun his professional activities in Australia a decade earlier than Alfred Walter Campbell. However, throughout Rennie's career, and sometimes in the same volume of the journals in which he published his neurological writings, there appeared his papers on topics such as the open-air treatment of acute pneumonia, tuberculosis, the ductless glands, deafness in children, and pernicious anaemia. Because of these publications, Rennie is probably more appropriately regarded as a physician with a strong neurological interest than as a man committed predominantly to neurology. There appears to be little evidence that his contributions to neuroscience would allow neurology to make any stronger claim for his inclusions in its ranks than that, meritorious though his life clearly was.

Sidney Sewell (1880–1949)

Sidney Sewell was born in Melbourne, educated at Caulfield Grammar School, and studied Medicine at the University of Melbourne from which he graduated MB ChB in 1906, subsequently taking that institution's MD in 1910 (White 1949). After a period on the resident staff at the Melbourne Hospital, he spent a year with the pioneer neurosurgeon and neurophysiologist Sir Victor Horsley at University College Hospital in London, and also worked at the National Hospital for Nervous Diseases at Queen Square, and with F W Mott. On his return to Melbourne, he commenced practice in Collins Street, and over some months held an appointment as Honorary Neurologist to St Vincent's Hospital before becoming Outpatient Physician to the Melbourne Hospital. Early in his consultant career in Melbourne he gave postgraduate lectures in neurology, and also lectured to medical students on the nervous system and, in 1913, published on the effects of transverse lesions of the spinal cord These activities led to his fairly rapidly building up a substantial neurological element in his consultant practice. However, after World War I, though he clearly retained his interest in neurology and was described as Neurologist to the Base Hospital in St Kilda Road, Melbourne (Sewell 1920), he became very concerned about the welfare of sufferers from pulmonary tuberculosis and devoted considerable energy to advancing their cause. Nevertheless, he returned to a neurological theme, the localisation of function in the cerebrum, in his Listerian Oration (Sewell 1937). Sewell also became involved in the activities of the Association of Physicians and was a major driving force in that body's development into the Royal Australasian College of Physicians, of which he was to become the second President. His example was a significant factor in Graeme Robertson's taking up of neurology. Sewell was knighted four years before his death.

Sewell's professional interests ranged well beyond neurology, and history would probably regard his main achievements as being in relation to the foundation of the Royal Australasian College of Physicians and the development of tuberculosis services in Victoria. Nonetheless, his own example and his endeavour to advance Graeme Robertson's career were significant factors in getting neurology underway as a specialty in Australia.

Henry Fitzgerald Maudsley (1891–1962)

Maudsley came from a distinguished medical lineage, his father being a knighted Melbourne physician who, in 1906, had published a detailed interpretation of what probably was red nuclear tremor, though he seemed unaware of Gordon Holmes' then recent work (1904) concerning the phenomenon. The younger Henry Maudsley was educated at Melbourne Grammar School and the University of Melbourne, graduating MB BS from the latter in 1915. He served in the Army during World War I and took the Melbourne MD in 1920 before going to London where he passed the Membership of the Royal College of Physicians and the Diploma of Psychological Medicine. During the inter-war years, he was Honorary Physician in Charge of the Neurology and Psychiatry Clinic at the Melbourne Hospital, and Honorary Neurologist to the Victorian Eye and Ear Hospital. He became a Fellow of the London College of Physicians in 1937 and a Foundation Fellow of the Australasian College of Physicians in the following year. During World War II he was consultant in Psychiatry to the Australian Army.

Although by all accounts Maudsley was competent in neurology, his main professional activity was in the field of psychiatry, and he was the chief founder of the Royal Australian and New Zealand College of Psychiatrists, of which he was elected President on two occasions. He did not publish a great deal in connection with neurology, though his name often appeared among the discussants at the neurological presentations in Melbourne that were recorded in the pages of the *Medical Journal of Australia*. He wrote in that journal on ocular signs in neurological diagnosis (1928), and on the consequences of encephalitis lethargica (1926). It seems possible that Maudsley's neurological abilities were a factor which delayed for some years the appointment of a dedicated neurologist at the Melbourne Hospital.

J Froude Flashman (1870–1917)

In Sydney, around the end of the first decade of the 20th century, whilst A W Campbell was practising as a neurologist, and George Rennie as a physician and neurologist, a third man appears to have entered the practice of neurology, though only for a short period. The advent of World War I, and premature death in it, cut short that man's neurological career. However, the evidence of his publications, and the testimony of the unnamed writer of one of his obituaries, leave little doubt that James Froude Flashman was a man of considerable talent and organising ability, a productive neuroscientist and a capable clinician. Had he returned from war service, who knows how Australian clinical neuroscience might have developed under his leadership, so long as his obvious gifts in that direction were not to be seduced into some other direction of professional life.

Flashman was born at Braidwood in New South Wales in 1870, and took, consecutively, first level degrees in Arts, Science and in Medicine from the University of Sydney, the latter qualification in 1894. He then proceeded to a Doctorate in Medicine in 1897. Near the end of his life, he took the Membership of the Royal College of Physicians of London whilst serving in Britain with the Australian Army Medical Corps. This latter qualification suggests his interest in continuing the clinical side of his career. Much of Flashman's professional life was spent in the service of the Lunacy Departments of the State of New South Wales where his major interest lay in pathology. In 1900 he became the first Director of the Pathology Laboratory of the State Lunacy Department, an institution whose sympathies clearly lay in the direction of the biological rather than the psychodynamic approach to psychiatry. Flashman arranged for the laboratory to be sited in the Medical School of the University of Sydney and there he and Oliver Latham carried out various neuropathological and clinical pathological investigations into the basis of insanity. They combined to publish the first account of pathologically confirmed multiple sclerosis in Australia (Flashman and Latham 1915). Flashman also worked on the comparative anatomy of the brain of the Australian Aboriginal people, though these particular studies were never completed. He instituted serological testing for syphilis – the old Wasserman reaction – in the inhabitants of the various institutions for the mentally retarded in New South Wales and published on this and various other clinical pathological topics, as well as on morphological pathological matters. Latham (1934), in his Beattie Smith Lectures, almost incidentally listed Flashman's published work (including some that is not readily accessible) and gave an account of his investigational interests. For a time, Flashman acted as *locum tenens* for the Professor of Pathology at Sydney University. In 1910 he entered private practice in neurology and pathology in Sydney, to better provide for the future of his family. He enlisted in the Army in 1915 and, with the rank of Lieutenant-Colonel, was sent to England. There he showed great foresight and organising ability in setting up arrangements and facilities for the care of the Australian wounded from the battlefields of France. Those who wrote his obituaries (Anonymous 1917; Maclaurin 1917; Mills 1917) concentrated heavily on this aspect of his career, perhaps in part reflecting the preoccupation at that time concerning men who were serving in a war. Nonetheless, it would seem that Flashman had made a very major contribution to the care of the Australian wounded, and that not enough time had elapsed for this to be officially acknowledged before death from pneumonia carried him off at Boulogne, in France, on 12 February 1917.

How much clinical neurology J Froude Flashman had practised in Australia, and what impact he had on that specialty, are not clear, partly because of the brevity of his time in its practice. Certainly, he deserves some mention in the record of the development of Australian neuroscience. Reading his obituary leaves one with a sense of regret for what might have been.

Oliver Latham (1877–1974)

Despite his being a well-known figure in Australian clinical neuroscience over more than half a century, details of Latham's career are hard to obtain. The difficulty seems to arise because he outlived not only his own generation but most of the succeeding one, so that by the time he died there was no one to write his obituary whose knowledge of him spanned the length of his whole career. In particular, his quite extensive publication record went almost completely unmentioned in the available accounts.

Latham was born in Dublin and educated there and at Harrow, where Winston Churchill was also a boy at the same time (Noad 1975). Latham graduated in Medicine from the University of Sydney in 1903, and soon joined Flashman in the Pathology Laboratory of the State Lunacy Department, where he continued to spend the remainder of his entire professional life. He seems to have been regarded as a learned and well-liked man whose life was devoted to the morphological neuropathology that was so important in his time. During his career, he published on a considerable variety of topics, often in the form of case reports to which he added detailed and beautifully illustrated neuropathological descriptions, but there were also studies on histological methodology and on clinical pathology. In the pages of the Australian medical journals of his time one can find his name associated with topics such as the Wasserman reaction in mental hospital patients, modification of the Widal test, methods for estimating glucose in urine and test meals in the insane, as well as more formal neuropathology topics as diverse as glial biology (1926), Friedreich's ataxia (Litchfield *et al.* 1917), the various encephalitides (Latham 1922, 1927, 1930, 1931), encephalomyelitis (Dawson and Latham 1931), dementia and other disturbances related to cerebral tumour (Wallace and Latham 1914; Nowland *et al.* 1924), multiple sclerosis (Flashman and Latham 1915), Australian `X' disease (Mathewson and Latham 1917), the general pathology of the cerebellum (Latham 1941), cerebello-olivary atrophy (Hall *et al.* 1945), olivo-ponto-cerebellar atrophy (Lambie *et al.* 1947), cerebellar degeneration with epilepsy (Minogue and Latham 1945), cerebellar laminar degeneration (Hagen *et al.* 1951), haematomyelia (Latham 1939), the reactions of the small calibre cerebral blood vessels (Latham 1938), acute haemorrhagic encephalomyelitis (Shallard and Latham 1945), dementia praecox (Dawson and Latham 1943), and Alzheimer's disease (Edwards and Latham 1943; Himmelhoch *et al.* 1947). Latham also carried out the studies on muscle histology mentioned earlier in this chapter in collaboration with John Irvine Hunter in the Anatomy Department at the University of Sydney (Hunter and Latham 1925). As well, on occasions, Latham provided the pathology reports appended to various published case studies e.g. to those of Mathewson (1921), Blackburn (1922), Hogg (1923) and Bell

(1928). His 1934 Beattie-Smith Lectures incorporated his vast experience of diverse types of morphological neuropathology and reveal something of his professional activities over the course of a third of a century. During his long career his publications in the pages of the *Medical Journal of Australia* covered a great deal of the recognised range of morphological neuropathology.

Latham may not have done a great deal of original experimental work in his lifetime, but that seems to have been the norm for a neuropathologist of his day. He constituted the main source of the pathological knowledge and experience which underpinned Australian clinical neurology for half a century. Clearly, it was he who, more than anyone else, carried Australian neuropathology forward from almost its earliest times to the emergence of the Australian Association of Neurologists, of which he was elected an Honorary Member in 1951, one year after the Association itself was founded.

Chapter 2

A W CAMPBELL – AUSTRALIA'S FIRST NEUROLOGIST

As mentioned earlier in this book, Alfred Walter Campbell's career and achievements in the international neurological science of his day constitute the major exception to the generalisation that, prior to the threshold of World War II, Australian contributions to the accumulating corpus of international neurological knowledge came from those who had not practised as neurologists.

CAMPBELL'S LIFE

Campbell's career was described in some detail in the obituaries written by his friend and physician L R Parker and by Professor W S Dawson, both published in the *Medical Journal of Australia* issue of 22 January 1938. Further information appeared in a later obituary written by John Farquhar Fulton in the American Medical Association's *Archives of Neurology and Psychiatry* (1938). The fact that this eminent Yale neurophysiologist, who also was Cushing's biographer, was motivated to write of Campbell as he did testifies to the international standing of the latter's reputation that persisted three decades after he had disappeared from the world scientific stage. Some additional biographical material and Campbell's photograph (see next page) became available as the outcome of a personal communication from Mrs Veda Hope, Campbell's older daughter. There is also the account of Campbell in the Dictionary of National Biography (Ford 1979), and, much more recently published, a major biography written by Malcolm Macmillan (2016), who painstakingly searched out original documents and, on that basis, corrected certain information contained in the earlier accounts while adding considerable further detail about Campbell's life and career.

Alfred Walter Campbell was the son of a pastoralist, David Henry Campbell, and his wife Amelia, née Breillat. He was born on 18 January 1868 at his parents' station at Cunningham Plains, near Harden, in New South Wales. His early education occurred at Oakland School, near Mittagong,

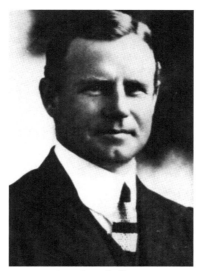

A W Campbell

where his headmaster was the son of Robert Southey, the English poet. Campbell apparently determined on following a medical career only three years after the University of Sydney had opened its Medical School, and before it had produced the first graduates from its own medical course, although the University of Melbourne had already done this, a few years earlier (Young *et al.* 1984). At the age of 18 Campbell followed a rather common practice among aspiring Australian medical practitioners of the time, entering the University of Edinburgh as a medical student. Four years later, in 1889, he graduated, taking the degrees MB, CM, though not with honours as some of his obituaries stated. During his time in Scotland, Campbell appears to have been a rather considerable sportsman, captaining both the cricket and the football teams at Edinburgh University. After graduation, he worked as an assistant in several British mental hospitals and seems to have attended the ward practice at the National Hospital for Nervous Diseases, Queen Square, London. There he had some contact as `a newly fledged graduate and ward follower' with John Hughlings Jackson, whose genius he recognised and to which he paid tribute long afterwards, near the end of his own life (Campbell 1935).

Campbell then proceeded to further his neurological studies in Europe, working for a time as assistant to Krafft-Ebing in Vienna. After that, he became a member of the staff of the State Asylum in Prague. He returned to England in 1892 and, at the age of 24, submitted a thesis entitled 'The Pathology of Alcoholic Insanity' and on that basis was awarded the degree Doctor of Medicine of the University of Edinburgh, not with the gold medal that his obituaries described, but with the award 'being deemed worthy of competing for a gold medal'. Holding this higher qualification, Campbell was appointed Resident Medical Officer and Director of the Pathology Laboratory at the Rainhill Asylum, Liverpool. He remained in that position till 1905. Over those 13 years in Liverpool, he carried out the series of investigations which brought him recognition as one of the foremost neurohistologists and neuropathologists in the world. In his obituary of Campbell, Parker (1938) stated that his laboratories 'became a place of visitation and study by specialists from all parts of the world'.

In 1904 Campbell had applied for the post of InspectorGeneral of the Insane in Victoria. His obituaries indicated that he withdrew his application when he knew that there was a local contender for the post. However, MacMillan found evidence that he remained in the competition as a very strong contender but was ultimately bypassed, perhaps because he had less administrative experience than the successful applicant. Also, his greatest scientific work was not yet in print. A year after that rejection, at the age of 37, and having lived overseas for a little more than half his life, Campbell finally returned to Australia, to live in Sydney. There he commenced practice as a specialist in neurology and mental diseases, though he described himself as a neurologist. He occupied rooms at 183 Macquarie Street for over 30 years, retiring in 1937. During his Sydney period he was appointed Honorary Neurologist to the Royal Alexandra Hospital for Children, the Coast Hospital and the Department of Repatriation, though he held no appointment to the longer established and more prestigious Sydney and Royal Prince Alfred Hospitals. The contents of the *Medical Journal of Australia* over a period of some three decades provide evidence that he played a significant part in the local medical affairs of the day, particularly in connection with neurology and, to a much lesser extent, with psychiatry. Over a number of years, he was responsible for selecting from the international literature the Abstracts on Neurology and Psychiatry which were a regular feature of the issues of the *Medical Journal of Australia* of those times.

One year after returning to Australia, Campbell had married Jenny Mackay, a childhood friend who had been brought up on 'Wallen Been', the pastoral holding adjoining that on which Campbell had spent his youth. According to Campbell's daughter, Mrs Veda Hope, Campbell's future wife and her mother had spent a considerable amount of time overseas and presumably had seen something of Campbell in Britain. The newly married couple went to live at 'Wallendoon', Rose Bay, Sydney, and subsequently had two children, both daughters. At the age of 46, at the commencement of the 1914–1918 war, Campbell enlisted in the A.I.F. He served with the Army in Egypt with the rank of Major before returning to Australia, where he resumed clinical practice. After retirement from practice in 1937, his health began to fail, and he died on 4 November 1937 from cancer which, judging from Parker's obituary, probably had spread to involve his central nervous system.

Campbell's personal characteristics are probably of some importance in any attempt to understand the pattern of his life. He was described as someone who said relatively little, though he spoke with careful diction and employed wellchosen words. He was fluent in French, German and Italian. Those who wrote or spoke of him on a basis of personal experience seem generally agreed that he was a rather reserved man. His daughter said that he was 'frightfully shy and reserved and loathed publicity'. Parker mentioned how Campbell once said that he could not have borne to be a teacher because 'It would have taken too much out of me, the constant dread that I should leave something out, or say something which might not be true.'

CAMPBELL'S SCIENTIFIC CAREER

Campbell's career in neurology fell into two reasonably clear-cut parts – the European, mainly Liverpool, years between 1889 and 1905, during which he did nearly all of the scientific work on which his international fame was based, and the Sydney years from 1905 to 1937 in which his main activity appeared to be that of a practising clinical neurologist.

The European Years

After his early studies on 'The Pathology of Alcoholic Insanity', which gained for him a doctorate from the University of Edinburgh in 1892, Campbell worked on various neuropathological subjects. In 1894, no fewer than three major papers appeared under his authorship, as well as several more minor works. In the *British Medical Journal,* constituting one of a pair with a paper authored by the London neurologist J S Risien Russell, Campbell provided a detailed description of the tract degenerations resulting from local lesions of the human cerebellum. He had studied five cases of recent thrombotic, embolic or haemorrhagic softening of the cerebellum and, in serial sections of the brain stem and spinal cord which he had stained by the Marchi technique, had traced the resultant tract degeneration. The *Journal of Mental Science* published his prizewinning essay 'A Contribution to the Morbid Anatomy and Pathology of the Neuromuscular Changes in General Paresis of the Insane'. In that paper he described peripheral nerve changes in 12 cases of general paresis of the insane. Campbell's third major paper for the year 1894 was entitled 'On Vacuolation of the Nerve Cell of the Human Cerebral Cortex'. It appeared in the *Journal of Pathology and Bacteriology* and was based on the histological examination of the brains of 47 cases of pulmonary tuberculosis and 13 cases of acute lobar pneumonia. Vacuolation, which was present in cortical neurons in nearly all these brains, was regarded by Campbell as a toxaemic phenomenon.

> ... with so much positive and direct evidence, is one, therefore, not justified in concluding that, in the case of the highly organised cortical nerve cell, so intrinsically dependent on a pure and untainted supply of blood for its healthy maintenance, such a harassing factor as toxaemia must not only play a most important pathogenic role, but actually induces the remarkable vacuolatory change in all these conditions.

In that prolific year, additional papers appeared on changes in the senile brain, on thrombosis of the inferior cerebellar artery and on the breaking strain of the ribs of the insane. Thereafter, Campbell continued to write on various neuropathological topics, and some nonneurological ones (e.g. acute pancreatitis, dysentery). As well, there were publications dealing with neuropathological technique (the use of formic aldehyde in the laboratory), spinal heterotopias, disseminated sclerosis, amyotrophic lateral sclerosis, the relationship between syphilis and general paresis of the insane, the anatomy and pathology of the pineal, the histology of cerebral tumours, and the effects of pernicious anaemia on the nervous system. It was a wide-ranging coverage of neuropathological territory, culminating in 1897 in a learned and detailed review 'On the Tracts of the Spinal Cord and Their Degeneration', which was published in the journal *Brain*.

In 1900 Henry (subsequently Sir Henry) Head's great work on the dermatomes appeared, also in *Brain*. The paper's title was 'The Pathology of Herpes Zoster and its Bearing on Sensory Localisation', and Head's co-author was Campbell, The latter's role in this investigation is sometimes passed over, though Head's is remembered. The paper comprised a lengthy (170 page) correlation of Head's clinical observations with Campbell's 21 autopsy studies. It remains one of the chief sources of our knowledge of the distribution of the dermatomes in humans.

As judged from his publication record, from 1900 onwards, Campbell's interests appear to have been increasingly focused on the anatomy and pathology of the cerebral cortex. In 1895 Charles Scott Sherrington had been appointed as Holt Professor of Physiology in the University of Liverpool. In 1901, Sherrington's studies on the physiology of the cerebral cortex in higher apes appeared. Campbell subsequently examined the brains of Sherrington's animals. This material formed part of his own investigation of cerebral cortical architecture. Campbell set down his reasons for undertaking his study of the microscopic structure of the cerebral cortex when he wrote:

> Particularly do I hope that those who, like myself, have pledged their energies to the apparently hopeless task of elucidating problems connected with mental disease will derive benefit from this research for it was only after several valuable years had been spent in the cause of scientific research in a laboratory attached to an asylum for the insane that I recognised that it was necessary for some worker to begin at the beginning, and attempt to piece together our disjointed knowledge of the cortex ... .

For his investigation of the microscopic organisation of the cerebral cortex, Campbell cut three complete normal human cerebral hemispheres into approximately 50 blocks, and embedded them in celloidin. A 25-micron thick section was cut every millimetre through each whole hemisphere. Alternate serial sections were stained for myelinated fibres by the WoltersKulschitzky technique and, for cellbodies, with thionin. The examination of each individual hemisphere occupied Campbell for six months. Three further normal complete hemispheres were cut in serial section and stained for nerve fibres only, whilst parts of another two normal hemispheres were cut in serial section and stained for both nerve cells and fibres. Campbell also cut in serial section the relevant regions of cerebral cortex from two cases of amyotrophic lateral sclerosis, three cases of tabes dorsalis, one case of internal capsule infarction, two cases of longstanding blindness and from seven patients who had an extremity amputated at least two years previously. The cerebral hemispheres of two chimpanzee and one orang monkey, and those of a cat, a dog and a pig were also studied in detail, employing the same meticulous neuroanatomical techniques. All of this enormous collection of material was examined microscopically, an undertaking which must have involved prodigious labour and the expenditure of a vast amount of time. Hand drawings were made of the sections with the aid of a special eyepiece, because the then available photographic techniques could not adequately display each individual section in its entirety.

On the basis of his histological examination of this material, Campbell considered himself justified in dividing the human cerebral cortex into some 12 major areas. He correlated these areas with what evidence of localisation of function he could derive from knowledge of comparative anatomy, experimental physiology and the consequences of human disease. His thinking was not purely in terms of morphology at a microscopic level but constituted an attempt to correlate neurohistology with localisation of function.

Sherrington communicated the outcome of Campbell's great investigation to the Royal Society in 1903, and it was published in an abstract in the Society's *Proceedings* (Campbell 1903). However, the work, *in toto*, was regarded as too extensive for publication in the *Philosophical Transactions of the Royal Society*. Instead, Sherrington, already influential in the councils of the Society of which he was later to become President, persuaded that body to provide a grant which resulted in Campbell's work appearing in 1905 as a separate monograph under the insignia of the Cambridge University Press. The volume, *Histological Studies of the Localisation of Cerebral Function*, comprised 360 pages, 11.5 by 9 inches in dimension, with 29 whole-page plates. Before the book was available in print, Campbell had resigned his post in Liverpool and returned to Australia.

The Sydney Years

Some additional papers on cerebral anatomy and pathology appeared in 1905, the year of Campbell's return to Australia. These papers (on the homologies of the Rolandic region, on the brain of the cat compared with that of man, on cerebral sclerosis and on cortical localisation) were probably

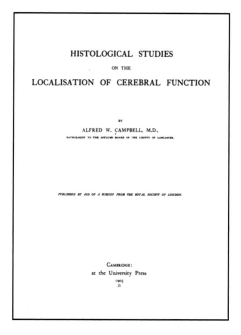

HISTOLOGICAL STUDIES
ON THE
LOCALISATION OF CEREBRAL FUNCTION

BY

ALFRED W. CAMPBELL, M.D.,
PATHOLOGIST TO THE ASYLUMS BOARD OF THE COUNTY OF LANCASTER.

PUBLISHED BY AID OF A SUBSIDY FROM THE ROYAL SOCIETY OF LONDON

CAMBRIDGE:
at the University Press
1905

The title page of A W Campbell's monograph

the results of work already carried out in Britain. Thereafter, as judged from the list of his 66 publications and presentations appended to his obituary which appeared in the *Medical Journal of Australia*, Campbell's research output seemed to cease for several years. However, there is good evidence that this was not the case. Despite the distractions of establishing himself in consultant practice and bringing up two young children, Campbell continued to do original investigational work during his first few years back in his homeland. The list of publications in Campbell's obituary is incomplete, at least for the period in question. It omitted a paper on the labyrinth (1924a), and another on the injection of alcohol into the trigeminal nerve and various of its branches for the relief of trigeminal neuralgia (1910), a technique he had learned in Paris from Ostwalt.

Much more importantly, in the *Transactions of the Ninth Australasian Medical Congress* held in Sydney in 1911, there is a description of a very considerable piece of Campbell's research which must have involved the expenditure of considerable time and effort. It went unmentioned in his obituary and seems to have escaped notice elsewhere. The publication's title was 'On the Localisation of Function in the Cerebellum'. Bolk, of

Amsterdam, had made use of a principle employed by Thomas Willis in his *De Anima Brutorum* (1683) and had drawn deductions about the function of parts of the cerebellum by correlating their degrees of development in different animal species with the capacities of these species to carry out certain motor activities. On this basis, Bolk had assigned responsibility for various parts of the body to particular areas of the cerebellum. Campbell had taken this type of approach further in an exhaustive anatomical and histological study of the cerebellum of the frog, lizard, albatross, turkey, platypus, native-cat, wallaby, rabbit, cat, dog, pig, gorilla, and man. It was a logical sequel to his work on the cytoarchitectonics of the cerebral cortex. As far as can be ascertained, this extensive investigation carried out by Campbell was never published except in the *Transactions* of what would have been regarded even at the time as a relatively obscure colonial medical society. For this reason, the study probably escaped the international notice that had been accorded to Campbell's work on the cerebral cortex.

None of Campbell's obituarists, including Fulton, mentioned the work on the cerebellum, yet its validity and worth are incontestable. Gordon Holmes in his 1922 Croonian Lectures on the cerebellum (Holmes 1956) devoted considerable space to refuting Bolk's views but seemed quite unaware that Campbell a decade earlier had arrived at, and published, a similar conclusion. Campbell's fellow Australian, Abbie (1941), in discussing the lack of validity of Bolk's deductions about localisation of function in the cerebellum, made no reference at all to Campbell's work on the matter. Campbell put the matter of localisation of function in the cerebellum thus:

> My conclusion, therefore, from an impartial consideration of all the evidence is that the surface of the cerebellum cannot be cut up into functional territories. I would subscribe to the belief that the cortex of the cerebellum subserves a function which is sensory in kind. I would regard it as a general receiving station for impressions from muscles, bones, and joints, and from the vestibulum. It is my belief that these impressions are not delivered at special stations, but are diffusely distributed in the cortex of each homolateral hemisphere. From the cortex these impressions are transferred to the intrinsic nuclei from which the efferent tracts lead to other parts of the nervous system, and thence again to the muscles, &c. so a great reflex arc is completed, the function of which is to regulate and co-ordinate movement.

Admittedly the outcome of Campbell's extensive investigation was a negative one, but it was nonetheless important. Regrettably, Campbell appears not to have been a man to put himself forward and, on this occasion, there was no Sherrington to ensure that the results of the investigation were published where they would be noticed by international science. Consequently, a great study seems to have wasted its sweetness on the desert air of a former British colony remote from the centres of northern hemisphere medical thought.

Campbell described a case of syringomyelia in the *Australasian Medical Gazette* in 1913 and gave an account of his examination of the gorilla brain in 1916 which was published in a relatively inaccessible report. In that same year he wrote on his experience of neurosis and psychosis under the stress of war (Campbell 1916). There was a case report of Friedreich's ataxia in the *Medical Journal of Australia* in 1917 (Litchfield *et al.*), one on probable myotonia congenita in that same journal in 1919 and one with N Dowling on nervous or hysterical fever in 1920. Campbell collaborated with JB Cleland, later Professor of Pathology in the University of Adelaide, in a series of investigations into the transmission of the poliomyelitis virus in 1918 (Campbell *et al.* 1918), and into the aetiology and pathology of Australian X disease (as mentioned in Chapter 1). He and Cleland defined the pathology of that condition and demonstrated very clearly that it was not an aberrant form of poliomyelitis (as had been suggested by Breinl in 1918) but was a novel type of encephalitis. These investigations were published in stages in the *Medical Journal of Australia* between 1918 and 1920, with a final major review paper in the *Journal of Hygiene* in 1920, and a report of the epidemic in the 1920 *Proceedings of the Royal Society of Medicine*.

After this, Campbell published no further scientific work, though he contributed to the clinical neurological literature from time to time in his later years, dealing with topics such as cerebral palsy (Campbell 1924b), childhood epilepsy (Campbell 1927a), nervous disease in childhood (Campbell 1927b), ocular signs in neurological diagnosis (Campbell 1928b), cerebrospinal syphilis (Campbell 1930), affections of peripheral nerves (Campbell 1931), the nervous child (Campbell 1933a) and the treatment of migraine (Campbell 1933b). Near the end of his life, in 1935, he produced a gracious account of the life and achievements of John Hughlings Jackson, whom he appears to have long admired (Campbell 1935).

The Significance of Campbell's Neuroscience

Campbell's range of investigations covered a goodly part of the territory of classical neuropathology. Much of the work was descriptive, but that does not detract from its value at a time when the corpus of available knowledge in the area was not as great as it subsequently became. And underlying a deal of it was a concern for reconciling morphology with normal and with disordered function. It was Campbell's investigation of the dermatomes, carried out in conjunction with Henry Head, and even more so his study of the cytoarchitectonics of the cerebral cortex, on which Campbell's reputation rests. His only real rival as a contributor to knowledge of the neuronal arrangements in the cerebral cortex was Korbinian Brodman, and at least some authorities preferred to accept Campbell's sober views on the matter.

Nearly a century after its publication, the validity of Campbell's great work on cerebral cytoarchitectonics stands unchallenged. His drawings of cerebral cortical histology still appear in textbooks of neuroanatomy. In his obituary of Campbell which appeared in the *Archives of Neurology and Psychiatry* (1938), John Farquhar Fulton, Sterling Professor of Physiology at Yale, paid a great tribute to a man who had long faded from the sight of the international scientific community when he quoted the words of Lorente de Nó.

> The only really good cytoarchitectonic pictures are those of Campbell, who — let me put it in capital letters — HAS BEEN THE ONLY CYTOARCHITECTONIST WHO HAS DESCRIBED FACTS AND ONLY FACTS. The German cytoarchitectonist has mixed facts with theory in such a manner that nobody can tell where facts end and theories begin. I must say that there are perhaps no more than a dozen photographs out of hundreds in which the layers of the cortex have been properly and consistently labelled. On the other hand Campbell's ink drawings, besides being good, are easily reproduced.

Von Bonin (1970) assessed the value of Campbell's work thus:

> Campbell's subdivisions of the primate cortex were not as fine as those of the German school, but modern architectonics has time and again decided in favour of his sober views.

When Webb Haymaker and Francis Schiller collected the biographies of those whom they regarded as the greatest 146 neurologists and neurological scientists of the past and published them in the most recent edition of *The Founders of Neurology* (1970), only two Australians were included. Both were contemporaries, and both New South Welshmen. One was Grafton Elliot Smith (1871–1937), who graduated in Medicine from the University of Sydney, but spent almost all the remainder of his life in Egypt and England, studying the comparative anatomy and evolution of the nervous system. The second Australian was Alfred Walter Campbell. When one considers the magnitude of Campbell's achievements in relation to the level of knowledge, the opportunities and the career expectations of the neuroscientists of his day, it is difficult to quarrel with Haymaker and Schiller's assessment. Moreover, it was a judgement that apparently was made in ignorance of Campbell's study of the comparative anatomy of the cerebellar cortex.

It could, of course, be argued that a substantial part of Campbell's original neuroscience, including the part of it which was of the greatest importance to posterity, was not carried out in Australia, and therefore should not be considered a contribution made by Australian neurology. There is some force in that argument, and judgement regarding the matter is left to the reader. Nonetheless, Campbell did live out his early life in Australia, served his country in a war, and in his homeland practised as a neurologist and carried out further neuroscientific work over more than three decades, including a great study of the cerebellar cortex which, had it become known internationally, must have enhanced the reputation of Australian neuroscience.

CAMPBELL AS A CLINICIAN

In practicing clinical neurology in Australia more than a century ago, Campbell was in various ways disadvantaged. Locally, there were almost no colleagues with similar interests with whom he could discuss matters or compare professional standards, and for the most part he had to depend on medical journals for contemporary information about neuroscience. For the greater part of Campbell's period in practice, neurology was an almost entirely clinical art, skull radiography and cerebrospinal fluid examination being the only relevant ancillary investigations. By the close of his career, ventriculography and pneumoencephalography had become available, but Campbell would have had to achieve diagnoses by purely clinical means throughout nearly all his professional life. Further, the therapeutic options available to him were distinctly limited.

Though his neuropathological knowledge would have been extraordinarily profound even by today's expectations, Campbell probably had not received as extensive a clinical neurological training as might have been desirable for someone engaging in a highly specialised area of clinical practice, and he lacked the imprimatur of Membership, let alone of Fellowship, of a Royal College of Physicians. It seems likely that, after graduation, he had intended to make his career in the area that was to become psychiatry, then called 'mental science', and that the move into neurology came after his return to Australia. From what can be gleaned from certain sources, Campbell's contemporaries and juniors seemed to have sensed that his clinical performance fell somewhat short of their expectations. Whether what they expected was realistic in the circumstances, and whether the limitations were his or theirs, or largely simply reflected the thoughts of their own seniors, are further and undeterminable issues. After the lapse of more than half a century, the late Sir Kenneth Noad recalled Campbell sometimes writing 'NYD' (not yet diagnosed) on the hospital records of children with obscure neurological illnesses, though Noad commented that Campbell took the histories of children with neurological illnesses in meticulous detail, although his physical examinations were perhaps more brief. Reading Campbell's clinical writings long afterwards gives the impression that they were produced by a judicious, well-informed and humane physician.

It could have been that Campbell's reticence and scrupulous intellectual honesty combined to prevent his being adept at the art of showmanship, to which clinical neurological practice can prove so well suited. Possibly this, and the inescapable diagnostic limitations of the times, prevented his example from persuading a younger generation of Australians to enter neurology. Campbell left behind him no clinical disciples, and he fathered no Australian school of clinical neurology, despite his extraordinary record of personal scientific achievement. The circumstances in which he practised in Sydney, and possibly his retiring personality, may have conspired against him, but that is no criticism of the merits of the man, or of the enduring greatness of his original contributions to neuroscience.

CAMPBELL – AN ASSESSMENT

From an overall point of view, Campbell's career was interpreted on one occasion (Eadie 1981) as presenting the paradox of a wonderful early scientific flowering which was abruptly and seemingly volitionally cut short, with a brief blooming again, years later. Subsequent recognition of the existence of his largely unnoticed investigation of the cerebellum rather invalidates this interpretation. It may be nearer the truth to see Campbell's career in terms of a profuse early flowering which gradually withered with time and relative scientific isolation and lack of opportunity, his earlier science gradually being replaced by a mixture of investigational and clinical practice, with the latter not having quite the impact on his potential successors that might have been anticipated.

But the question still remains as to why the collaborator of Henry Head and the protégé of Sherrington chose to return to the former colony he apparently had not seen for almost 20 years, and there take up a new, seemingly less intellectually stimulating and satisfactory pattern of professional existence. The available written records provide no persuasive reason, and in later life it appears that Campbell gave some wistful hints that he would have preferred to remain more heavily involved in scientific work. One might speculate about all manner of possibilities, but one needs to take into account not only the fact that Campbell had applied unsuccessfully for an appointment in his home country a year before his return, but that Malcolm Macmillan discovered the hitherto unnoticed information that Campbell had been a strong contender for appointment to the Foundation Chair in Pathology in the University of Sydney in 1901.

The answer to the change in Campbell's career site and direction may simply be that he married a fellow Australian, and their family and financial interests lay in their homeland. Campbell, with his sense of responsibility, may have also believed that the post he occupied in Britain, whatever the prospects it held for his personal scientific advancement, would not enable him to keep his future wife in the style to which she was accustomed, for she had been in a position to be able to travel extensively for some years before the marriage. A return to Australia, and clinical practice in that country in a major city, near the family properties (but not on them, for his daughter said her mother hated country life), may have offered much more realistic financial and lifestyle prospects.

If this was the basis of the decision, Campbell's failure to find some appointment which would have enabled him to engage in neuropathological and neuroanatomical work in Australia still needs explanation. Campbell, apparently a reticent man, had already failed to compete successfully for two Australian senior positions for which he was both well qualified and exceptionally strongly recommended. One might suspect that when he returned to Sydney and found Flashman and Oliver Latham already established in neuropathology posts in the Mental Health Service in that city he chose to avoid another potentially competitive situation. As it happened, Latham long outlived Campbell and continued to work in neuropathology, so that no place in that specialty became available in Sydney at any stage for Campbell to occupy.

Sadly, as its first practising neurological clinician, Campbell seemed to have had relatively little enduring influence on the further development of Australian clinical neurology, yet when his original scientific achievements are seen in relation to the circumstances of his times he must stand as arguably the greatest neuroscientist his country has ever produced.

Chapter 3

THE FOUNDING GENERATION of AUSTRALIAN NEUROLOGISTS

As Alfred Walter Campbell's career in Sydney drew to its close, and no disciple or successor to his role emerged in that city, another man, Leonard Bell Cox, began to practise in Melbourne as a clinical neurologist. Like Campbell, his career was intertwined to a considerable extent with neuropathology, and his very considerable recognised original achievements lay in the latter area. As early as 1934, Cox received formal appointment as an Honorary Neurologist to a Victorian teaching hospital, the Alfred Hospital, where his brother-in-law, Hugh Trumble, set about developing the specialty of neurosurgery. In that same year another Melbourne graduate, Edward Graeme Robertson, returned to his home city after several years of clinical neurological training in London, where he had occupied junior consultant posts in neurology at St Bartholomew's Hospital and at the Postgraduate Teaching School in Hammersmith. Robertson practised clinically as a neurologist in Melbourne, but his formal appointment at the Royal Melbourne Hospital was that of Honorary Physician to Outpatients. It was to be several years before he was to be accorded the title of Honorary Neurologist to the (Royal) Melbourne Hospital, and to the Children's Hospital. Thus, in the years just prior to the outbreak of the second World War, at a time when the only neurologist practising in Sydney was near the end of his career, two men in Melbourne had begun to practice purely in clinical neurology. In Sydney, at the same time there were then practising two younger general physicians with strong interests in clinical neurology. However, neither of these men ever restricted his practice purely to the specialty. K B Noad was Physician to Sydney Hospital and E L Susman Physician to the Royal Prince Alfred Hospital. In Perth, Gerald Moss, despite appointment as an Honorary Physician to the Royal Perth Hospital, in private practiced predominantly, though not exclusively, as a neurologist. At the time, there were no medical practitioners in the other State capital cities of the Commonwealth of Australia who practiced purely, or even mainly, in clinical neurology. Thus, at the eve of World War II, there were in the whole of Australia two full-time practising clinical neurologists and three physicians with major neurological interests. Campbell had died shortly before.

It should be mentioned for the sake of completeness that there was another man apart from Leonard Cox and Graeme Robertson who had practised in Melbourne as a neurologist for a short period after 1939. This man was the Austrian émigré Arthur Schüller.

ARTHUR SCHÜLLER (1874–1957)

Schüller had been born in Czechoslovakia as long before as 1874. He had graduated in Medicine from the University of Vienna in 1895 and, although trained in neurology and psychiatry, and practising in the former area, had involved himself in aspects of the specialty of radiology almost from the time of its beginning. Schüller had been appointed a Professor in the University of Vienna in 1909 and continued to hold his Chair until 1938. He and his wife, both of Jewish ancestry, then fled from Nazism in Austria. By the following year they had made their way to Australia, their possessions, their two sons and their whole previous way of life abandoned.

In his time, Schüller was probably the world's greatest authority on skull radiology and is often remembered as the 'father of neuroradiology'. His name is preserved in the Hand-Schüller-Christian syndrome. He was a prolific writer and, according to Frank Morgan's moving obituary of him (1958), a most admirable and gifted man of very great genius and most considerable learning. Though not a surgeon, during his life he had devised new neurosurgical approaches to brain lesions as well as making numerous contributions to neuroradiology more generally. In addition, he was a competent clinical neurologist.

In his old age, Schüller's brief foray into clinical neurology practice in Melbourne, mainly in relation to neurosurgical patients in St Vincent's Hospital before John Billings returned to become that institution's first neurologist, seems to have had little influence on the further development of clinical neurology in the country. Nevertheless, his contacts with St Vincent's Hospital that continued to the end of his life seem to have had an effect in enhancing that institution's neuroscience and radiology, and also in enriching its culture. A recently available biography contains further details of his long and distinguished career in international neuroscience (Henderson and Henderson 2021).

During the war years (1939–1945) there was no further recruitment to the ranks of Australian clinical neurologists until, in 1948, a Melbourne medical graduate, John Billings, began to practise neurology in his home city after neurological training in London. A little later, an Adelaide medical graduate, John Game, who had also received postgraduate neurological training in Britain, commenced full-time neurological practice in Melbourne. Billings was appointed to St Vincent's Hospital, and Game at the Alfred Hospital as junior to Cox. As well, again in Melbourne, the youthful Professor of Anatomy at the University of Melbourne took an interest in peripheral nerve disorder. As a medical student, Sydney Sunderland had collaborated in research with Cox, and during the war years had been responsible for a nerve injury clinic. As result of this accumulation of neurologically concerned personnel, in the immediate post-war years Melbourne undoubtedly became the centre of Australian clinical neurological practice. It was the only Australian city with a potential critical mass of neurological clinicians large enough to permit the speciality to develop further in the immediate future. At least in Melbourne, Australian clinical neurology seemed to have begun to take root.

None of the men who belonged to this founding generation of Australian neurologists is still living. Their obituaries have appeared in print in various places and, together with personal knowledge when it is available, form the basis of the following accounts of their careers. In these accounts the emphasis has been placed on the parts they played in the development of Australian neurology, often to the relative neglect of their achievements outside neurology, and outside medicine. No attempt has been made to provide any complete listings of their publications.

LEONARD BELL COX (1894–1976)

When the first edition of this book was written, information regarding Leonard Cox was available in the obituaries written by Russell and Bradley (1977) and Schwieger (1994), and in an essay by Sydney Sunderland (1994). Subsequently, a full biography has become available, written by Cox's son-in-law, Volkhard Wehner, and an abbreviated version of much of the neurologically relevant content of that volume has been published in the paper of Bladin *et al.* (2004).

Leonard Bell Cox was born in Melbourne, the son of a clergyman. After attending Wesley College, where he formed a lasting friendship with the future Australian Prime Minister, Sir Robert Menzies, Cox graduated in Medicine from the University of Melbourne in 1916. Almost immediately afterwards, he became a medical officer in the Australian Army. After World War I ended, he took the Membership of the Royal College of Physicians of Edinburgh in 1919 (he appears never to have become a Fellow of that College). Cox returned to Melbourne in 1920 to take up the position of Beaney Scholar in Pathology in the University of Melbourne, which awarded him an MD in that year. After a period of illness, he married Nancy, sister of Hugh Trumble, in 1925 and began to build a consultant practice as a neurologist in Melbourne. At the same time, he continued to do neuropathological research at the University and at the Baker Research Institute, as well as in his own garage (Billings – personal communication).

In 1934, at the age of 40, Cox became Honorary Neurologist to the Alfred Hospital, and Lecturer in Neuropathology in the University of Melbourne, being appointed Stewart Lecturer there three years later. At the Alfred Hospital a Department of Neurology was opened, where Hugh Trumble, at his brother-in-law's urging, began to develop the specialty of neurosurgery. As well as continuing to be involved in neuropathological work, Cox lectured to medical students on clinical neurology. He became a Foundation Fellow of the Royal Australasian College of Physicians in 1938.

With the growth in the number of neurologists practising in Melbourne in the immediate post-war years, Cox became the driving force in founding the Australian Association of Neurologists. He was its first President, holding that office from 1950 to 1957. After retiring from the Presidency, he continued to serve on the Association's Council until 1961. By this time, he was in his later sixties, and his days as a clinical neurologist and neuropathologist were coming to their close. It seems that his last appearance at a Meeting of the Association was in Melbourne, in May 1965, at the Ordinary General Meeting held in the building of the Royal Australasian College of Surgeons. In 1968 the Association that he had founded elected him an Honorary Member Emeritus.

Well before his retirement from professional practice, Cox had found a consuming interest in collecting Chinese ceramics and art, and also

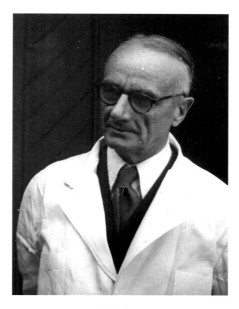

L B Cox

developed an interest in Chinese history. He played a major role in the affairs of the National Gallery of Victoria over a long period, and in later years to some extent sacrificed his neurological practice to serve the interests of the Gallery. This aspect of Cox's life was brought out by Schwieger (1994) in his obituary. It was principally for his contribution to the development of culture in Australia that Cox was awarded a CMG in 1968. He had written a much acclaimed history of the Gallery whose welfare and advancement had become a major concern of his life: *The National Gallery of Victoria 1861– 1968: A Search for a Collection.*

From the perspective of one who had never spoken with Cox, or indeed recalls seeing him more than once (in Sydney at a Scientific Meeting of the Association of Neurologist held in the Maitland Theatre of Sydney Hospital in June 1963, where Cox sat alone in the front row listening to the papers being presented with the afternoon sun streaming through the stained glass windows and casting a coloured pattern at his feet), it would seem that Cox made four main contributions to Australian neurology. While these contributions are individually identifiable, the effects overlapped harmoniously. Cox's role as founder and first President of the professional association for Australian neurologists was obviously of the greatest importance to the development of the specialty. His vision, organising ability, and professional reputation were crucial for setting the fledgling organisation on a sound footing from which it could grow in a relatively untroubled fashion, as it subsequently did. Secondly, there was the example that his career provided in demonstrating that it was practicable to work purely as a clinical neurologist under the conditions of Australian life of his day. His third significant contribution lay in the fact that he led others to the practice of clinical neurology, and into neuroscience. He saw to it that John Game became first his junior at the Alfred Hospital, and later his successor there. While Sydney Sunderland was still a medical student in Melbourne, Cox perceived his talent and introduced him into the neuroscience research in which he was to make so great a career. There were also men such as the neurosurgeon Kenneth Jamieson and the neuropharmacologist David Curtis whose career directions were at least partly influenced by Cox and his example. A small Australian school of basic and clinical neuroscience emanated from Leonard Cox. His influence was therefore an ongoing one, unlike that of Campbell in Sydney who, though probably a greater genius and no less worthy or likeable a man, for reasons which can no longer be clear was unable to ensure that there was someone to whom he could hand on the torch that he had lit. Fourthly, as one gets more distant from the times when Cox lived, his original investigational work takes on an increasing significance among his numerous achievements. He was not merely a pioneer clinical neurologist or a routine neuropathologist. He did scientific work of international calibre over much of his professional life, and he did it in relative intellectual isolation far away from the research centres and research facilities of northern hemisphere countries. He does not seem to have ever received any extended period of formal training in neuropathological research, or to have obtained special funding to support his studies. Yet from his energy, genius and initiative there came at least three very significant original contributions to neurological knowledge. His work on the cytology and classification of intracranial tumours, guided by the behaviour of their cellular elements in tissue culture, resulted in the publication in 1933 in the *American Journal of Pathology* of 'The cytology of the glioma group with special reference to the condition of cells derived from the invaded tissue'. This work became a widely used reference source for neuropathologists for a number of years. He also wrote on various aspects of cerebral and spinal tumour for the consumption of a local readership in a series of papers (Cox

1932a, 1934, 1935, 1939a,b; Cox and Trumble 1939) which could easily have been reworked into a monograph on tumours of the nervous system. Secondly, Cox investigated the neuropathology of cryptococcal infection of the nervous system, and in collaboration with the microbiologist Jean Tolhurst wrote *Human Torulosis,* a substantial monograph which appeared in 1946 under the imprint of the University of Melbourne Press. Thirdly, his synthesis of his own observations and various data obtained from the literature in the paper 'Tumours of the base of the brain: their relation to pathological sleep and other changes in the conscious state', published in the *Medical Journal of Australia* in 1937, anticipated the post-war interest in the role of the reticular formation of the brain stem in maintaining alertness in higher animals. Had work of such calibre and critical insight, written in clear and cautious language, been published in the medical journal of a more populous and more affluent northern hemisphere country, and had its author been better known at a personal level there, he probably would have received much more considerable academic acclamation for his synthesis. Early in his consultant career Cox had also had interests in other neurological topics e.g. Sluder's spheno-palatine neuralgia (Cox 1931; 1932b), the formation of syringomyelic cavities (Cox 1938b), whilst after the end of World War II he took up the matter of the clinico-pathological correlations of the effects of head injury (Cox 1949b).

Melbourne's first professional neurologist, and the Australian Association of Neurologists' founder, was a home-grown neuroscientist of considerable genius, something that succeeding generations of Australian neurologists have sometimes appeared a little slow to appreciate, even if they have not lost sight of the fact entirely.

Edward Graeme Robertson (1903–1975)

A number of accounts of Graeme Robertson's life and career are available. These include the obituaries by Game (1976) and Lance (1988), the recollections of Critchley (1990) in his *The Ventricle of Memory* (which contained a few inaccuracies), and certain preliminary remarks made by some of those who at Meetings of the Australian Association of Neurologists have delivered the annual lecture named in Graeme Robertson's honour, and especially in the initial one that was given by his cousin and Royal Melbourne Hospital surgical counterpart Reginald Hooper (1978). In addition, in the

Preface to the first edition of his work *Pneumoencephalography* (1957), Graeme Robertson wrote almost lyrically of his own neurological apprenticeship and the men and influences that helped shape his subsequent career. There is also available a very recent biography written by his son (Robertson 2023).

Graeme Robertson, like Cox a Victorian, was educated at Scots College Melbourne before undertaking medical studies at the University of Melbourne. He graduated MB BS with honours from Melbourne University in 1927. He spent the next three years in various capacities at the then Melbourne Hospital, where he came under the influence of Sidney Sewell. After taking the Melbourne MD in 1930, Robertson spent several years in London 'on the house' at the National Hospital at Queen Square, during this time becoming a Member of the London Royal College of Physicians. During those years he collaborated with the New Zealander, Derek Denny-Brown, who later was to become the J Jackson Putnam Professor of Neurology at Harvard, in an investigation of the innervation of the sphincters in humans both in health and in spinal cord and cauda equina disease (Denny-Brown and Robertson 1933a,b; 1935; Robertson 1935). He also published other investigative work during these years in Britain, e.g. on the effects of frontal lobe lesions (Walshe and Robertson 1933) and on oligodendrogliomas (Greenfield and Robertson 1933). His period of neurological apprenticeship in London was followed by appointment to the consultant staff of St Bartholomew's Hospital as Assistant to C M Hinds Howell, and also as First Assistant to Francis (later Sir Francis) Fraser at the London Postgraduate Teaching Hospital at Hammersmith. In 1934 Sewell persuaded Graeme Robertson to return to Melbourne, to what it was hoped would be a neurological appointment at the Melbourne Hospital. For some years prior to that time, it appears that neurology at that Hospital had been partly the province of the psychiatrists, notably H F Maudsley (1891–1967), who possessed the qualifications of a physician as well as those of a psychiatrist. As it happened, for a decade Robertson had to work at the Hospital as Honorary Physician to Outpatients before a Department of Neurology was created, at which time he became Honorary Neurologist to the Hospital and also to the nearby Children's Hospital. He also held consultant neurological appointments to various Victorian institutions, to the Royal Australian Navy, and to the Tasmania Government. He was a Foundation Fellow of the Royal Australasian College of Physicians and became a Fellow of the Royal College of Physicians of London in 1946.

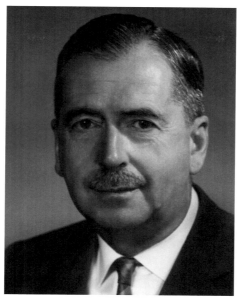

E Graeme Robertson

Graeme Robertson engaged in private consulting neurological practice from rooms in Collins St, Melbourne. He was an Originating Member of the Australian Association of Neurologists, and its second President (from 1957 to 1965). From 1965 to 1972 he was the Editor of the Association's annual publication *Proceedings of the Australian Association of Neurologists,* which he saw through the difficult period of its establishment and some rather precarious financial times.

In his later years Graeme Robertson held several prestigious positions e.g. Vice-President of the Royal Australasian College of Physicians and President of the Second Asian and Oceanian Congress of Neurology which was held in his home city. Throughout his career he travelled frequently, mainly to Britain, where he maintained contacts with his old alma mater at Queen Square and with English neurologists, in particular his old mentor Gordon Holmes. In the 1970s Robertson's health began to fail. His last attendance at an Australian Association of Neurologists' Meeting was at Canberra, in May 1974, and on that occasion his public appearances were brief. He died at Christmas 1975, the news of his passing being broadcast over the national radio network since he had become a rather well-known community figure. He had achieved this status not so much because of his neurological achievements as because of the series of books on old cast-iron and Australian colonial furniture which he had authored and illustrated, e.g. Robertson (1984). For many years he had combined his urge for perfectionism, his photographic talents, and his love for old cast-iron in a consuming hobby which produced a number of superbly illustrated books, the final one written in combination with his daughter Joan. These books dealt with the colonial ironwork from earlier years that was fast disappearing from Australian cities and country towns. In his last years he was also co-author of an illustrated work on colonial furniture which, from conversation with him, was a more recently acquired interest that he had hoped to take further.

When Graeme Robertson visited another Australian city, it often became the lot of one of the younger neurologists from that city to drive him from site to site to allow him to inspect, and photograph, the local cast-iron. On such expeditions, members of the Australian neurological community now in their own twilight years came to know something of the man. He appeared in dress and in manner a highly conservative person, diffident and almost shy. He was invariably courteous and considerate except when any circumstance threatened to interfere with his opportunity to photograph an item of ironwork under conditions which he was determined to make as ideal as feasible. In that situation he would suddenly become quite assertive, and almost irascible, though he would soon enough become apologetic for his period of out-of-character behaviour. He was happy enough to try to educate his companion about iron work and photographic technique, but he seemed more guarded in talking of neurological matters and the personalities and deeds of neurologists. Possibly he may have behaved differently in the company of his contemporaries.

Among the Australian neurologists of his day, Graeme Robertson's fame was perceived not so much to depend on his works on ornate cast-iron or on his other artistic contributions as on his reputation as the world's greatest living authority on the procedure of pneumoencephalography. This was the radiological technique which, in his day, more adequately than any other, permitted the display of the structure of the brain in the living patient. For his work on this subject, he had been elected to Honorary Fellowship of the College of Radiologists of Australasia. He published his experience with pneumoencephalography in a series of amply, indeed almost lavishly, illustrated monographs of increasing size: *Encephalography* (Robertson 1941); *Further Studies in Encephalography* (Robertson 1946a);

Pneumoencephalography (Robertson 1957, with a second edition in 1967) as well as in a book chapter (Robertson 1974) and several research papers (e.g. Robertson 1947, 1949a). It is rather sad to reflect that, by the end of his life, he must have realised that the investigative technique to which he had devoted so much of his effort was fast being superseded by the much more comfortable, safer and more informative method of computed tomography, and that it was fated to soon disappear entirely from use in neurological practice.

Over the years following his return to Australia, Graeme Robertson published on several topics other than pneumoencephalography, though this was probably the main subject with which he dealt in his later years. There had been aspects of his work on the innervation of the sphincters, and during his period in waiting for a formal neurological appointment at the (Royal) Melbourne Hospital, he did some research on poliomyelitis at the Walter and Eliza Hall Institute (Robertson 1940), some of it in collaboration with Macfarlane Burnet. There were also writings on topics such as cerebral aneurysm (1936, 1949b), spinal arachnoiditis (Robertson 1938), toxoplasma encephalomyelitis (Robertson 1946b), photogenic epilepsy (Robertson 1954) and other aspects of epilepsy (Robertson 1934, 1959), the neuropathology of Murray Valley encephalitis (1952), and historical essays on James Parkinson (Robertson 1955) and on John White. The latter had been the Surgeon General with the first fleet which came to settle New Holland in 1788, and continued to live for several years in the infant colony at Sydney before returning to Britain (Anderson 1933; Robertson 1968).

Graeme Robertson played a major role in establishing the stature of Australian neurology not only in Australian eyes, but in the eyes of world medicine. He was thoroughly steeped in the great Queen Square neurological tradition and had gone a significant way towards establishing himself professionally in the London neurological scene before he chose to return to his homeland. There he attempted to transplant the Queen Square tradition to Australian soil and, by and large, succeeded in doing so. His existence and his personal contacts linked the neurology of the parent institution in Britain with that of its offspring in its former colony. Critchley's (1990) conclusion that 'we remember him not only for putting neurology on the map in Australia, but for his unique artistic achievements', seems a fair summary of the way in which his influence and achievement were perceived internationally. Throughout his career he had continued to publish at a rate at least comparable with that of most of his British and American neurological contemporaries. As well, he achieved an international reputation for his mastery of a particular diagnostic method. All this was enhanced by his notable contributions to an aspect of non-neurological cultural life in his own country. The Australian neurology of his time saw him as its leading exponent. It could take pride in him, and realise that, through his example, it could appropriate some of that pride for itself. Graeme Robertson was Australian neurology's figurehead and, to a major extent, its inspiration.

There can be little doubt that, a quarter century ago, many Australian neurologists considered him to be a much more significant figure than Leonard Cox. However, with the passage of time there may be occasion for some reassessment of the relative merits of the two men. Australian neurology over the years since Graeme Robertson's death has acquired the maturity and independence which would allow it to appreciate better its comparability to the neurological standards of other advanced countries. It would probably no longer see a single hero figure as being so important to it. Although Graeme Robertson did ensure a clinical neurological succession at the Royal Melbourne Hospital, those he trained tended to remain neurological clinicians and did not branch into investigational neuroscience to the extent that Cox's intellectual progeny did. It may be that the Queen Square tradition, so important for establishing embryonic Australian neurology, tended to encourage convention in practice, and to stifle the urge towards innovative curiosity-driven inquiry. Therefore Cox, to a greater extent neurologically self-educated than Robertson, may have been capable of greater original contributions to the knowledge of nervous system disease and to the advancement of Australian neuroscience. Undoubtedly, they were both very great men, and in their lives and achievements Australian neurology found a sure foundation on which to begin building.

ERIC LEO (GUS) SUSMAN (1896–1959)

Even at the time of the first edition of this book, few who knew Susman well were still living and active. Consequently, the following account necessarily is based on obituaries (Kempson Maddox 1959; Larkins 1959; Selby 1988) and on recollections of several conversations with the late George Selby more than half a century ago.

Susman was a Sydney man, educated at the Church of England Grammar School in that city. Service in World War I, where he was wounded at Gallipoli and repatriated to Australia, delayed commencement of his medical studies at Sydney University. War intervened in Susman's medical career a second time, when he served in the Royal Australian Navy throughout World War II.

After graduating in Medicine in 1921, Susman was a resident medical officer at the Royal Prince Alfred Hospital where he was George Rennie's last house physician. Susman then spent time in London where in 1924 he took the Membership of the Royal College of Physicians. He was house physician at the Westminster Hospital (to James Purves-Stewart), and then at the National Hospital at Queen Square before returning to Sydney in 1925. In the following year he became Honorary Assistant Physician to the Royal Prince Alfred Hospital, and from 1945 to the end of his life was Honorary Physician to that institution. He became a Foundation Fellow of the Royal Australasian College of Physicians in 1938. While he never held a formal appointment as a neurologist to the Royal Prince Alfred Hospital, there is little doubt that he was, *de facto,* that institution's neurologist. He also provided a neurological consultant service to the nearby Royal Alexandra Hospital for Children, and with his war service connections was involved in the affairs of the Northcott Neurological Centre. He was one of the Originating Members of the Australian Association of Neurologists and remained a member of its Council from the outset until his death some nine years later.

By all accounts, Susman was a man of some style, wit and character. He was able to live largely as he pleased, and his happy qualities of personality and eccentricities reputedly endeared him to many with whom he had dealings. He became something of a local legend in his own lifetime, and memories of the man and his influence and generosity lingered long in his old hospital and in the Royal Australasian College of Physicians.

Susman was not a researcher into neurological phenomena, nor was he a prolific writer on neurological matters, though he and Kempson Maddox reported a series of cases of the Guillain-Barré syndrome in 1940. In 1949, in a racy style, he addressed in print the treatment of neurosyphilis.

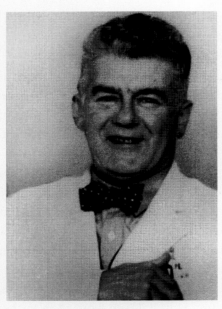

Gus Susman

His main role in neurology was that of a clinician, and his contribution to Australian neurology lay in his establishing a role for that specialty in the main teaching hospital of the University of Sydney, in maintaining its existence in Sydney after Campbell's death, and in stimulating younger men to enter it. These included George Selby, to whom Susman with characteristic generosity left his Zeiss ophthalmoscope and his collection of classical neurological texts.

KENNETH BEESON (BOB) NOAD (1900–1987)

Susman's fellow New South Welshman, and slightly younger contemporary, K B Noad, outlived him, and also most of his own contemporaries. Noad's death occurred at the time when the *Medical Journal of Australia* had, sadly, ceased to publish detailed obituaries, even those of the great figures of Australian medicine. Fortunately, Wolfenden's account of Noad's life (1994) is available, and a few members of a generation survive who remember him, at least as he was in his later years.

K B Noad was born at Maitland, in New South Wales, and graduated in Medicine from the University of Sydney in 1924 with the old MB ChM qualification. After residency at the Sydney Hospital, he spent the years 1928 and 1929 in London, where he became a Member of the Royal College of Physicians. On his return to Sydney, he was taken under the wing of the senior physician Alan Holmes à Court at Sydney Hospital where, in 1935 he was appointed Honorary Assistant Physician, later becoming Honorary Physician there. On the eve of World War II, he became one of the Foundation Fellows of the Royal Australasian College of Physicians. After war service in the eastern Mediterranean theatre and in New Guinea he returned to practice in Sydney as a consultant physician. Fellowship of the Royal College of Physicians of London followed in 1948, and he was awarded a Doctorate of Medicine by the University of Sydney in 1953, for a thesis that dealt with infectious disease as he had encountered it while on war service in the Middle East.

Noad became increasingly involved in the affairs of the then youthful Royal Australasian College of Physicians. In time he became its Censor-in-Chief and, soon afterwards, its President (1962–1964). In the latter capacity, he foresaw the possibility of the College coming to play a significant role in postgraduate medical education in South-East Asian countries and expended considerable effort and time in advancing this cause after his Presidency of the College ended. During the later stages of his career, Noad continued to be involved at a high level in many aspects of medical and educational affairs in Australia. He received further academic and professional honours, and in 1970 was knighted.

Noad always remained a general physician at heart and by his own acknowledgement, though he was responsible for the development of neurology as a specialty at Sydney Hospital. During his time in Britain early in his career he had made neurological contacts and gained neurological experience, and over his career he published a number of observational-type studies on various neurological matters. These publications included descriptions of cerebral tumour simulating cerebral vascular disease (Noad 1933), head injury (Noad 1943), uncinate epilepsy (Noad 1944), the details of a family with cerebello-olivary atrophy (with Hall and Latham, 1945), the ocular manifestations of carotid artery disease, and the neurological features of tsutsugamushi fever (Noad and Haymaker 1953). He had been one of the Originating Members of the Australian Association of Neurologists and served on its Council between 1950 and 1959. He was elected an Honorary

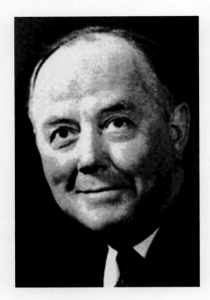

K B Noad

Member Emeritus of the Association in 1968, and occasionally after that time was present at its scientific meetings when they were held in Sydney.

As he grew older, Noad gradually faded from the clinical scene. His last years were blighted by failing health and on one occasion he confided that the onset of dyslexia deprived him of the pleasure he had always found in reading. Despite this, on the occasion of that confidence, he pretended to read a long address to a major medico-political meeting in Melbourne, though he had already committed the entire substance of his address to memory. He was able to get through the occasion without significant apparent difficulty. Noad, despite his distinction and seniority, always appeared kindly and helpful in his relations with younger colleagues, though his later years may have been lonely for want of contact with professional contemporaries. Some years after he had ceased to appear at meetings of the Association of Neurologists, I approached him to seek his help in trying to obtain information about A W Campbell. On more than one occasion after that, he went well out of his way to help me, and ultimately presented me with his copies of the two volumes of Haymaker and Adams' massive work on *The Histology and Histopathology of the Nervous System* which he said had been given to him by his old friend Webb Haymaker.

Like Susman, Noad played a key role in initiating the development of neurology in one of the two major Sydney teaching hospitals of the day.

There it continued to flourish after his time until the hospital itself ceased to exist as a viable entity, because of a Government decision reflecting the effects of local geography and demography. Noad's role in the Royal Australasian College of Physicians, given the circumstances and professional attitudes of his time, virtually precluded him from practising purely in neurology. Nevertheless, in the guise of a physician, he made contributions to neurological knowledge that were at least as substantial as those of many neurologists of his time in other lands.

GERALD CAREW MOSS (1901–1972)

Gerald Moss was the first man to ractise neurology in Western Australia. Details of his career are available in obituaries written by Gillett *et al.* (1973) and Sadka (1988).

Moss was educated Guildford Grammar School and, after commencing medical studies in Perth, completed his undergraduate medical studies in Melbourne (in 1925). At that time there was no full medical course in Perth. He then entered general practice in Claremont, and later went to Britain where, in 1936, he took the Membership of the Royal College of Physicians of London. When he returned to Perth, he practised in St George's Terrace as a physician with a particular interest in neurology. During the 1939–1945 War he served in the Army Medical Corps in the Middle East and back in Australia. He had become one of the Foundation Fellows of the Royal Australasian College of Physicians (in 1938).

Moss was Physician to the (Royal) Perth Hospital for a number of years prior to 1955, when he resigned his hospital appointment after becoming Neurologist to the Mental Health Service. He had also held appointment as Senior Honorary Neurologist to the Fremantle Hospital. At the Perth Hospital he had fulfilled the role of neurologist, functioning as the medical counterpart to the neurosurgeon James Ainslie, though he was never formally appointed as the institution's neurologist. He was one of the Originating Members of the Australian Association of Neurologists and a Member of its Council from 1961 to 1970, becoming an Honorary Member Emeritus of the Association in 1971.

In 1956, with a now more easily regulated pattern of professional life in his new appointment, Moss began part-time studies for a Bachelor of Arts degree at the University of Western Australia. In 1960 he graduated with

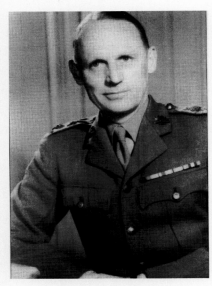

Gerald Moss

first-class honours in Greek. After this, he continued to delve into the classic world, taking up matters such as disease and drugs in the ancient world and the mentality and personality of the Julio-Claudian emperors (Moss 1968), publishing original works of scholarship in these areas (Gillett *et al.* 1973). The latter part of Moss's life appears to have been more concerned with such explorations of the classics than with clinical neurology, though he seems to have retained some medical professional interests.

During Gerald Moss's time in practice, travel between Perth and the eastern seaboard of Australia was neither particularly easy nor convenient. Consequently, Western Australian medicine tended to develop somewhat in isolation from medicine of the rest of the country. Moss's importance to the development of Australian neurology would appear mainly to have been local. He was the first to raise the neurological flag in Perth, and placed before his contemporaries and juniors in that city an example of professional competence and wider scholarship, but he also did provide the early link between neurology in West Australia and that in the Eastern States. He made no major original contributions to neurological knowledge, though he published accounts of subacute and chronic meningococcal infection in 1941, and of encephalitis and encephalomyelitis in 1949, though neither broke much new ground. Nonetheless, his presence and activities in Perth created a situation that his successors were not unhappy to avail themselves of when they followed in his pioneering neurological footsteps.

Sir Sydney Sunderland (1910–1993)

It could be argued that Sydney Sunderland was an active clinical neurologist (and even then, only a part-time one) for no more than a relatively short portion of his long career, so he does not merit inclusion in the company of those of the other men discussed in the present Chapter. However, he was one of the eight Originating Members of the Australian Association of Neurologists, and over many years his name was among the few Australian ones that were readily recognised in international neuroscience.

Sydney Sunderland was born in Brisbane and received his earlier education in that city (Ryan 1993). He completed the first year of a science degree at the University of Queensland but, because at that time there was no full medical course in Brisbane, he then entered on medical studies at the University of Melbourne. As has already been mentioned, during his undergraduate years he was invited by Leonard Cox to collaborate in work on the culture of cerebral tumour tissue, and this brought him to the notice of the Professor of Anatomy, Frederick Wood Jones. As soon as Sunderland graduated MB BS in 1935, he was appointed to a Senior Lectureship in Anatomy in the University of Melbourne. He continued his investigations in the Anatomy Department there in collaboration with Leonard Cox and with the latter's neurosurgical counterpart Hugh Trumble at the Alfred Hospital. In 1938 Sunderland worked in the Department of Human Anatomy at Oxford, and from there applied for, and was appointed to, the Chair of Anatomy in the University of Melbourne which had been vacated by Wood Jones. After gaining further experience overseas, Sunderland took up his Chair in 1940. During the war years, as well as carrying out his University duties, he was in charge of an Army peripheral nerve injury unit in Melbourne. He became interested in the anatomy and biology of the peripheral nerves and in the surgical repair of severed nerves. This interest continued through his professional life and he wrote two major textbooks on the subject, the massive *Nerves and Nerve Injuries,* first published in 1968 with a second edition 10 years later, and the smaller *Nerve Injuries and Their Repair: A Critical Approach,* which appeared in 1991, when he was already an octogenarian.

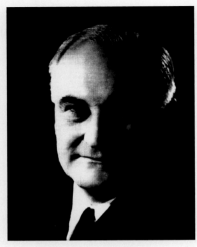

Sydney Sunderland

From 1939 to 1961, Sunderland remained Professor of Anatomy in the University of Melbourne. His University title then became that of Professor of Experimental Neurology. He continued in the latter position until 1975, maintaining his research whilst becoming increasingly involved in highest level administrative tasks in his own University and in the wider Australian university system and community. During his career he acquired two 'earned' doctorates (in Medicine and in Science) from University of Melbourne, and in addition several honorary doctorates from various universities and also Honorary Fellowship of the Royal Australasian College of Surgeons. He was also a Fellow of the Royal Australasian College of Physicians and of the Australian Academy. Within the Australian Association of Neurologists, he remained an Ordinary Member until elected to Honorary Membership in 1964, one assumes in recognition of his already great distinction and the fact that he had become very much a part-time clinical neurologist, while remaining a very considerable and very active neuroscientist.

Whilst a great deal could be written about Sydney Sunderland's service to medicine and to the Australian academic and scientific communities, in the present context the main interest lies in his place in the development of Australian clinical neurology. Very clearly, he was a great authority, probably the greatest authority of his time in the world, on peripheral nerve tissue and its injury. The knowledge that this was the case was important for the self-esteem of Australian neurology and neuroscience in their infancies. Long after Sydney Sunderland ceased to attend meetings of the

Association of Neurologists one could judge from conversation with him that he maintained a benevolent concern for that body and an interest in local neurological affairs more generally, though his clinical activities had inevitably become more remote as the passage of the years increasingly involved him in the highest levels of national academic administration. He remained enviably alert and active well after most men are no longer able to make any intellectual contribution to the life of their communities. Though he trained no clinical neurologists and founded no school of clinical neurology, the contemporary Australian neurological community of his day understood well that, in Sydney Sunderland, it possessed within its ranks a very considerable neurological scholar.

JOHN AYLWARD GAME (1913–1995)

John Game, a Tasmanian by birth, received his schooling in Adelaide at St Peter's College and obtained his basic medical qualifications from the University of Adelaide, graduating there in 1938 (Gilligan 1996). After service in the Royal Australian Air Force during World War II he spent the following two years with the rank of Group Captain and was the commanding officer at the Heidelberg Repatriation Hospital. During this time, he took an MD (presumably by examination) from the University of Melbourne. He then worked for some time at the National Hospital for Nervous Diseases at Queen Square in London, returning to Melbourne in 1950 to take up a consultant neurological position as junior to Leonard Cox at the Alfred Hospital. He became Honorary Neurologist to that institution in 1955 after Cox retired. After John Game's return to Melbourne, he had become a Member of the Royal Australasian College of Physicians, and subsequently was elected to Fellowship of that body. In the years after his return to Melbourne, his publication record suggests an interest in the newly developing field of percutaneous cerebral angiography, and in the general question of cerebral tumour (Game 1951). Earlier, he had published on polyarteritis nodosa (Game 1946). Game resigned his appointment at the Alfred Hospital in 1963, to devote himself to private consultant practice. Over the last decade his life, or rather longer, he was increasingly limited by chronic illness which did not continue to respond satisfactorily to the available treatments. He struggled to remain active for as long as he could, and was cared for with great devotion by his wife Barbara over many difficult years.

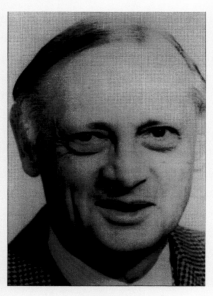

John Game

Although he was always very conscious of the importance of research for the advancement of neurology, and for the desirability of the specialty receiving academic recognition, John Game was neither by nature nor by talent a researcher, and he published relatively little during his career. Rather he was a fine clinical neurologist and, perhaps as a consequence of his Air Force experiences, an excellent organiser and far-sighted planner. When the Australian Association of Neurologists was founded in 1950, he was the first Honorary Secretary and Treasurer of the body. He continued in the former capacity until 1963, when he became the Association's third President. He occupied that office for a term of nine years, during which time he organised a thorough revision of the Association's original Constitution and led it patiently through complex negotiations with the governments of the day and with certain outside bodies, in an attempt to establish the status and improve the financial remuneration of clinical neurologists. During the same period he conceived, and moved to put in place, his vision of an Australian Neurological Foundation. This body was intended to advance neurological education, research and patient care throughout the country. He served as the Foundation's first President from its inception until 1980.

John Game was a man of strong principles, courteous and distinguished in manner, but firm when he considered that he needed to be. Occasionally his sense of principle may have led him into decisions and situations which became a little impracticable in their operation, but his vision played a very significant role in shaping the development and organisation of Australian neurology for some two decades. His memorial is the Australian Association of Neurologists, and the affectionate memory in which he is held by those of a generation fortunate enough to have known him.

John Billings (1918–2007)

Melbourne born, John Billings was the youngest of the eight Originating Members of the Australian Association of Neurologists, and their last survivor. He was educated in Melbourne at Xavier College and the University of Melbourne, from which he graduated MB BS in 1941. After a two-year residency at St Vincent's Hospital in his home city, he spent three years in Papua-New Guinea with the Australian Army before returning to Melbourne to take the local MD and the Membership of the Royal Australasian College of Physicians. He then went for two years to London, to the National Hospital for Nervous Diseases at Queen Square, becoming a Member of the Royal College of Physicians of London during this time. He returned to Melbourne in 1949 and began his long period in the practice of neurology at St Vincent's Hospital. There he worked in collaboration with the neurosurgeon Frank Morgan over so many years, both of them seemingly ageless, whilst younger men came, stayed a while, and seemed to disappear again.

From 1950 to 1984 Billings was Head of the Department of Neurology at his old hospital, St Vincent's, subsequently becoming Consultant to that Hospital where, from 1974 to 1983, he was also Dean of the Clinical School. He had, in the course of time, become a Fellow of both of the Royal Colleges of Physicians of which he had previously been a Member. From 1961 to 1975 he was a member of the Australian National Health and Medical Research Council.

Outside clinical neurology, John Billings, together with his wife Evelyn, herself a medical practitioner, had a close and continuing involvement in promoting family planning achieved by exploiting knowledge of the expected time of ovulation. They advocated what came to be called the `Billings' method in many countries throughout the world, a service for which John Billings received a Papal Knighthood in the Order of St Gregory the Great in 1969, an AM in 1991, and honorary doctorates from four universities.

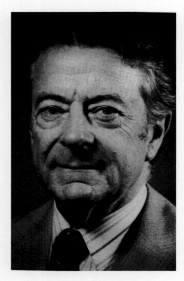

John Billings

As a neurologist, John Billings was a clinician rather than a researcher, though he published a number of articles on neurological phenomenological topics during his career, e.g. paraplegia following chest surgery (Billings and Robertson 1955). His professional life spanned almost the entire first half-century of the existence of Australian clinical neurology, and his activities played a very significant part in the growth of the specialty. He also played a distinguished role in the wider Australian medical scene, and an influential international one, in conjunction with his wife, in relation to promoting family planning. At a later stage of life, when most men would have felt justified in leisurely and perhaps contemplative inactivity, John Billings remained energetic and vigorous, his mental capacities undimmed, his physical appearance largely unchanged, with his strong sense of duty toward society undiminished. His well-lived life came to its end in 2007.

Chapter 4

THE FOUNDATION OF THE AUSTRALIAN ASSOCIATION OF NEUROLOGISTS

On the 23 October 1948, Leonard Cox recorded in his diary:

> Today at 10 am Robertson, with Noad and Sussman [sic] of Sydney met with me to discuss the formation of an Australian Neurological Society. We were all in agreement & R[obertson] and I will now get down to business on the constitution. This may be an important step in Australia neurology.

This appears to be the initial record, albeit a private one, that a seed had been sown that, over the next year and a half, was to grow into the seedling Australian Association of Neurologists.

The Royal Australasian College of Physicians had met in Melbourne on that Saturday, and on the preceding two days. The Saturday morning College meeting was scheduled to occur at St Vincent's Hospital, but whether Cox and his three compatriots met there is not certain. In fact, there is no easily obtainable proof that they as much as attended the College meeting, but the circumstantial evidence and timing are quite suggestive. None of the participants at that preliminary occasion is still living, and the further stages of the gestation processes are unlikely to ever become known with any certainty, though it is recorded that, at some stage, perhaps at that time of origin, an *ad hoc* Council for the proposed new Society comprised of the above-named men was set up.

However, it is possible that the sowing of the seed may have begun a little earlier. At the British Medical Association's Congress held in Perth in August 1948, when Cox was President of the Section on Neurology and Psychiatry, both Noad and Gerald Moss were present and both presented papers. Perhaps the three also talked together there. Many years later, when speaking privately about the Association's foundation, Sir Sydney Sunderland gave no indication that he had himself played any significant role in the early Melbourne events, and he had worked with Cox at the relevant times. Of the other Melbourne-based men who might have played a part in the inception, John Billings probably was too junior and too recently on the scene after overseas training to have had any influential role. Billings's fellow Melburnian, John Game, at least as one knew him later, certainly had the ability to have contributed, but he was still undergoing neurological training in Britain over much of the relevant period and was recruited into the new Association's membership only at the time of its actual inauguration, and then perhaps because a Secretary and a Treasurer were needed.

Perusal of the Minutes of the first Meeting of the body, which was to be named the Australian Association of Neurologists (Appendix I), also suggests that Leonard Cox was the driving force in guiding the emerging organisation through its period of gestation and its delivery into the world. In doing this, Cox would have had available for his assistance the examples of at least two comparatively recently formed professional medical specialist organisations in his own country, viz. the Royal Australasian College of Physicians and the Neurosurgical Society of Australasia. The former had been constituted in the years immediately prior to the outbreak of World War II. It provided a focus for the scientific and professional interests and aspirations of consultant physicians, but it was also intended to function as an examining body to determine those medical practitioners who were worthy of the status of physician. From the outset, the College of Physicians had a reasonably sizeable corpus of Foundation Fellows. It seems unlikely that the mere handful of neurologists then practising in Australia, almost all of whom had relatively recently been accepted into the Australasian College of Physicians, would at that time have had any serious thoughts about setting up a rival examination mechanism to determine suitability to practise clinical neurology. The small group of neurologists probably regarded their situation as much closer to that of the eight neurosurgeons who, in 1940, had set up an Australasian body which was to become the Neurosurgical Society of Australasia (Simpson *et al.* 1974; Curtis *et al.* 1980). Both the College of Physicians and the Neurosurgeons had included New Zealanders within their ranks from the outset. The neurologists did not do likewise. It seems a strange rejection of a sensible precedent. For some years after 1931, Ivan Allen had practised in New Zealand exclusively as a neurologist, the only one in that country (Burns 1963). He has been the subject of a recent biography (Anderson 2016). Allen had received a thorough neurological training in Britain at Queen Square and had a significant record of personal neurological publication, e.g. on aseptic meningitis (Allen and Spencer 1935), reflex epilepsy (Allen 1938) and grasping and tonic innervation (Allen 1939) which had appeared in the *Medical Journal of Australia*. It is therefore most unlikely that the small Australian neurological community was unaware of Allen's existence. Possibly the Originating Australian Members envisaged that their Association, unlike the Royal Australasian College of Physicians, would in the future be required to play a medico-political role and not mainly a scientific and educational one. If so, an Association that was Australian rather than Australasian may have seemed better suited to deal with an Australian government.

THE INAUGURAL MEETING

The first gathering of the Australian neurologists took place on 25 October 1950 on what could be regarded as comparatively neutral ground in Melbourne, in Sydney Sunderland's University Department of Anatomy, rather than in the professional rooms or homes of one of the Melbourne neurologists. However, the site of the meeting may really have been determined by the fact that it was to be followed by another meeting, a scientific one, which would probably have required a more public and larger venue with appropriate facilities. The Original Meeting and its attendance have been described by Game (1975), though Sydney Sunderland in private conversation once gave a slightly different account of the meeting. From the Minutes, it seems that originally six people were invited to the Inauguration Meeting, and that these six constituted the proposed `Originating Members'. However Gerald Moss, one of this six, was not present on the day and apologised for his absence. Sunderland and John Game were also in attendance at the meeting, presumably by invitation, and while there were admitted as additional Originating Members. Therefore, the Original Meeting involved seven Originating Members physically present, and the absent Gerald Moss. Cox opened the meeting, and Graeme Robertson, seconded by Noad, proposed that Cox be elected President. Cox then suggested that the posts of Honorary Secretary and Honorary Treasurer be combined, and Robertson and Noad nominated John Game for that combined office. There was obvious convenience in this arrangement, as Game was the junior to Cox at the Alfred Hospital. The two would be likely to see a considerable amount of each other in the course of their ordinary work. Once the office-bearers were in position, the newly appointed President submitted a draft constitution of the Association for discussion. The name suggested for the association was the Australian Association of Neurologists. However, Susman suggested the alternative title `The Association of Australian Neurologists', but it was pointed out to him that this title would have excluded from the Association's membership neurologists who were not Australians. This settled, the draft Constitution appears to have been accepted without difficulty, and with some alacrity. It was realised that the Constitution might later require modification after it underwent legal scrutiny, and that this process was a necessary preliminary to the Association's being registered.

A Council comprising Cox, Robertson, Noad, Susman and Game was decided on at the Meeting, the initial annual subscription was set at one guinea, and plans were made concerning the principles to be applied in meeting the costs of future social functions of the infant Association. Susman raised the important issue of whether the criteria for membership of the Australian Association of Neurologists might make it too exclusive and so deny general physicians with some interest in neurology the possibility of becoming involved. However, Cox and Robertson took the view that the membership needed to be reasonably exclusive, and of high standard, to allow the objectives of the Association to be achieved.

This first Meeting commenced at 10 a.m. and concluded some 55 minutes later. Clearly there had been some very careful and thorough preparation beforehand, and a good measure of prior agreement must have been achieved. Whilst the philosophy underlying the Association's aims needs to be examined further, a potentially important issue had already arisen at the Initial Meeting, viz. the question of the exclusivity of the Association's membership.

Those present at the Meeting then seem to have moved on to the initial Scientific Meeting of the Australian Association of Neurologists, also held in the same Anatomy Department of the University of Melbourne. It appears that certain guests were present at the Scientific Meeting for, beside papers by Sunderland, Susman, Robertson and Cox, a paper was read by the Melbourne anatomist and neurosurgeon Keith Bradley, and a joint paper by Game and Luke, the latter a Melbourne radiologist. The contents of the program are shown in Appendix II.

THE ORIGINAL CONSTITUTION OF THE ASSOCIATION

The full text of the original Constitution of the Australian Association of Neurologists is reproduced in Appendix III. Those possessed of a legalistic turn of mind may find interest in perusing it in its entirety, but certain aspects of the document appear to hold the key to how the Association was intended to function and to the role envisaged for it in Australian medicine.

The stated 'objects' i.e. objectives, of the Association were to bring together neurological clinicians and neurological scientists with the broad aim of facilitating their interaction and thereby advancing knowledge of the normal and diseased nervous system. The document defined four classes of membership of the Association and provided for members of all classes to attend the Annual General Meetings and Scientific Meetings of the Association but accorded voting rights only to Ordinary Members. The criteria for the various classes of membership were not very tightly defined at that stage, but it was made very clear that the Council had the right, and the responsibility, to determine the class of membership to be offered to any given person. The criterion for Provisional Membership, viz. to practise neurology but not to hold a senior neurological appointment to an approved hospital, and in the opinion of the Council to possibly not adhere to the practice of neurology, may seem somewhat contradictory at first sight. However, in practice it seems that persons who would have been qualified to practise neurology but who, by virtue of their professional circumstances, were not yet committed fully to its practice were admitted to this category of membership. The status of each provisional member was to be reviewed after three years in that category of membership. By this time, it would have been expected that the person concerned would either have demonstrated a commitment to practise fully as a neurologist or would have moved into some other area of medicine. In the latter case there would not have been much point in his or her maintaining a relationship with the Association. The powers of Council were clearly defined and were considerable, and the composition of its membership was made explicit. In effect, the Council controlled the Association, and it was only the Ordinary Members who had the power to elect the Council. As a result, the Association was to be very much a body controlled by professional clinical neurologists. Those with an interest in clinical neurology, but who did not appear to have made a commitment to carry out their dominant or exclusive pattern of practice in

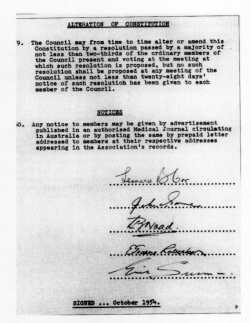

ALTERATION OF CONSTITUTION

9. The Council may from time to time alter or amend this Constitution by a resolution passed by a majority of not less than two-thirds of the ordinary members of the Council present and voting at the meeting at which such resolution is proposed, but no such resolution shall be proposed at any meeting of the Council unless not less than twenty-eight days' notice of such resolution has been given to each member of the Council.

NOTICES

10. Any notice to members may be given by advertisement published in an authorised Medical Journal circulating in Australia or by posting the same by prepaid letter addressed to members at their respective addresses appearing in the Association's records.

SIGNED ... October 1954.

Signatures on the Constitution of the AAN

the specialty, could only with some difficulty reach even the fringes of the Association. However, non-clinical neuroscientists had a place in it. In being an association dominated by clinical neurologists, rather than being a body which embraced on a more or less equal footing all those in the country who had some neurological interest, the Australian Association of Neurologists differed from most of the other bodies which were later set up to cater for the interests of physicians engaged in other sub-specialties of internal medicine. Its exclusivity of membership resulted in the Association of Neurologists being numerically smaller than other sub-specialty professional bodies for a long time, but simultaneously made it very much more cohesive and internally stronger. Its smaller numbers tended to encourage its members to make friendships and alliances across State boundaries and to develop more easily a national rather than a more parochial attitude.

In a generally far-sighted and well-drafted document such as the original Constitution, even though the initial membership of the Association was so small, the quorum for the Ordinary General Meeting, which was to be held once each year, was to comprise at least 30% of the ordinary members present in person or by proxy. This wording seemed to allow of the possibility that the entire physical attendance at the meeting could comprise of one person, who held sufficient proxies. In fact, the third General Business Meeting of the Association, which was to have been held in March 1953, did lapse for want of a quorum.

At the second General Business Meeting of the Association held in the Boardroom of Sydney Hospital on 10 April 1951, only six of the Originating Members were present (Sunderland and Moss being absent). At that time the draft Constitution was still in the hands of the lawyers. The Constitution achieved its definitive form and was then signed by the members of Council in October 1954, though no actual day, but only the month of signing was shown on the document itself. However, when the fourth Ordinary General Meeting of the Association was held in the Boardroom of Sydney Hospital on 12 October 1954, the Minutes of that meeting indicated that the final draft of the Constitution was to be confirmed by Council later on that day. Hence that date probably was the day of the signing.

The original Constitution remained in force over the first decade of existence of the Australian Association of Neurologists, but some modification was put into effect in 1961. The main change was that the mechanism for nomination of new members was made very much more specific. Each prospective member was to be nominated by two Ordinary Members of the Association, and a Council Member, briefed by one of the nominating members, was to sponsor the application for its consideration by the Council. The academic and professional training, and the qualifications, required for Ordinary and Provisional Membership were set out in detail. Basically, the possession of a medical degree from a recognised university was required, plus Membership or Fellowship of the London or the Australasian Colleges of Physicians, or of one of the other Royal Colleges of Physicians, as well as at least one year of approved neurological training and, in the case of Ordinary Members, at least three years of experience in a consultant neurological role. For Provisional Members the latter requirement was not necessary, but in practice if it had not been met within the next three years the Provisional Membership was likely to lapse. The specific criteria are reproduced in Appendix IV. For many years they in practice determined who would, and who would not, be likely to be admitted to the Association's membership. They have also tended to define, in the eyes of the Commonwealth Government, those persons in the country who were to be regarded as clinical neurologists.

THE ASSOCIATION'S FIRST DECADE

During the period between 1950 and 1954 the Minutes of the Annual General Meetings (sometimes called Business Meetings) of the Australian Association of Neurologists and those of its Council suggest that there was very little activity within the Association. However, the tempo had increased by 1954.

Membership

At the Council Meeting held in April 1951 at Sydney Hospital, Drs Fisher (of Perth), Rail and Selby (both of Sydney) became Associate Members of the Association, while the neuropathologist Dr Oliver Latham and the then Professor of Anatomy at the University of Sydney, Norman Birkett, were elected the Association's first Honorary Members. At the Council Meeting held in March 1953, held in the Anatomy School of the University of Melbourne, Dr Macdonald Critchley of London was elected to Honorary Membership, thus becoming the Association's first overseas Honorary Member. At the following Council Meeting on 12 October 1954 there was still more activity. Drs Rail and Selby were appointed Ordinary Members of the Association after their periods of Associate Membership were served, and Drs W G Burke (of Sydney), J Gordon (of Adelaide) and A Schwieger (of Melbourne) were appointed directly to Ordinary Membership without spending any qualifying period in Provisional or Associate Membership. Why Selby and Rail had been required to go through the preliminary period of Associate Membership whereas their three contemporaries had not, is unclear from the Minutes. Possibly Selby and Rail were victims of the lack of clear definition of the membership criteria in the original Constitution. It may be that realisation of this lack of clarity led to the constitutional changes referred to above which came into effect a few years later. These changes clarified the whole membership criteria matter for the future. At the same 1954 meeting, the Melbourne neuropathologist Ross Anderson and John Tyrer, Professor of Medicine in the University of Queensland, who had received neurological training under Russell Brain at the London Hospital, were appointed Associate Members, and Sir Charles Symonds of London was given Honorary Membership. Thus, by late 1954, the original Ordinary Membership category had increased in number from 8 to 13 persons. The number of Ordinary Members then remained stationary until 1957, when a further Ordinary Member, A Fisher, of Perth, was appointed from the ranks of Associate Membership and the first batch of Provisional Members, 9 in total, was added to the Association. From the time that the Provisional Membership category began to be employed, it is not unreasonable to regard the total of the Ordinary plus Provisional Members as being the measure of the clinical neurological component of the membership of the Association, since the Provisional Members were potential career neurologists who after three years in the category nearly always moved into the Ordinary Member category. If this interpretation is accepted, by the end of 1960 the Association had a total of 26 members, 18 being Ordinary Members. Hence the number of neurologists in Australia had a little more than trebled over the decade since the inauguration of the Australian Association of Neurologists.

In the first decade of the Association's existence, Council Meetings were nearly always held in conjunction with the Ordinary General and Scientific Meetings of the Association. The composition of the original Council was unaltered until 1957, when Graeme Robertson succeeded Leonard Cox as President, Cox reverting to the role of Council member. At the same time Billings was added to the Council as Honorary Treasurer, Game relinquishing that component of his previous dual office. Two years later there were further changes in the composition of the Council. Rail and Selby became members, replacing Susman, who had died recently, and Noad, who had become overburdened in his office as Censor-in-chief of the Royal Australasian College of Physicians. With the new appointments, two Council members continued to come from New South Wales, though there is no suggestion in the Minutes that considerations of State representation were involved in the appointments.

Scientific Meetings

Until 1959 all the Scientific Meetings of the Association were held in Melbourne or Sydney, tending to alternate between the Anatomy School of the University of Melbourne and the Maitland Lecture Hall of Sydney Hospital. In 1959 the Meeting was held at the Medical School of the University of Adelaide and, later in that year, in conjunction with a session of the Royal Australasian College of Physicians, there was a Meeting in the Australian Academy conference chamber in Canberra. The Scientific Meeting in 1960 returned to the Anatomy School in the University of Melbourne. The programs for these meetings, and several subsequent ones, are contained in Appendix II. Between 1950 and 1957, the number of papers presented at each meeting varied between 5 and 7, but for the next three years averaged 10 per meeting. The Council Meeting in October 1958 discussed the possibility of tape recording the proceedings of the Scientific Meetings. Two years later there was a proposal to have a stenographer record the papers given at future Scientific Meetings. The prospects of publishing these papers were subsequently discussed, and the possibility considered of seeking from the Royal Australasian College of Physicians an agreement to allow the papers to appear annually as one of the issues of the College's journal *The Australasian Annals of Medicine.* The possibility of publishing the papers in conjunction with the Australian Psychiatrists was also raised, as well as that of the Association in its own right publishing the papers. At that time, only a decade after the inauguration of the Association, Council found itself needing to discuss whether the length of the Scientific Meeting should be extended from one to one and a half days, with the individual papers being of 30 minutes duration, each being followed by 20 minutes of discussion.

There thus is evidence that, over the first decade of the Association's existence, an increased amount of scientific material had become available for presentation by its members at its Scientific Meetings, and that its members sensed that this material was worth preserving in some durable form. The nature of the material presented at the Scientific Meetings indicates that, from the outset, the presentations tended to deal more with particular neurological topics of contemporary interest than to provide individual case reports. In fact, in 1958, the Council decided that no case reports would be presented at Annual Scientific Meetings unless they were of 'unusual interest'.

Financial Affairs

After mention that the original annual subscription for Ordinary Members was set at one guinea, the Minutes of the Ordinary General Meetings remained silent regarding financial matters until 1954, a time when the Association had a credit balance of £3-12-9. By 1958 the credit balance was £38-1-2; two years later it had grown to £46-11-0. Two years after that the credit balance was reported as about £60. In 1958 the annual subscription had been increased to £2-2-0.

Other Matters

In 1957 the Council had discussed the possibility of including New Zealanders in the membership, but did not seem to reach any decision. By the end of the decade increasing amounts of time at Council and Ordinary General Meetings were being spent in discussing the relationships between the Association and outside bodies such as Government departments, lay groups interested in specific neurological disorders and the Royal Australasian College of Physicians, as well as the British Medical Association in Australia. Clearly the Association was becoming recognised and influential in the Australian medico-political arena.

At the 1954 Ordinary General Meeting, the President drew the attention of those present to a wooden gavel which had been presented to the Association as a gift from Macdonald Critchley. The gavel had been made from wood salvaged from the area of the National Hospital, Queen Square, which had been bomb-damaged during World War II. The gavel was inscribed:

> To the Australian Association of Neurologists from the President of the Section of Neurology, Royal Society of Medicine, London, 1953.

The first decade of the Australian Association of Neurologists' existence saw it grow in membership numbers, begin to establish itself financially, start to become influential both within and beyond the Australian medical profession, expand its academic activities and begin thinking about enlarging its educational role, at least within Australia.

Chapter 5

THE YEARS OF INCREASING CLINICAL AND ACADEMIC GROWTH

By 1960, the efforts of the founding generation of Australian clinical neurologists had provided the specialty with a reasonably sure footing in the contemporary Australian medical scene. The ensuing six decades have seen Australian clinical and academic neurology grow progressively in a relatively steady and largely undisturbed fashion on the basis of that footing. The number of those practising the specialty has increased steadily, and they have become more widely distributed throughout the larger centres of population outside the State capital cities where clinical neurological practice had begun in the country (also see Chapter 8). The specialty has increased in academic status, with senior academic appointments in neurology being made in most Australian medical schools and with academic titles being bestowed on clinical neurologists in many teaching hospitals in recognition of their educational and sometimes research activities. New investigational and therapeutic approaches have been embraced as they became available, and confidence gained that the country has become capable of training its own neurological professionals without the virtual necessity, as distinct from the desirability, of their obtaining overseas experience. Overall, the sense has developed that contemporary Australian neurology has achieved a stature sufficient to enable it to hold its own in the international setting.

NEUROLOGIST NUMBERS

As can be inferred from some of the data in the previous chapter, by 1960 there were full-time neurologists practising in all the Australian State capital cities apart from Hobart, though there was none in the national capital of Canberra, itself situated only a comparatively short distance from Sydney, or in the Northern Territory with its comparatively small population. Since that time, the number of neurologists has increased in all of these places, though very few are based in the Northern Territory.

As well, neurologists have increasingly found places to practise in most of the larger Australian provincial cities, for the most part the coastal ones. Furthermore, intermittent consulting services have often been provided to population centres too small to sustain the full-time activity of a neurologist. There has also been a more recent tendency for an increased proportion of newly trained neurologists to remain in full-time or near full-time hospital appointments, and from these positions to undertake only a quite limited amount of extramural consulting work. Over the past 60 years, demographic and economic factors and numbers of available neurologists have largely determined the pattern of extension of Australian neurological services and the manner of clinical neurological practice, while the perceived professional advantages and relative security associated with predominantly hospital-based appointments have increasingly shaped how and where neurologists choose to practise.

The combined earlier categories of Ordinary and Provisional Members of the former Australian Association, and the equivalent category of Full Members of the subsequent Australian and New Zealand Association of Neurologists, largely coincide with the clinical neurologists who practise in Australia (after excluding the New Zealanders). Hence a plot against time of the number of the persons in these categories provides a measure of the numerical growth of the specialty in Australia (Figure 2 – see Chapter 8). A similar plot can be constructed on an Australian State-by-State basis (Figure 3, Chapter 8). Up to the end of the last century, the publication of Morris (1994a) provides information on the distribution of neurologists and the available investigational facilities within the individual Australian States (and the areas of research strength and expertise that had developed, at least in the major centres, in the States). Although the present book attempts to preserve a national perspective throughout, there is some logic (and convenience) in dealing with the growth in Australian clinical neurology on a state-by-state basis. However, listing anything like complete details of the expansions and other changes at the various individual institutions within each State in recent decades would inflict a rather overwhelming mass of material on the reader: a more general approach to such matters seems both more practical, and hopefully more tolerable, to a readership. In particular, there has been no intention to provide a currently contemporary account of the sites of practice of individual neurologists.

New South Wales

To his time of writing, Allsop (1994) provided an account of the development of neurology in New South Wales that is the basis for the earlier part of the following material.

At the time of the foundation of the Australian Association of Neurologists in 1950, there was no full-time neurologist practising in Sydney. In 1951 George Selby commenced private consulting practice in that city, working exclusively as a neurologist. However, his formal major hospital appointments, first and but briefly held, as a Clinical Assistant at the Royal Prince Alfred Hospital, and subsequently over many years at the Royal North Shore Hospital, were as a physician. Under this designation, he provided a consultant neurological service to the latter institution. Selby's was a pattern of professional practice within the New South Wales hospital system that resembled that which K B Noad had followed at Sydney Hospital, and E L Susman at the Royal Prince Alfred Hospital. Soon after Selby, William Burke was appointed as an Assistant Physician to the Department of Neurosurgery at St Vincent's Hospital in Sydney, making it possible for him to provide the medical neurological input required by the Neurosurgical Clinic which Douglas Miller (later Sir Douglas) had established at the Hospital. A little while afterwards, John Allsop received an Assistant Physician appointment at the Royal Prince Alfred Hospital, where he was to inherit the role left vacant by the death of Eric Susman in 1959.

The Children's Hospital and some of the lesser Sydney hospitals had created Consultant Neurological appointments at rather earlier stages of their developments, prior to World War II, e.g. for Alfred Walter Campbell at the Coast and the Children's Hospital, for John Irvine Hunter at the Lewisham Hospital (though the latter may have been more or less a token role), while Selby later was to hold a designated consultant neurology appointment at the Hornsby Hospital. However, it was to be rather a long wait before formal consultant neurological appointments and departments of neurology appeared at the major senior University of Sydney teaching hospitals of the day (the Royal Prince Alfred Hospital, Sydney Hospital, St Vincent's Hospital, and the Royal North Shore Hospital). The Sydney physicians, including those who played a very influential role in setting up the Royal Australasian College of Physicians, seemed to see little necessity, let alone desirability, in openly acknowledging neurology as a discrete sub-specialty within the general province of the physician. The notion that the consultant physician should be competent in every area of internal medicine appeared slower to disappear in Australia's oldest city that in much of the remainder of the country.

The first specifically designated neurological unit to be set up in a major Sydney teaching hospital was in the Prince Henry Hospital. In a way, that unit was the resurrection and expansion of Campbell's old position at the Coast Hospital which, re-named in the interval, had become a principal teaching hospital of the newly inaugurated University of New South Wales. When the Department of Neurology within the Division of Medicine of that University was opened at the Prince Henry Hospital, James Lance took charge of the Department. Other appointments to the Department soon followed (Fine, Preswick, Lethlean, Anthony), with further ones as time passed (e.g. Gillies, Burke, Mellick). The history of the earlier years of this particular Department has been described in some detail in the book *Mind, Movement and Migraine* (Lance 1987).

The Royal Alexandra Children's Hospital, which had appointed Campbell as its neurologist well before World War II, had used Susman as a *de facto* neurologist in the years immediately following that war. Donald Hamilton subsequently conducted a Seizure Clinic there, but Don Hamilton would never have seriously considered himself as a neurologist. Leonard Rail, a neurologist with a major interest in electroencephalopathy, developed the facility for that investigation at the Hospital after the untimely death of Geoffrey Trahair in 1950. It was to be 1968 before Robert Ouvrier was appointed as Staff Neurologist to the Hospital, followed in 1973 by a similar post for Peter Procopis. Additional neurologists subsequently received appointment to the institution (Jane Anthony, Elisabeth Fagan, and P Grattan-Smith). At the Prince of Wales Children's Hospital at Randwick, affiliated with the University of New South Wales, Graham Wise became the first Paediatric Neurology Consultant, and other appointments followed.

The status of William Burke's *de facto* Neurological Unit at St Vincent's Hospital became formally acknowledged by the Hospital in 1962. The unit's consultant staff grew to include O'Sullivan, Coffey, O'Neill, Darveniza and Brew. A neurological unit was established at the Royal North Shore Hospital in 1964, George Selby being appointed to its charge. Over the ensuing years its staff numbers increased (Davis, Williamson, Terenty, Herkes). At Royal

Prince Alfred Hospital, John Allsop's neurological activities were finally legitimised in a titular way in 1970, his general medical unit then becoming purely neurological in its pattern of practice. A formal Department of Neurology was established at the Hospital in 1978, with Professor James McLeod as its head. Allsop continued his activities within this unit, and a number of neurologists came to be associated with it, e.g. Walsh, Pollard, Halmagyi, Leicester. Neurology at the venerable Sydney Hospital was never able to develop far. Demographic realities condemned it to wither, with the needs of the growing population in the western part of Sydney requiring the development of the local Westmead Hospital as an additional major teaching hospital of the University of Sydney. In the 1960s and 1970s a number of neurologists who worked at Sydney Hospital (Wolfenden, Lorenz, McLeod), transferred their hospital allegiances elsewhere as Sydney Hospital progressively closed down. From the outset, Westmead Hospital had its own Department of Neurology, headed by John Morris. By the end of the 20th century smaller neurological units had also opened at the Concord Hospital, and at the Lewisham and St George's Hospitals, all within the city of Sydney.

Soon after the end of World War II, the Northcott Neurological Centre had been opened in Sydney to provide neurological facilities for the needs of ex-servicemen. The existence of this Centre openly acknowledged the status of neurology as a medical specialty at a relatively early stage in Australia. Beginning with George Selby, several neurologists worked as its Director, usually until they became better established at other sites. However, the expansion of neurological services in the Sydney teaching hospitals and the increasing recognition of neurology as a specialty within the local medical community saw the role of the Northcott Centre progressively diminish in importance.

Within the State of New South Wales, Newcastle was the first city outside the metropolis at which neurology developed. There, by 1965, Adrian Dawson had begun to provide a neurology service to the Royal Newcastle Hospital. He was later joined at that hospital by Terence Holland, who continued to head the Hospital's neurological services when they moved in 1991 to the new John Hunter Hospital. The latter, by 1994, had a total of six neurologists on its staff.

As well, by the 1990s, within the State of New South Wales there were neurologists living and practising in certain major country towns, for example Orange, Tamworth and Goulburn and in the Bowral area. Further expansion of neurology into provincial cities, e.g. Armidale, has continued in the 21st century.

Victoria

By 1960, in Melbourne there were well-established neurological units at the Alfred Hospital, where Leonard Cox was already beginning to fade from the clinical scene, though John Game was active, at the Royal Melbourne Hospital, where Graeme Robertson had been joined by Arthur Schwieger, and at St Vincent's Hospital, where John Billings worked. Neurologists seem to have been accepted as a respectable species by their physician colleagues in Melbourne at a rather earlier stage than in Sydney. In 1963, John Game resigned from the Alfred Hospital to practise purely as a private consultant, though he continued to play a major and ongoing role in the affairs of the then Australian Association of Neurologists. Cox came back for a short time to cope with the neurological situation at the Alfred Hospital until 1965, when Bernard Gilligan, after completing neurological training at Queen Square, returned to Melbourne. He thereafter provided the Alfred Hospital with its consultant neurological service. As time passed, he was joined at the Hospital by others, beginning with Richard Stark, and later Elsdon Storey, who was subsequently appointed to a Neurology Chair there. At the Royal Melbourne Hospital, Peter Ebeling joined Robertson and Schwieger and on Robertson's retirement became head of the Hospital's Department of Neurology. Schwieger moved to Prince Henry Hospital where he undertook responsibility for the development of the neurology service. At Prince Henry Hospital he was joined by John Balla. However, the latter subsequently became interested in educational questions and for a time moved to Hong Kong. Ultimately the unit at Prince Henry Hospital was closed down. That institution, and the Queen Victoria Hospital, situated almost in the centre of Melbourne (where Barrie Morley had become neurologist), met the fate of Sydney Hospital, and for the same reason, viz. the need to shift hospital facilities to areas of population growth nearer to the periphery of an expanding city.

At the Royal Melbourne Hospital, Robert Hjorth had joined the Department of Neurology as Ebeling's junior, and he was followed successively by John King, Stephen Davis and Christine Kilpatrick. By 1994 the numerical strength of the Department at that Hospital included 9 neurologists, with Ebeling in an Honorary Consultant role.

In the early 1960s, Peter Bladin was appointed as junior to John Billings at St Vincent's Hospital, but by the middle of that decade had moved to the Austin Hospital to found a neurological unit there. As John Billings grew older, and increasingly devoted his energies to the non-neurological activities in which he has served the local and international community so long and so well, St Vincent's Hospital moved to import Edward Byrne, who was subsequently appointed Professor of Neurology in the University of Melbourne and thereafter increasingly moved into more purely academic activities.

Bladin spent many years establishing neurology at the redeveloping Austin Hospital, and devoted much energy to developing programs directed towards the management of stroke and epilepsy. Associated with his initiatives, neurological staff numbers increased, with Frank Vajda, followed by Merory, Symington, Donnan and Berkovic, becoming members of the Department. On Bladin's retirement in 1994, Donnan became his successor, with Berkovic developing the epilepsy area. Both were subsequently appointed to Chairs in Neurology within the University of Melbourne. Vajda transferred to St Vincent 's Hospital in the late 1990s to take up a Professorial Fellowship and the Directorship of the new Australian Centre for Clinical Neuropharmacology which was established there. Heidelberg Hospital, close to the Austin Hospital, developed its own neurology service which came to be staffed mainly by those with a background in Austin Hospital neurology (Chambers and Merory).

The Monash Medical Centre was developed in proximity to Monash University. In a sense this Centre replaced, on a different site, the inner-city Melbourne hospitals closed down by the Victorian State Government, as mentioned above. At first, the Monash Medical Centre absorbed some of the neurological consultants displaced by the closure of the older hospitals, but with the passage of time a new generation of neurologists had come to provide its staffing, which included Malcolm Horne, who came to hold a Chair of Neurology at Monash University.

For a time, the Royal Children's Hospital in Melbourne obtained its neurology consultant service from the nearby Royal Melbourne Hospital, but in the 1960s Ian Hopkins was appointed to it as its first paediatric neurologist. Subsequently he was joined at the institution by dedicated paediatric neurologists such as Lloyd Shield and Kevin Collins.

Unlike the situation in New South Wales, there was less tendency, or need, for Victorian neurologists to reside and practise outside the State capital, simply because of geographical considerations. By Australian standards, Victoria is a comparatively small state, and much of its population is concentrated in and around Melbourne. Hence the demography and economic geography of the State tended to delay dispersion of neurological personnel to the provinces, because it was practicable to provide neurological services to rural centres from a base in the state capital. However, as time passed men such as Peter Gates, at Geelong, based their practices in larger peripheral cities and towns.

Queensland

During the 1950s a Queensland medical graduate, Peter Landy, returned from neurological training in London to be appointed as neurologist to the Mater Hospital in Brisbane, but this was a relatively small institution at the time. For several years Landy also held appointments at Royal Brisbane Hospital, but as an Outpatient Physician rather than a neurologist. Prior to his return to the city, neurology in Brisbane had been within the province of the psychiatrists, notably Vincent Youngman. Ellis Murphy (later Sir Ellis), a physician, had some neurological experience in the United Kingdom but never intended to practise exclusively in the specialty in Brisbane. Shortly after Landy returned, John Tyrer took up an appointment as the first full-time Professor of Medicine in the University of Queensland. Tyrer had received neurological training at the London Hospital, under the then Sir Russell Brain, but the demands of his academic post, and the fact that he at first had no academic colleagues at all in his department, precluded his practising purely as a neurologist. In fact, he had to devote much of his time and energy for many years to building up his Department rather than to advancing neurology in the Queensland hospital system. However, in late 1956 he appointed John Sutherland as a Senior Lecturer in Medicine. Sutherland had been trained in neurology at Glasgow under Douglas Adams, and soon began to provide a neurological consultant service at the then Brisbane General Hospital, where he collaborated with the recently appointed neurosurgeon Kenneth Jamieson. When Sutherland resigned his University position in 1960 to enter private practice as a neurologist, an appointment was created for a Senior Visiting Neurologist at the Brisbane General Hospital, soon to be named the Royal Brisbane Hospital. Sutherland received the appointment. Originally the Hospital's neurological beds were in the neurosurgical unit, but later separate neurological beds were allocated. In 1961 Eadie was appointed as junior to Sutherland, and with Sutherland also supplied neurological consultant services to the adjacent Children's Hospital.

Within the city of Brisbane, on the south side of the Brisbane River, the large Princess Alexandra Hospital began to open from 1956 onwards, and Landy was among the former Royal Brisbane Hospital consultant staff who in stages transferred to the new institution. There he was at first nominally a physician, though formally appointed as its Neurologist in the early 1960s. He was also, for some years, Neurologist to the Repatriation Hospital at Greenslopes in the inner southern suburbs of Brisbane.

The two large hospitals, the Royal Brisbane and the Princess Alexandra, became the main sites of development of neurology in Queensland. John Sutherland continued to head the neurological unit at the former institution until 1977. He then moved to the country city of Toowoomba to semi-retirement, though continuing some private neurological practice. At almost the same time Eadie accepted a full-time academic research appointment in the University of Queensland, whilst remaining as Neurologist to Royal Brisbane Hospital. By this time younger neurologists had been appointed to the Hospital and they continued the neurology services (Edwards, Mann, Ohlrich, Banney, Bradfield and Lander, and for a time John Corbett). Later two academic appointees to the University Department of Medicine joined the Hospital's neurology service (Michael Pender and Pamela McCombe, both subsequently achieving professorial status in the University Department of Medicine,). Sutherland and Eadie had continued to serve as neurological consultants to the Royal Children's Hospital in Brisbane until 1972, when both resigned, making way for a trained paediatric neurologist Barry Appleton, who was subsequently joined at the Hospital by Christopher Burke and James Pelekanos, and later by additional paediatric neurologists.

At the Princess Alexandra Hospital, Peter Landy built up his Department of Neurology, coming to be joined in it by a number of colleagues as his own activities diminished to some extent with the passage of time (Boyle, Cameron, DeWytt, Read, Sandstrom and Staples, and later Silburn and younger people).

After some years of working at the Mater Hospital, Landy resigned from its staff, being replaced there by Noel Saines, later to be joined for a short time by Daniel McLaughlin.

Unlike Victoria, and even New South Wales, Queensland is a very large State. Along its east coast and in the south-east corner there are scattered, often at a considerable distance from one another, a number of population centres, each containing upwards of 50,000 people. From the 1960s, Peter Landy had provided an intermittent visiting neurology consultant service to Toowoomba, some 100 km west of Brisbane. Other neurologists from Brisbane later provided the same type of service to that city until John Sutherland moved into residence there in 1977. J Barrie Morley, displaced from the Queen Victoria Hospital in Melbourne when it closed, moved to Toowoomba in the early 1990s. After being trained in neurology in Melbourne, Gamini Jayasinghe in the later 1970s and the 1980s provided a consultant neurological service in North Queensland, based in Townsville. In the 1990s he moved to Brisbane and was replaced in Townsville by John Reimers, whilst Geoffrey Boyce from time to time provided neurological services in Cairns, even further north, and John Archer lived and worked in that city for a number of years before returning to Melbourne to pursue his interest in epilepsy, with others being appointed in his stead after an interval. Three neurologists (Adams, Corbett and Maxwell) came to live in various parts of the Gold Coast, south of Brisbane, and practised in the local area with its rapidly growing population (and expanding numbers of newer neurologists). Vivian Edwards moved his practice from Brisbane to Ipswich where he worked till retirement, after relinquishing his neurological appointment at Royal Brisbane Hospital. Various Brisbane neurologists visited the so-called Sunshine Coast area a short way north of Brisbane and one neurologist (Schapel) resided and practised there before Peter Patrikios and others based themselves in that growing area. Thus, as time has passed, the distribution of neurologists and neurological services in the State has followed the distribution of the major centres of population, as has been the case in other parts of Australia.

South Australia

In 1953, after several years of postgraduate training at Guy's Hospital with Sir Charles Symons and at the National Hospital at Queen Square, John Gordon returned to Adelaide to practise neurology. Prior to this time, except for the short period between 1920 and 1924 when H V Fry had been appointed Honorary Assistant Physician in Neurology at the Royal Adelaide Hospital (Rischbieth 1994), neurology had been the province of the general physicians and the Adelaide neurosurgeons (Lindon and Dinning). Gordon's consultant career at the Royal Adelaide Hospital began with appointment as a Physician, though he also acted as Clinical Assistant to the Neurosurgical Unit. In 1959 his appointment was changed to that of Honorary Neurologist to the Hospital. He held a similar appointment at the Adelaide Children's Hospital until 1969. As well, he provided an electroencephalography service to both of these institutions.

Just before John Gordon received his formal neurological appointment at the Royal Adelaide Hospital, Rischbieth returned to Adelaide from Queen Square to become Consultant Neurologist to the Queen Elizabeth Hospital. Richard Burns, after neurological training at Cleveland in the United States, joined Gordon in the Department of Neurology at the Royal Adelaide Hospital in 1967. In the mid-1970s there was some turnover among the Royal Adelaide Hospital neurologists. The Medical Centre attached to the new Flinders University opened, and Burns moved there in 1977 as its Associate Professor of Neurology. In the following year John Gordon himself resigned and moved to the United Kingdom to pursue his musical interests. Peter Rice took over responsibility for neurology at the Hospital, being joined there by Jeremy Hallpike. Subsequently Burrow, Kneebone and Heather Waddy received consultant neurological appointment to that institution. Later Thompson took up a Chair of Neurology there, with a further generation of neurologists progressively receiving appointments as time passed.

In the meanwhile, the number of neurologists at the Queen Elizabeth Hospital grew, Paul Hicks (in 1972) and Andrew Black (in 1975) joining Rischbieth. Later Purdie (1983) also became a member of the unit, and further consultant neurological staff were recruited, whilst Rischbieth and Hicks retired with the efflux of time.

John Gordon's resignation in 1969 from his neurology post at the Adelaide Children's Hospital was quickly followed by the appointment to that institution of its first paediatric neurologist, James Manson. Later Abbott and Hardboard joined Manson as the neurological consultant staff of the Hospital.

At the Flinders Medical Centre, Burns developed a neurological unit which came to include John Willoughby and William Blessing, both neuroscientists as well as clinical neurologists.

As is the case in Victoria, in South Australia the population tends to be concentrated in and around the state capital city, Adelaide. As a result, almost the entire neurological workforce of the State has tended to be based in that city, and to provide for the State's neurological needs from that base.

Western Australia

Like Victoria and South Australia, the population of the vast State of Western Australia is mainly concentrated in one region, in the south-west around the State capital of Perth and its neighbouring port of Fremantle. The remainder of the State remains sparsely settled, and nowhere is there a sufficient number of persons to warrant the continuing presence of a neurologist.

In the account of the career of Gerald Moss (Chapter 3) it was pointed out that, though he provided the Royal Perth Hospital with a neurology consultative service both before and after World War II, he never received the title of neurologist to that institution. However, after his resignation in 1955 to become Neurologist to the West Australian Mental Health Service, the Hospital began to develop neurology as a medical specialty, though slowly. Ernest Beech became Senior Honorary Neurologist in 1957, with Anthony Fisher, a Melbourne graduate, as Assistant Honorary Neurologist. Beech also functioned as a Physician to the Hospital. In the latter capacity he retained his general medical beds in which the neurological patients were accommodated. In 1959 Mercy Sadka, Australia's first female neurologist, returned to Perth after training in Boston to take up a position of Clinical Assistant Neurologist at the Hospital and to establish an electroencephalography service there. She also developed a rehabilitation service which became one of her great and continuing professional interests.

When the Sir Charles Gairdner Hospital opened in 1963, there was some redistribution of the neurological personnel in Perth. Mercy Sadka moved to the new institution as Honorary Consultant Neurologist. In 1968 Beech abandoned neurology to pursue other professional avenues. Fisher replaced him as Senior at the Royal Perth Hospital, Sadka became Assistant Neurologist there and Sonny Gubbay was appointed Clinical Assistant Neurologist. Frank Mastaglia, after training under John Walton (later Lord Walton) at Newcastle-upon-Tyne, returned to a Senior Lectureship in Medicine at the Sir Charles Gairdner Hospital in 1971. During the next two years the Western Australian neurologists and neurosurgeons came to an arrangement whereby they all had dual appointments to the two major adult hospitals in Perth. This led to the need for some readjustment in affiliation, especially since University units transferred from the Royal Perth to the Sir Charles Gairdner Hospital at much the same time. In effect Sadka and Fisher changed places, Gubbay succeeding the former as head of neurology at the Royal Perth Hospital in 1977, there being joined by Stewart-Wynne and Edis, and later by Dunne after Sadka retired in 1987, and subsequently by Hankey. In 1978 the University of Western Australia appointed Frank Mastaglia to a Personal Chair in Neurology which he held at the Sir Charles Gairdner Hospital. There the neurological consultant staff over time came to include Scopa, Grainger, Carroll, Day, and Stelle, with Anthony Fisher, after his official retirement in 1989, continuing to maintain an interested role.

After 1981, at the Repatriation Hospital in Perth a Senior Lecturer in Medicine at the University of Western Australia, Louis Herzberg, was responsible for providing a general neurological service, with a minimal quota of visiting sessions being provided by Fisher and later by Day.

From around 1960, paediatric neurology in Perth was in the hands of Peter Silberstein who worked at the Princess Margaret Hospital. Harvey Sarnat was appointed to the neurology staff of that Hospital in 1976, but left after a little more than one year. A few years later Walsh joined the neurological consultant staff of the institution.

For a time, neurology consultant services were provided to Fremantle Hospital by Anthony Fisher on a visiting basis. Subsequently Bajada and later Knezevic became that institution's neurologists.

Tasmania

In Tasmania until comparatively recent times, Hobart was the only city large enough to sustain the practice of a clinical neurologist (in the form of Keith Millingen). However in 1981, Siejka began practice in the specialty in Launceston, and PT Yeo received the second neurological appointment at the Royal Hobart Hospital, as Clinical Assistant in Neurology. Prior to 1952, neurological services in Tasmania had been provided from Victoria, principally by Graeme Robertson, who would visit the island (and its old ironwork and furniture) from time to time.

The late Keith Millingen, after obtaining neurological experience at the National Hospital at Queen Square, commenced practice in Hobart in 1952 and was later appointed Neurologist to the Royal Hobart Hospital. In time he accepted a Senior Lectureship and subsequently a Readership in the University of Tasmania's Department of Medicine, but continued to work as a neurologist at the Hospital until his retirement in 1987.

As in other Australian States, neurologist numbers have grown with time in the main Tasmanian cities.

Australian Capital Territory

Prior to 1973, neurology in Canberra either was handled by the local general physicians or by referral to neurological specialists in Sydney. Then Colin Andrews, who had recently taken a Doctorate in Medicine from the University of New South Wales whilst working in James Lance's unit, moved to Canberra to practise neurology. He became Consultant Neurologist to both the Royal Canberra Hospital and the Woden Valley Hospital. Soon afterwards Gytis Danta joined the staff of the Woden Valley hospital as a full-time neurologist, heading the unit there, with Roger Tuck later joining the neurological consultant staff. With the closure of the Royal Canberra Hospital, neurology in the Australian capital came to be centred on the Woden Valley Hospital.

Northern Territory

For over two decades, a single neurologist lived in Darwin, and from there serviced the Northern Territory's neurological needs.

As one looks at the development of clinical neurology services in the Australian States over the past 60 years, it becomes clear that neurologists have tended to enter practice where there were sufficient numbers of people who lacked the convenient availability of neurology services, and where a neurologist could obtain a consultant appointment to a local hospital. Professional survival without such an appointment appears to have often been difficult, though certainly not impossible. In the longer established hospitals, neurosurgical demand for congenial and effective neurological support to deal with the non-operative aspects of surgical practice often proved a significant stimulus to making the initial neurological appointment to the institution. Once that appointment was put in place the addition of one or more neurological colleagues usually proved desirable to maintain continuity of service and to cope with demand. Under Australian conditions of relative geographical isolation except in the larger cities, the solo neurologist practising at a distance from colleagues functioned under difficult conditions professionally and tended not to be as productive as those who were able to work in proximity to other persons with similar interests. When new hospitals have been opened in Australia in recent times it has nearly always been recognised that neurology and neurosurgery should be developed side by side, intellectually and, as far as feasible, physically.

These factors, plus population growth and movement, increasing community affluence and the quality of Australian clinical neurological practice, have over almost three-quarters of a century allowed the number of neurologists in the country to grow from seven (Sydney Sunderland being excluded from the original count because clinical neurology was not his dominant mode of activity), to some one hundred times that number.

INVESTIGATIONAL FACILITIES

Within comparatively short periods of time after they became commercially available internationally, various types of investigational equipment potentially useful for neurological purposes began to appear in one or two hospitals in the larger Australian cities. If they proved their clinical value, they then progressively became more widely available. The more notable items were concerned with imaging, first computed tomography, then magnetic resonance imaging and positron emission tomography. Equipment for clinical neurophysiology studies became fairly widely disseminated, electroencephalography facilities increasingly became available outside the larger cities, with video EEG monitoring occurring in specialised centres. There was parallel expansion in the ability to conduct biochemical and genetic laboratory investigations that was provided by various pathology services, and the development, particularly at the Royal Prince Alfred Hospital in Sydney, of investigational facilities to study balance disorders.

New Diseases

Kuru

From the standpoint of neurobiology, the recognition of kuru was an event of very considerable importance. It provided the stimulus for the set of investigations which led to the realisation of the existence of a new class of human infective disease, that due to prions. This concept brought together, and explained, a number of hitherto ill-understood nervous system disorders.

Kuru occurred on Australia's northern doorstep, its presence being restricted to the ancestors of today's inhabitants of an isolated area of the eastern highlands of Papua-New Guinea. At the time when the existence of kuru became known to the world, Papua-New Guinea was an Australian protectorate. There is no question that the major scientific discoveries in relation to kuru were made by Americans, notably the Nobel Laureate Carleton Gajdusek. Therefore, the propriety of associating Australian medicine with the kuru research may at first sight appear doubtful. However, the fact that the existence of kuru was first recognised by a medical officer employed by the Australian authorities should not be forgotten. This man was Vincent Zigas. In the course of his work, he became aware of the presence of kuru and, soon after, in December 1956, reported the existence of the disorder to his local medical seniors. Zigas also persuaded Gajdusek to study the matter (Gajdusek 1981), and thereafter collaborated in its investigation in the field.

The whole set of correspondence and field notes relating to the investigation of kuru was published in a volume under the editorship of Farquhar and Gadjusek in 1981. Zigas, after coming to live in Brisbane near the end of his life, gave the present author his own copy of the volume, one given to him by Gadjusek and bearing the latter's signature.

Zigas' report dated 26 December 1956, directed to his superior in Port Moresby, read:

I have to inform you that on 22/10/56 I left station for Moke area to investigate a form of encephalitis amongst the Okapa people - returned on 12/11/56 with preliminary brief report which reads below.

A number of people were found suffering from a probably new form of encephalitis attributed by inhabitants to sorcery and called `kuru', the prominent clinical symptoms of which are as follow:-

Disease originally started with fever, somnolence, muscular pain and weakness, headache (mostly occipital), vertigo, occasional vomiting. As course progresses condition becomes far more pronounced giving the well-known condition of Parkinsonism with its mask-like face, flexed arms and wrists, and unsteady walk, ocular disorders such as diplopia, strabismus, nystagmus, tremors of fingers and hands giving a cigarette rolling movement. In the late stage – no control of sphincters, increased W.B.C. and C.S.F under increased pressure. Duration of disease approximately from seven to nine months, slowly progressive and usually ends in death.

During my stay at Moke no more than 27 cases were under my close observation for three weeks, during which time two cases died in coma. I also visited surrounding villages and found another 11 cases. I observed that no age is immune, female more affected than male and I would say in ratio 3 to 1. I sent 22 samples of blood sera and a brain to Dr Anderson of Eliza Hall Institute in Melbourne and am anxiously awaiting the results of tests.

Zigas had come from the Baltic states as a post-war refugee and his medical qualifications were considered inadequate to allow him to be registered to practise in Australia, though they were deemed sufficient for him to work as a medical officer in Papua-New Guinea. He appeared to be a very modest, indeed humble, man who was extraordinarily cheerful and who, after he left New Guinea, worked at the Queensland Institute of Medical Research in Brisbane for a time prior to his death.

Australians were also involved in some of the earlier laboratory investigations on kuru, though the critical studies were later carried out in the United States. Anderson, of the Walter and Eliza Hall Institute in Melbourne, was responsible for the earlier virological studies which failed to reveal any organism. Graeme Robertson provided the initial neuropathological data with subsequent reports by Ross Anderson, and with electroencephalographic studies being carried out by Leonard Rail, of Sydney. The New Zealand neurologist Richard Hornabrook, at a slightly later stage, played a role in documenting the clinical features of the disorder.

In retrospect, the Australian contribution to the investigation of kuru was more in the nature of opportunistic research that of a deliberately planned investigational program. However, had the disorder not been recognised when it was, the understanding of a whole new factor in the pathogenesis of nervous system disease would have been delayed, and possibly might not have happened.

Reye's Syndrome

In 1963, the pathologist Douglas Reye (1912–1977) and certain of his colleagues from the Royal Alexandra Hospital for Children in Sydney described an apparently novel illness, instances of which they had observed between 1951 and 1962. The disorder comprised a fairly rapidly progressing illness which proved fatal in 17 of the 21 affected children. It involved increasing depression of consciousness, convulsions, vomiting, a disturbed respiratory rhythm, and altered muscle tone and reflexes. There was hypoglycaemia and biochemical evidence of disturbed liver function during life. At autopsy, the brain was swollen, the liver a little enlarged with a bright yellow colour, and the renal cortex pale and a little widened. Microscopically, the brain showed evidence of neuronal abnormality, and the glia were swollen. There were extensive fatty changes in the liver.

Reye *et al.* (1963) remarked on the similarity between the condition they described as `Encephalopathy and fatty degeneration of the viscera' and the disorder Jamaican vomiting sickness, though they did not then consider the two conditions identical. The illness has usually been referred to as Reye's syndrome since the original description. As experience of the disorder accumulated, it became clearer that a failure of mitochondrial metabolism was involved, and that it was a syndrome with a number of possible causes e.g. inherited metabolic defects, exposure to various toxic substances including a chemical in the Jamaican akee fruit, salicylates and the antiepileptic agent valproic acid, and that sometimes infections seemed to precipitate its onset.

Reye's syndrome stands as an example of a neurological and metabolic disorder first described in Australia, and to which an Australian's name is attached.

HIV Infection

While the investigation and management of HIV infection and its possible neurological consequences generally remained within the province of the Australian physicians specialised in infectious disease, at St Vincent's Hospital in Sydney, an institution that serviced the needs of a population with a particularly high incidence of the disorder, Bruce Brew and his colleagues took a particular interest in the neurological aspects of the infection. In 2018 Brew edited a volume of the Vinken-Bruyn *Handbook of Clinical Neurology* series concerned with the matter of HIV infection.

NEUROTOXICOLOGY

Since the end of World War II Australians have been involved in reporting, and sometimes in investigating, several patterns of chemically induced neurotoxicity.

Thallium Poisoning

Thallium was introduced into Australia as a rat poison in 1937. Instances of thallium poisoning in humans followed. Allsop (1954) described 18 instances of such poisoning admitted to Royal Prince Alfred Hospital in Sydney and provided a very thorough review of the topic. The poisoning produced a polyneuritis which could involve the cranial as well as the peripheral nerves, and sometimes caused a retrobulbar neuritis and an encephalopathy with depressed consciousness, delusions, hallucinations and involuntary movements. There was also gastro-intestinal disturbance, severe tachycardia and, if the sufferer survived long enough, alopecia.

Bismuth Subgallate Encephalopathy

Burns *et al.* (1974) encountered five patients who developed a novel and characteristic neurological syndrome involving confusion, tremulousness, clumsiness, myoclonic jerking and gait difficulty. All had undergone abdomino-perineal resection of the rectum and were taking bismuth subgallate as a de-odourising agent for their colostomies. The disorder resolved when bismuth subgallate intake ceased. The clinical picture was not the one previously associated with bismuth toxicity.

Ciguatera Poisoning

Outbreaks of a toxic food poisoning associated with the eating of tropical fish have occurred in Queensland coastal communities for well over half a century. A similar toxicity has been reported in other tropical countries. The topic was reviewed in some detail by Gillespie *et al.* (1986). The first report in the Australian medical literature was probably that of Cleland (1942). The symptoms usually commence within 18 hours of eating the culprit fish. At the outset, paraesthesiae and numbness occur around the lips and tongue and there is a gastro-intestinal disturbance lasting up to 24 hours. However, the sensory symptoms may last for several days and less well-defined ill health may persist for months afterwards. The toxins responsible for the condition are thought to originate in a dinoflagellate which has been eaten by fish. Investigators, including Lewis, in Brisbane, one of the co-authors of the review cited above, have shown that ciguatoxin produces its effects by prolonging the opening of voltage-dependent sodium channels in cell membranes. The Brisbane neurologist, John Cameron, carried out clinical neurophysiological investigations on patients and experimental animals affected with the toxicity (Cameron *et al.* 1991; Cameron and Capra 1993).

Clioquinol Neurotoxicity

Instances of clioquinol-associated subacute myelo-optic neuropathy occurred in Australia (Selby 1972) at much the same time as they occurred elsewhere in the world. As well, Ferrier and Eadie (1973) added to the mere handful of reports in the world literature two further instances of an acute amnesic syndrome which followed the ingestion of a single large oral dose of clioquinol. Interestingly, after an interval of several years, both their Australian cases developed partial epileptic seizures of temporal lobe origin, an event not previously recorded (Ferrier *et al.* 1986).

ACADEMIC NEUROLOGY

Seven decades ago, when neurology was first becoming established in Australia as a clinical specialty, academic clinical medicine was not itself particularly well developed. There was a long-established Chair of Medicine in the University of Sydney, a more recent one in the University of Adelaide, and a half-time Chair in the University of Queensland, whilst the University of Melbourne had its Stewart Lectureship in Medicine. In the eyes of clinicians, this latter post was equivalent in status to that of a professorship, but in University eyes it lacked the titular recognition accorded to a Chair. In general, the occupants of these four positions were expected to be first and foremost clinicians and teachers – research (if any) and a role in university politics were very much subsidiary expectations at that time. In such a situation it is not surprising that the founding generation of Australian neurologists at first appeared to see little advantage, or practicability, in having academic aspirations for the specialty. Rather, the eyes of at least some of them tended to become fixed on a vision of transplanting not only the Queen Square neurological culture to Australian soil, but of creating a Queen Square-like physical facility somewhere on that soil. That vision, probably never explicitly and publicly enunciated, though mentioned in the Minutes of the 1970 Annual General Meeting of the Australian Association of Neurologists, took many years to fade away completely, yet in retrospect it would appear to have never been practicable. The Australia of that time simply did not have a sufficient population to sustain such an institution. Moreover, the population of the country was scattered over a very much greater land mass than that of the total area of Britain, there was no single incontestably predominant population centre, and neither of the country's two major cities was the national capital. Nor was there any well-developed tradition of private charity such as that which initiated and supported the early development of the National Hospital at Queen Square. At the time in question, Australia was still recovering from the effects of a recent major war. Sydney possessed the only institution in the country specifically dedicated to neurology, the Northcott Neurological Centre, but by virtue of the purposes for which it had been set up access to that Centre was open only to a distinctly limited section of the general community. On the other hand, Melbourne had much more experience of established neurological practice, but that practice was subdivided between two, and arguably three, major hospitals, without any one institution clearly being the preponderant centre.

As the earlier-touted possibility of an Australian Queen Square became increasingly unlikely, partly because of geographical factors, some Australian neurologists in the 1960–1969 decade began to foresee another, probably more achievable, goal: that of the creation of a Chair (or Chairs) of

Neurology in one or more of the Australian universities of the time. By 1960 the Australian university system was expanding. Staff numbers, particularly at the sub-professorial level, in the academic clinical departments were increasing, Queensland and Melbourne had recently created full-time Chairs in Medicine, research was being done in the university departments and research funding was becoming available in increasing amounts. At least in the minds of a few of the more senior neurologists of the day, notably John Game, there seems to have arisen the idea that neurology might find its way to a place in the sun through being acknowledged academically (specifically in the form of at least one professorial appointment in the area). By this means, neurology might also gain access to funding to conduct its own research (though the particulars of that proposed research were always left nebulous). Certainly, such ideas were recorded in the Minutes of the Australian Association of Neurologists' Annual General Meetings on at least two occasion (1969, 1970), though to the present-day reader the concepts always seemed to lack particularity. Nonetheless, these ideas did ultimately come to realisation through various means, and in the end probably did achieve something of what had been hoped of them.

Whilst such notions were beginning to form, John Tyrer in 1954 had been appointed to the Mayne Chair of Medicine in the University of Queensland. Although the research for which he had obtained his MD from the University of Sydney had been in the cardiovascular area, he had subsequently spent a year at the London Hospital with Russell Brain acquiring neurological knowledge. Thus, almost before the idea dawned of having a Chair of Neurology created somewhere in Australia, a person with neurological training had come to occupy one of four chairs of Medicine then existing in the country. It could, of course, be argued that at that time, in the person of Sydney Sunderland, the Australian university system already possessed someone with a professorial-level appointment and considerable neurological knowledge. However, Sunderland was primarily a neuro-anatomist, and a very great one, and the Australian neurologists of the times regarded him in that light. For many years, rather than being considered a neurologist, Tyrer was perceived as a physician who probably would have been a neurologist if he was not also, by virtue his academic appointment, required to take responsibility for the teaching and clinical practice of internal medicine as a whole. It was only after his department had accumulated sufficient academic staffing, with expertise in other areas of medicine, that he achieved conditions in which he was able to practise more exclusively in clinical neurology. However, well before that time, Tyrer had imported to Brisbane in 1956 a Scottish-trained neurologist, John Sutherland. Yet, Sutherland also had to function clinically outside his specialty for a few years until he resigned from his University position to enter full-time consultant neurological practice. He then received a part-time appointment as Lecturer and Research Consultant in Neurology in the University of Queensland, his appointment perhaps constituting the first recognition in a titular sense of clinical neurology as an academic discipline in an Australian university.

James Lance resigned from a neurological consultant appointment at Sydney Hospital in 1961 to become Senior Lecturer in Neurology in the University of New South Wales. As mentioned earlier, this new University had from the outset created a Department of Neurology, though as a section within its Division of Medicine. Lance, by virtue of his scholastic and research achievements, not only built up the Neurology Department, but was promoted first to Reader and, in 1976. was appointed to a Personal Chair in Neurology. By this time, his Department also contained academic appointees in neurology at sub-professorial levels. With Lance's appointment to a designated Chair in Neurology, a two-decade-old dream of the founding generation of Australian neurologists was transformed into reality.

Prior to this time, another academic neurologist in Australia had come to hold a professorial-level appointment, though in Medicine, not Neurology. James McLeod, a former Sydney Rhodes scholar, had returned to his home city to a Senior Lectureship in the Department of Medicine at Sydney University in 1960, and worked as a neurologist at Sydney Hospital. He later became the second Professor in the University of Sydney's Department of Medicine. In this position, unlike Tyrer more than a decade earlier, he was in a situation where his Department contained a sufficient range of professional expertise for him to be able to continue to practise predominantly as a clinical neurologist. At a later date, McLeod was also able to combine his Chair of Medicine with the newly created Bushell Chair of Neurology in the University of Sydney. However, shortly before this happened, the second Australian professorial-level appointment in neurology had occurred, this time in Brisbane. There Sutherland had first become part-time Reader in Neurology and Eadie was appointed to the part-time Lectureship in that discipline which Sutherland had vacated. In 1972 Eadie's appointment was changed to that of a half-time Readership and in 1977 to a half-time Professorial Fellowship in Neurology. Later in the same year he was appointed to a named chair in Clinical Neurology and Neuropharmacology in the University of Queensland.

In 1983 Frank Mastaglia, who had held an academic appointment in Medicine in the University of Western Australia, and who had recently deputised for John Walton in the Chair of Neurology in the University of Newcastle-upon-Tyne, was appointed to a personal chair in Neurology in his home institution.

In these ways, the decade 1975 to 1984 saw the creation of professorial appointments in neurology in four of the Australian medical schools, with Richard Burns being appointed to an associate professorship in the discipline in the new Medical School at Flinders University in 1976. John Game had the satisfaction of knowing that his goal had been reached, not once, but four times and in four separate places within Australia, over a comparatively short period. And the medical schools of his home city of Melbourne were to follow suit later, with Chairs in Neurology being created at St Vincent's Hospital (for Edward Byrne), at the Austin Hospital (for Geoffrey Donnan), where Peter Bladin previously had held a Professorial Fellowship, at the Royal Melbourne Hospital (for Stephen Davis) and at the Alfred Hospital (for Elsdon Storey) and at the Monash Medical Centre (for Malcolm Horne), with Samuel Berkovic later (1998) being appointed to a Personal Chair in Neurology at the Austin Hospital, and Frank Vajda to a Professorial Fellowship at St Vincent's Hospital. Sydney too was not idle in making further professorial appointments in neurology. David Burke was appointed to a chair in the University of New South Wales and later John Pollard to a Personal Chair in the University of Sydney at Royal Prince Alfred Hospital and later succeeding to the Bushell Chair, whilst John Morris received an associate professorship at Westmead Hospital. The University of Adelaide appointed Phillip Thomson to a Chair of Neurology, and John Willoughby became the second Associate Professor in Neurology at Flinders University. As well, two neurologists were appointed to Chairs in Geriatrics, Robert Helme in Melbourne and Anthony Broe in Sydney. Thus, in Australia from 1976 onwards, professorial appointments in neurology, and academic neurology itself, expanded more rapidly than the development of the remainder of the clinical specialty. But did this luxuriant and continuing growth achieve what John Game and his generation had hoped would flow from the creation of senior academic appointments in neurology?

The answer is probably a mixture of `yes' and `no', though predominantly `yes'. There can be little argument with the assertion that the research done by many of the academic neurological appointees, both prior to their formal appointments and subsequently, has contributed more than any other single factor to making Australian neurology known internationally for its achievements and its quality. The existence of the academic appointments has meant that Australian medical students have learnt their neurology from neurologists rather than from physicians, and this has tended to bring home to them early in their professional lives the stature and the importance of neurology within the discipline of internal medicine. It has also provided neurology with a platform on which to build within a learned community which is more wide-ranging intellectually, less restricted in its vision, and less service-orientated, than the hospital one. It is also a community in which neurology's influence is more readily perceived internationally. Where the effect of the academic appointments in neurology has probably fallen short of the earlier expectation is that, when the idea of Chairs of Neurology was first mooted, it was anticipated that such chairs would be associated with the headships of established university departments of neurology. That is, it was expected that the Chairs of Neurology would be so-called establishment ones. Instead, over the intervening years the circumstances of professorial appointments have changed somewhat within universities in Australia. Nearly all the chairs of neurology that have been created have in essence been personal ones, or ones based in hospitals and funded by them, rather than being primarily university based and university funded. As such, the Chairs of Neurology may have become subservient to other academic or hospital considerations to a greater extent than would have been envisaged a generation or more earlier. It is easier for a university to suppress, or leave unfilled, a personal chair than it is to deal similarly with an established chair, or an established department, though their extinctions certainly are not impossible. Therefore, the changed basis of the foundation of many university chairs and sub-professorial appointments over more recent years has meant that neurology still does not have as secure a home in the academic world in Australia as might appear at first sight, despite the reality that, so far, neurology certainly has not been made unwelcome in that world.

Neurological Training

Once the stage was reached when at least one neurologist had begun to practise in each Australian city with a medical school, it became possible in theory for universities to have their undergraduate medical students taught neurology by professional neurologists. Such a state of affairs had been achieved by 1960, and the subsequent appointment of academic neurologists simply enhanced the opportunity for undergraduate medical education in neurology to be carried out in the hands of those practising solely in the specialty and having particular knowledge of it.

In the earlier years after the foundation of the Royal Australasian College of Physicians, postgraduate training for practice as a clinical neurologist involved acquisition of the Membership of the College (in general medicine). This was followed by at least one, and usually more, years of supervised, exclusively neurological, practice with some exposure to neuropathology and neuroradiology, and experience in the common investigational techniques then carried out by neurologists, mainly lumbar puncture, electroencephalography and clinical neurophysiological studies. However, in 1970 the Royal Australasian College of Physicians formalised a pattern of medical sub-specialty training such that Membership of the Royal Australasian College of Physicians was replaced by an examination for the first part of a Fellowship of the College. Success in this was followed by what was in essence a three-year apprenticeship in the specialty, undergone in at least two specialist centres somewhere in the country. If desired, one of these three years could be spent in research relevant to the specialty. Following that, and subject to satisfactory reports from supervisors, Fellowship of the College was conferred, so that registerable specialist status could be attained.

The customary pattern of Australian neurological training in the 1950s and 1960s had involved the trainee in spending one or more years in neurological posts overseas, usually at the home of British neurology, the National Hospital at Queen Square, London. During this time, the Membership of the Royal College of Physicians of London was often obtained. The trainee then returned home, with admission to the Membership of the Royal Australasian College of Physicians having occurred either before or after the time overseas. There was in those times a perception that Australia could not offer an aspiring neurologist full training in his homeland, if it could offer any adequate training at all. There simply was not a sufficient number of neurologists available in any one centre, or a sufficient number of neurological training positions, for the possibility of a sufficiently varied experience of neurology to be obtained in a single city. The time spent overseas, preferably whilst undergoing Queen Square training, was in those days seen as being virtually obligatory by a profession not yet confident enough in its own educational capabilities.

This situation could change only when one or more of the major Australian cities contained a sufficient number of practising neurologists to provide variety in training, when there was adequate local neurological research underway to allow exposure to the research ethos, if not actual participation in research activity, and when Australian neurology had become convinced of its ability to train its own people. From a purely minimal numerical point of view, Melbourne had probably reached this state by 1950, though the research options there at the time were relatively limited. Brisbane probably achieved this situation next, because of the university connections and the research activities of Tyrer and Sutherland. Sydney did not appear to reach it until a little later when James Lance's research became established. However, in practice, achieving these minimalist criteria did not mean that Australia began to produce its own totally home-grown neurologists in the early 1960s. Greater numbers of practising neurologists and a great diversity of research in the major cities seem to have been needed, but more than this a realisation that Australian neurological research and scholarship in at least several areas had achieved international respectability. Such a situation probably began to apply by 1970. From about that time, some neurologists who met Australian accreditation criteria began to practise in Australia prior to, or without ever, receiving overseas neurological training experience. However, the tendency to complete neurological training overseas, or to gain overseas experience after completing neurological training in Australia, continues at the present time of writing.

However, the increased maturity of academic neurology and of its training capacity meant that, in recent years, young Australian neurologists, or would-be neurologists, have tended to go overseas relatively later in their careers than in the past. Consequently, they have sometimes been rather too senior for some of the available training posts there. Because of this, they have tended to find their way into overseas neurological research positions. Accordingly, they have returned to Australia with acquired research skills and with research publications to their names. Although this experience may have been of considerable educational value to them, it has sometimes proved to have been wasted from the point of view of advancing Australian neurological research. The type of research they had been trained to do overseas did not fit into the patterns of, or accord with the facilities available for, neurological research that were extant in the city in Australia to which they returned. Overall, by recent times, Australian neurological research has come to cover a reasonably wide spectrum of investigative activity. However, in a city where a clinical opportunity for a neurologist may have existed, research possibilities and facilities compatible with a given individual's overseas research training often did not. The expense and the difficulty of then setting up the required facility often proved prohibitive. Clearly it would have been desirable to have achieved better co-ordination of local Australian neurological research with research training opportunities overseas, or else to have organised for prospective appointees to neurological posts in Australia to begin to obtain research experience in their own country before going overseas. With such experience, they should have been in a better position to understand what types of overseas research would be practicable for them to transfer back to Australia on their return. The largely haphazard arrangements in relation to overseas training that have applied in the past appear to have wasted some of the potential that could have been obtained from overseas research training and experience.

There was also the desirability of possessing some easily discernable evidence of research achievement as an indication of medical qualification in addition to graduation degree(s) and Membership or Fellowship of Colleges of Physicians. In earlier times, possession of an Australian or British Doctorate of Medicine qualification served this purpose, but Australian university MD degrees varied considerably between institutions in their standard and requirement, and sometimes also changed within the one institution as time passed. The latter difference substantially increased in very recent years as Australian universities began to award the MD as a graduating degree, a so-called professional doctorate, equivalent in standard to the former Masters' degree, so that the MD was no longer considered a higher doctorate. As a result, increasing numbers of those doing neurological research have chosen to follow the more uniform standards of the pathway leading to a PhD qualification, using it as a further commendation for appointment to the staff of teaching hospitals and academic institutions.

The various factors discussed above probably prompted the Australian Association of Neurologists in 1996 to set up a committee in each State to undertake responsibility for the coordination of the training of prospective neurologists and for the accreditation of neurological training posts in that State. By that time, the situation had become such that Australia was also in a position to train prospective neurologists from overseas countries. However, the Australian pattern of training, under the constraints of the formal Royal Australasian College of Physicians' requirements, possibly would have been regarded by overseas graduates as unnecessarily cumbersome for their needs and their country's registration standards. Hence there has been a tendency for overseas graduates, intending to practise neurology in their home countries, to make use of the educational capacities of Australian neurology more as a finishing school than as a full training facility.

Chapter 6

THE YEARS OF INCREASING RESEARCH AND SCHOLARLY ACTIVITY

Prior to around 1950, as mentioned earlier, much of the neurological research in Australia seems to have been prompted by local issues for which appropriate overseas solutions were not available, or not readily applicable. There were, in addition, some attempts to set up investigational programs into unsolved, or unsatisfactorily understood, global problems, e.g. the Hunter and Royle work on spasticity, Campbell's studies on cerebral and cerebellar architectonics. By the time the founding generation of Australian neurologists was fading from professional activity, the investigation into the known peculiar local neurological problems in Australia had become a fairly well-tilled field, though a few new local problems were to arise in the future and warrant investigation.

With this relative exhaustion of local neurological issues as research subjects, Australian neurological research in the past 70 years has moved increasingly into studying more global problems, in doing so often in competition, and sometimes in cooperation, with investigators from elsewhere in the world. Such studies have often involved the activities of research groups rather than the solo investigator, and increasingly have required sophisticated and expensive facilities likely to be available only in universities, research institutes or larger and more amply funded hospitals. Rather than discuss such research over the years on a purely chronological basis, which inevitably leads to discontinuity in tracing the progress of the understanding of particular matters, it has seemed better to discuss each major individual topic as a whole before proceeding to the next. The studies to be mentioned below fall well short of the sum of all the Australian investigations carried out in the relevant areas. The account merely attempts to pick out the major research areas that have engaged the efforts of Australian neurological scholarship over a period of rather longer than the past half-century.

RESEARCH FIELDS

Headache

James Lance seems to have taken the decision to involve himself in headache research at a relatively early stage in his postgraduate career, and to have remained a very significant figure in the area throughout his professional life. He had worked in Boston after the then traditional (for a would-be Australian neurologist) period of training at the National Hospital at Queen Square in the mid-1950s. In Boston he was probably influenced by Graham, one of the Americans who took up the legacy of headache research which remained from Harold Wolff's pioneering studies in the 1950s. After Lance returned to Australia and received an academic appointment to the University of New South Wales he took up two main lines of clinical and laboratory investigation into headache. The first line was a dominantly neuro-anatomical one, with which he seems to have maintained a close association over the years and which has continued in the country, albeit perhaps at a slower pace, after his departure. The second was a biochemical one in which he was soon joined by Michael Anthony and, for a time, by the biochemist Herta Hinterberger, and which has tended to fade away with the passing of time. Lance's overall attempt developed into a broad-ranging and sustained program of investigations into the basis of headache and, in particular, the basis of migraine. It yielded an ongoing series of publications, came to receive very considerable international recognition, and gave birth to a generation of Australian headache researchers.

Before his headache studies began to pay scholarly dividends Lance, in collaboration with George Selby, his predecessor at the Northcott Neurological Centre, published a detailed analysis of the clinical features of migraine (Selby and Lance 1960). Selby, though his main research and clinical interests lay elsewhere, later produced a monograph on migraine, one with a dominant clinical orientation (Selby 1983). Lance also produced his own book, though one on the more general topic of *The Mechanism and Management of Headache*. This work ranged over a broader territory than merely that of migraine, and the text was based on a more detailed scientific background. The first edition of Lance's book (Lance 1969) appeared to provide, relative to the bulk of the second edition of Wolff's classic *Headache and Other Head Pain* (1963), a concise but competent account of the subject. With Wolff's death and the later and smaller-sized multi-authored editions of the book still bearing his name, the subsequent editions of Lance's monograph, each a little larger than its predecessor and, after the fifth, co-authored by Peter Goadsby, increasingly took on the stamp of very considerable authority. Throughout its evolution, the book retained its characteristics of clarity, balance and thoroughness, and a sense of homogeneity produced from originally being written by a single author who had made himself into a great authority on his subject. It would probably not be unfair to regard the book as, in the eyes of many, the world's leading text on the subject of headache, the symptom which provides the bread and butter for much clinical neurological practice. Lance's own pre-eminence in the headache field was recognised internationally in a number of other ways, but his book stands as a consistent and continuing reminder to the world of an Australian's contribution, and that his colleagues, to a major global neurological problem.

The studies on the neuroanatomical background to headache carried out under Lance's leadership attempted to trace the central connections of the pathways whereby pain impulses from various structures in the head and neck reach the levels of the brain at which they are responsible for the experience of pain. The studies were linked to investigations of cranial vascular behaviour and its response to various forms of stimulation and treatment. The associated biochemical investigations stemmed from Sicuteri's observation of increased 5-hydroxyindoleacetic acid excretion in urine during migraine attacks, a finding that has rather faded from present-day medical awareness without ever being disproved. Lance with his colleagues defined the changes that occurred in whole plasma concentrations of serotonin, the metabolic precursor of 5-hydroxyindoleacetic acid, around the time of migraine episodes. The work on serotonin later extended to cluster headache, where the role of histamine was also explored. Under Lance's supervision, members of his school studied other various headache-related matters. Brian Somerville probed the relation between female sex hormonal changes and migraine attacks, a laboratory and patient-based investigation that would have been difficult to carry out because of logistic problems in obtaining patient co-operation at the appropriate times. Bogduk took up from an applied anatomical perspective the rather unfashionable and previously largely ignored aspect of the role of neck structures in the pathogenesis of headache, and Drummond and Lambert also carried out anatomical studies relevant to headache pathogenesis.

Associated with these scientific investigations into headache mechanisms, there were clinical trials of the efficacy of various drugs in particular varieties of headache. Such studies may perhaps not be perceived as constituting highly innovative science, but nevertheless they have been of considerable value to clinicians grappling with the difficulties in treating headache sufferers.

The multifaceted headache program initiated and directed by James Lance at the University of New South Wales considerably enhanced the international standing of contemporary Australian neuroscience, and also yielded real benefit for patients. It provided the venue for Michael Anthony's own headache studies and enabled the training in medical research of a number of younger Australian neurologists, of whom at least two have built up their own empires in headache studies, Andrew Zagami at St George's Hospital in Sydney and Peter Goadsby at various academic institutions in London and the United States. Goadsby, in particular, has achieved a considerable international reputation, partly by enunciating the valuable and increasingly accepted unifying concept of the headache category of trigeminal autonomic cephalalgia (Goadsby and Lipton 1997), embracing a number of overlapping and obviously mechanism-related headache syndromes.

Apart from the Lance group in its ramifications, there was relatively little headache research elsewhere in Australia over the last four decades of the 20th century, though a monograph considering *The Biochemistry of Migraine* emanated from Brisbane (Eadie and Tyrer 1985), and an investigation into the absorption of orally administered aspirin during migraine attacks, and the effect of orally administered metoclopramide on this, was carried out in that city (Ross-Lee *et al.* 1982). However, in the early decades of the present century headache interest groups have appeared in other State capital cities, so that the fire that James Lance lit in Australia has not been extinguished by his departure from the scene.

Epilepsy

Research into epilepsy has gone on in a number of centres in Australia ever since the practice of neurology began in the country. As early as 1905,

George Rennie in Sydney had chosen to ventilate the question as to what was epilepsy, and whether it could be cured? However, he dealt with the matters more at a philosophical than at an investigative level. After an interval of 40 years, N V Youngman (1945), a Brisbane psychiatrist, returned to the question of the curability of epilepsy. He concluded that epilepsy could not be cured because it was the expression of a tendency inherent in the sufferer. However, he considered that it could be controlled, as it was in some 50% of his patients treated with the then available antiepileptic agents. It should be noted that, to him, 'control' of epilepsy could exist though epileptic auras continued to occur in a patient. Cade (1947), famous for his discovery of the efficacy of lithium in the prophylaxis of mania, reported a personal investigation in which he showed that creatinine protected against pentylenetetrazole-induced seizures in experimental animals.

In the mid-1960s Peter Bladin, in the then newly opened Neurology Unit at the Austin Hospital in Melbourne, began to develop a clinical investigative program into epilepsy, in conjunction with certain laboratory studies which were carried out under his aegis. The work, which had its major emphasis on improving patient management, has flourished ever since. Others joined the investigations and, as Bladin increasingly moved towards retirement, one of his protégés, Samuel Berkovic, after gaining experience in epilepsy research at the Montreal Neurological Institute, took over the direction of the Austin Hospital epilepsy program until his own recent retirement, and continued to expand its horizons, particularly in relation to epilepsy genetics, partly by virtue of forging local and international collaborations.

To the outsider, the original main thrust of the Austin Hospital program, at least until the end of the last century, would probably have appeared to be the attempt to relieve medically intractable epilepsy by surgical procedures. This attempt made it necessary for the Austin Hospital neurologists to assemble the facilities to allow them to investigate the presence of epileptic seizures and to determine the site of epileptogenesis in their patients undergoing assessment for surgery. Beginning with video-EEG monitoring, they developed and then utilised single proton emission computed tomography scanning, positron emission tomography, depth electrode studies and neuropsychological assessment to help locate the site of epileptogenesis. All these investigative technologies have since become more or less commonplace in specialised epilepsy centres in the larger Australian cities, following in the footsteps of Bladin's pioneering ventures, but their most extensive use for research purposes has occurred in Melbourne. Over earlier years, the concentration of patients with epilepsy, and often difficult-to-control epilepsy, that occurred at the Austin Hospital permitted the study of the features of particular epileptic syndromes, e.g. tonic seizures, the Lennox-Gastaut syndrome, the myoclonic epilepsies. It also permitted the delineation of several new epileptic syndromes, e.g. nocturnal frontal lobe epilepsy. Underlying the epilepsy work at the Austin Hospital appears to have been a continuing awareness of the social implications of the disorder, and this aspect has been studied sympathetically in a variety of ways. As well, Berkovic in various investigations, probed the genetic basis of various epileptic syndromes through a number of means, including twin studies, some in conjunction with the paediatric neurologist Ingrid Scheffer from the Melbourne Children's Hospital. This continuing program of genetically-based investigations has led to Berkovic's achieving a most distinguished international reputation, and to the receipt of a most unusual honour for an Australian clinician, the Fellowship of the Royal Society of London, a distinction which, a little later, also came to Ingrid Scheffer.

In collaboration with overseas investigators, Berkovic and local colleagues at an early stage defined the molecular abnormalities in the nicotinic acetylcholine receptor which are present in nocturnal frontal lobe epilepsy (Bertrand *et al.* 1998) and then proceeded to define the genetic backgrounds for other epileptic syndromes. In passing, while carrying out these studies, Berkovic recognised the existence of a syndrome of inherited familial temporal epilepsy, a finding that calls into question the universal validity of the previously widely accepted principle that focal epilepsies are the results of localised cerebral cortical pathology, rather than being genetically determined.

Among others associated with the epilepsy work in Melbourne, some of whom currently hold appointments in more than one university or hospital or research institute, at least Graeme Jackson warrants mention for his ongoing investigations into the magnetic resonance imaging and electrographic detection of cortical epileptogenic lesions of various natures, and the anatomy and volume of the hippocampus and other temporal lobe structures (and in correlating these volumes with matters such as the outlook after epilepsy surgery).

At the time of writing, advanced imaging technology is being applied in relation to epilepsy in Brisbane under the direction of David Reutens, but it is rather early to assess where it may lead.

There also is the initiative of Bladin's close friend, Frank Vajda, who in the late 1990s set up a national register of the outcomes of intrauterine exposure to antiepileptic drugs in relation to foetal malformation and seizure control. This Australian Pregnancy Register continues to function at the time of writing and contributes its data to the corresponding European Register. Analysis of the Australian material itself yielded early and persuasive evidence of the dose-related teratogenic hazard from exposure to valproate during pregnancy (Vajda and Eadie 2005), leading to a progressive alteration in antiepileptic drug prescribing practice before pregnancy. It also demonstrated a lesser degree of heightened teratogenic hazard in relation to intrauterine exposure to carbamazepine and topiramate. As well, it produced the first evidence that continued pre-pregnancy freedom from epileptic seizures was strongly associated with the prospect for continuing seizure control throughout pregnancy (Vajda *et al.* 2008).

The Austin Hospital epilepsy program also provided the initial medical impetus for the formation of the Epilepsy Society of Australia, which as it grew came to provide a forum for discussion and action in relation to numerous matters connected with the disorder. The earlier scientific meetings of this Society took place at the Austin Hospital. Members of Bladin's Department in those times edited the proceedings of these meetings to produce a series of small volumes which reflected the contemporary Australian thinking about various aspects of the disorder.

In Adelaide, at Flinders University during the early 1990s, John Willoughby abandoned his previous research area of neuroendocrinology and took up the experimental study of the generalised epilepsies, in particular absence seizures, and electrical aspects of seizure genesis in animal models and the human EEG.

In Sydney, for some years Beran paid attention to the population and social aspects of epilepsy, and to the legal implications of suffering from the disorder. Eadie (1994), in Brisbane, published an analysis of the clinical features of some 1900 patients with epileptic seizures who presented to a neurological consultant practice over a 30-year period. Earlier, he had collaborated with Sutherland and, initially, also with Tait, to produce a small student-level textbook on epilepsy *(The Epilepsies. Modern Diagnosis and Treatment)* which ran to three editions (Sutherland and Eadie 1980).

The clinical pharmacological approach to the management of epilepsy was opened up in Brisbane in the late 1960s and early 1970s in the wake of the investigation of an outbreak of phenytoin intoxication which will be described later in this chapter. Vajda shortly afterwards began utilising the same therapeutic drug monitoring approach in Melbourne. It was subsequently applied throughout the country and led to research of some practical significance for a time, but has subsequently declined in activity, partly because of lack of interest from the pharmaceutical industry in supporting the relevant and clinically desirable studies. This topic will be described further in relation to the section on neuropharmacology research, though logically it could have been dealt with in the present context.

Involuntary Movement Disorders

Reports of instances of, and of families afflicted with, Huntington's disease had appeared in the pages of local Australian medical journals by the turn of the 19th century. Brothers (1964) traced the history of the disorder in the comparatively enclosed population of the island state of Tasmania, and also in Victoria. Several workers examined aspects of the disorder in various other Australian communities (e.g. Parker 1958; Wallace 1972; Pridmore 1990) without breaking ground of any fundamental importance. In comparatively recent times a very unusual Queensland family was reported in which biochemically proven Wilson's disease was present together with clinically diagnosed Huntington's disease in other family members (Parker 1985). In at least one such member without evidence of abnormal copper metabolism, the movement disorder was more suggestive of a torsion dystonia. The family was reinvestigated by Wilcox *et al.* (2011).

As mentioned earlier, Parkinsonism was reported in the wake of the outbreak of encephalitis lethargica in Australia though, with a possible solitary exception (Burnell 1922), it did not follow Australian X disease which occurred at much the same time in eastern Australia. There was relatively little interest in Parkinson's disease in Australia until the various types of basal ganglia and thalamic stereotaxic surgery came into vogue for its treatment in the late 1950s and early 1960s, prior to the advent of levodopa therapy but following Cooper's serendipitous discovery of the benefits obtained from surgical injury to the inner part of the globus pallidus in patients suffering from the disorder. Parkinsonian patients with inadequate responses to the then relatively ineffective available medical therapies began to accumulate in neurosurgical clinics, where they became available for investigation. In Brisbane, Eadie (1963) studied the medullary pathology of the disorder in such patients, and the contribution these brain stem changes might make to the alimentary tract dysfunction present in Parkinson's disease, in a sense accidentally studying the anatomical background to the Braak hypothesis of four decades later (Braak *et al.* 2003), though interpreting the events the wrong way round in terms of the hypothesis.

In the 1960s and later, Selby, at the Royal North Shore Hospital of Sydney, carried out his own stereotaxic procedures to alleviate the symptoms of Parkinsonism after his neurosurgical colleague Mr John Grant had made appropriately placed burr holes in the patient's skull. Over the years Selby amassed a considerable number of Parkinsonian patients, and quantified matters such as the clinical features of the disorder, the presence of cerebral atrophy in patients suffering from it, and the long-term prognosis following therapy with dopaminergic agents. At a later date, John Morris at Westmead Hospital in Sydney, undertook the study of involuntary movement disorders in general, using quantitative methodologies, and also was concerned with the therapeutics of these conditions. These interests have continued in the hands of his successors. There have been several large-scale collaborative trials of various agents in the treatment of Parkinson's disease involving neurologists in the Australian State capitals. Blessing and colleagues at Flinders University re-examined aspects of the brain stem pathology of the disorder, using more refined investigational techniques than those employed in earlier studies of this brain region, but arrived at conclusions similar to the earlier ones.

Stereotaxic surgery for the relief of Parkinsonian symptoms fell from favour after the advent of levodopa and other dopamine agonist therapy in the early 1960s, but after an interval of some years began to be employed again as the late-stage problems attendant on prolonged use of dopaminergic drug therapy began to appear. However, stimulatory rather than tissue-destructive procedures were by then available, and continue to be employed in several Australian cities where a group of investigators, including Peter

Silburn in Brisbane, are publishing research observations made during and following such procedures, sometimes in collaboration with international colleagues, in particular ones at Oxford in Britain.

Demyelinating Disease of the Central Nervous System

The early history of multiple sclerosis in Australia was described in chapter 1. There was relatively little Australian interest in the disorder in Australia until the second half of the decade 1951–1960. Then John Sutherland emigrated from Scotland, fresh from the research he had done in his homeland into the aetiology of the disease and its prevalence in Scots people of different racial backgrounds, e.g. Celts, Norsemen. His work was responsible for the subsequent recognition that he had been the first to demonstrate evidence of a genetic basis for susceptibility to multiple sclerosis. This had followed earlier investigations into the disease which had obtained for him the degree of Doctor of Medicine from the University of Glasgow. Sutherland, whose life story is recounted in his autobiography *A Far-off Sunlit Place* (1989), proposed carrying out epidemiological studies in Queensland similar to those he had already done in Scotland. His main aim was to see if the increasing prevalence of the disease with increasing distance from the equator, already shown to apply in the northern hemisphere, also applied in the southern. This he proposed to do in an Australian State where the general belief at the time was that the disorder of multiple sclerosis did not occur in native-born Queenslanders. Sutherland, with co-investigators, proceeded to carry out a field survey of the main population centres along the lengthy eastern coastline of Queensland (Sutherland *et al.* 1966). He demonstrated not only that multiple sclerosis did indeed occur in Queenslanders, but that it became more prevalent the further south one went within the State. Heartened by the outcome of this study, he then proceeded to organise a prevalence study of the disorder throughout the whole Australian continent.

This investigation, carried out in conjunction with colleagues in the other States surveyed, confirmed the increasing prevalence of the disorder with increasing south latitude (McCall *et al.* 1968, 1969). After this, Sutherland carried out some smaller investigations into the relationship between multiple sclerosis and certain factors which correlated with latitude, viz. the prevalence of poliomyelitis and sunlight exposure and various geophysical factors, the latter carried out in collaboration with a geologist, William Layton (Layton and Sutherland 1975).

Peter Landy, the neurologist who began practice in Queensland at much the same time as John Sutherland, also had a continuing interest in multiple sclerosis and clearly recognised that it did occur within the state. His particular interest lay in the relation of optic neuritis to the disorder.

Sutherland's work on the epidemiology of multiple sclerosis in Australia was later developed further by James McLeod, of Sydney. With a team of co-investigators, he carried out a more detailed survey of the prevalence and clinical features of the disorder throughout Australia. The conclusions from the study (published in stages in a number of places) proved to be reasonably similar to those of the earlier work, though the prevalences were found to be roughly 50% greater (Hammond *et al.* 1987, 1988a, 1988b, 1989; McLeod *et al.* 1994). This result was possibly partly attributable to more thorough case ascertainment, in part to a greater medical awareness of the disorder which had been prompted by the earlier survey, and partly by the increasing availability of more advanced diagnostic technology. A therapeutic trial of the effects of transfer factor on the progress of the disease was also carried out under McLeod's aegis, and suggested that this substance did indeed have disease-modifying properties (Basten *et al.* 1980; Frith *et al.* 1986).

Following on from Weston Hurst's studies in Adelaide in the years around 1940, work on the pathology and pathogenesis of central nervous system demyelination and its animal model experimental allergic encephalitis was carried out in Australia by research groups in Canberra (Willenborg and Danta), in Melbourne (Bernard, and Carnegie, though the latter subsequently moved to Perth) and in Brisbane by Michael Pender. For a time, there was controversy over a possible feline virus found in central demyelinative lesions in multiple sclerosis brains by Cook, from Perth (1981, 1986), while Pender (2012) expended considerable effort in amassing evidence concerning the possible role of Ebstein-Barr virus in the pathogenesis of the disorder. However, in more recent years, the main activity of the increasing number of Australian neurologists who have become particularly concerned with multiple sclerosis has been in relation to immunological aspects of the disorder, and evaluation of the therapeutic efficacies of the increasing number of recently introduced agents that have become available for treatment of the condition.

Spino-Cerebellar Degenerations

This now somewhat outmoded nosological category still provides a convenient designation under which to discuss work carried out in Australia on a number of progressive central nervous system disorders of genetic or uncertain aetiologies. Earlier classifications of the disorders, with their often eponymous titles, began to be undermined by Anita Harding's work that led to a proliferation of numerical classificational types, with genetic advances making further reclassification almost inevitable. It probably would be fair to say that none of the Australian work on these conditions has achieved more than to add further descriptive data to the world stockpile of such information. No major contribution to the understanding of their fundamental natures appears to have been made on Australian soil.

As mentioned in Chapter 1, quite convincing clinical descriptions of Australian families afflicted with Friedreich's ataxia were recorded late in the 19th century and subsequently. The neuropathological changes in an instance of the disorder were described by Litchfield *et al.* (1917), though the two neuropathologists associated with this particular publication (Latham and Campbell) appeared to have had reservations about the precise classification of the pathological abnormality that was present. Hall *et al.* (1945) recorded a family with the uncommon degenerative disorder formerly designated cerebello-olivary atrophy (Greenfield 1956), and Lambie *et al.* (1947) described a family with the manifestations of olivo-ponto-cerebellar atrophy.

Tyrer and Sutherland (1961), in Brisbane, documented a substantial case series of the various spino-cerebellar degenerations that they had traced in Queensland. They also analysed the mechanisms involved in the production of pes cavus when it occurred in these disorders. Later, each of these authors, and also Eadie, wrote as individuals on particular varieties of cerebellar and spino-cerebellar degeneration for Volume 21 of the Vinken-Bruyn *Handbook of Clinical Neurology* (1975).

Late in the 20th century, a peculiar form of progressive neurological disorder involving a bilateral neo-cerebellar degeneration was described as occurring in the Arnhem Land region of the Northern Territory. Originally this condition was suspected to be a manifestation of manganese poisoning. Ultimately, after further data had accumulated and genetic studies had been carried out, it proved to be due to the Machado-Joseph disease. Presumably it was a legacy from the voyages of Portuguese navigators more than two centuries earlier and of their contacts with the local Australian Aboriginal women (Burt *et al.* 1993, 1996).

In more recent years, there has been little further Australian publication in the area.

Amyotrophic lateral sclerosis

In recent years, research groups in Sydney (Kiernan) and Brisbane (Henderson and colleagues) have taken a particular interest in amyotrophic lateral sclerosis and related disorders which, based on previously existing knowledge, at first sight may have seemed not particularly rewarding areas for exploration. New insights into disease patterns and prognostic factors have been obtained and, as a dividend, better support for those affected by the conditions.

Cerebral Vascular Disease

In Australia, the specialist management of stroke remained for a long time within the province of the general physician, a territory relatively impervious to invasion by neurologists. In more recent times neurologists have increasingly made inroads into the area, bolstered by knowledge of the research that some of their members have carried out into the phenomenology of the disorder, particularly the ischaemic variety. The physicians' defences were first broached by Peter Bladin in Melbourne, though he probably always remained more interested in epilepsy. In the 1960s, initially at St Vincent's Hospital and then at his unit at the Austin Hospital in Melbourne, Bladin instigated an attempt to diagnose varieties of stroke more reliably and to trace their natural histories and devise better management strategies to mitigate their consequences. He recruited more junior colleagues to his investigations and organised collaborations with specialists in other relevant area of medicine e.g. neuroradiologists, neurosurgeons and vascular surgeons. As an outcome of his type of work, some of the old syndromes of occlusion of the various individual cerebral arteries which were described in textbooks of neurology, and which seem to have been defined more on the basis of theoretical expectation than clinical actuality, began to disappear from neurological thinking in Australia. They were replaced by a smaller number of syndromes which could be recognised empirically and correlated with arteriographic and neuroimaging studies in the patient (Donnan *et al.* 1991, 1993; Read *et al.* 1998). One of Bladin's protégés, Geoffrey Donnan, had become increasingly involved in the field, and took over the area, and also Bladin's former Department, when Bladin reached his date of retirement. Donnan had by then organised, and conducted, a number of studies attempting to define risk factors for various stroke syndromes in the hope of identifying targets for the prevention of ischaemic stroke (You *et al.* 1995). In particular he showed for the first time the role of tobacco smoking in increasing the hazard of such events (Donnan *et al.* 1989; You *et al.* 1995), although the role of smoking in coronary and peripheral arterial disease had been established earlier, by others. Donnan formed collaborations with Stephen Davis, of the Royal Melbourne Hospital, and others in Melbourne to expand the stroke studies and extend their sites of conduct. He left behind him an ongoing stroke program at the Austin Hospital when he moved into the Directorship of the Florey Institute in Melbourne. Davis's interest at the Royal Melbourne Hospital seems to have been particularly in stroke outcome and cerebral blood flow studies. Other Austin stroke protégés have made their careers elsewhere, or have followed somewhat peripatetic career courses, like that taken by Mark Parsons with his numerous publications.

In Perth, Hankey and Stewart-Wynne in the 1990s devised and carried through a program of investigations into stroke, including a stroke survey of the city of Perth intended to define the demographics and other features of the condition (Stewart-Wynne *et al.* 1987). Hankey's activities in the area continued after Stewart-Wynne's retirement.

During recent years, centres for stroke research and treatment have appeared in the remaining Australian State capital cities and in some larger provincial cities, in particular Newcastle.

Multi-centre Australian trials of various interventions in ischaemic stroke e.g. thrombolysis, and participation in international stroke studies have been carried out, or are in progress at the time of writing, though in these centres the main emphasis has been on management aspects.

Over the past half-century cerebral aneurysm, ruptured or unruptured, and cerebral vascular malformation have largely remained the clinical territory of the neurosurgeons, who are in the position of being able to offer potentially definitive management for these disorders. However, interventional radiological procedures are increasingly replacing operative surgery in some situations. More effective therapy for arterial hypertension in the hands of general practitioners and physicians has reduced the frequency of intracerebral haemorrhage. Unfortunately, once such a haemorrhage has occurred the treatment options continue to be rather limited, but increased information has become available.

While all this Australian neurological activity in recent years related to stroke has been going on, and has resulted in a significant record of publication, it is hard to identify any single outstanding original contribution that has been made to relevant contemporary knowledge, meritorious and valuable though the local work has been.

Peripheral Nerve Disease

The development of clinical neurophysiological techniques and nerve and muscle biopsy procedures opened up the area of peripheral nerve and muscle disease in the decades following the end of World War II. Although Peter Ebeling was probably the first to bring electromyography and clinical neurophysiological studies back to Australia, it was James McLeod in Sydney who initiated the first large-scale program of investigation into peripheral nerve disorder in the country. By progressively accumulating sufficient numbers of cases and studying them by electrophysiological and biopsy techniques, including electron microscopic examination, he and those who worked in his research group at various times (e.g. Pollard, Tuck, Fitzsimons, McCombe, Walsh, Nicholson) made a series of contributions to the knowledge of various types of peripheral polyneuropathy (for example the Guillain-Barré syndrome, chronic inflammatory demyelinating polyneuropathy, alcoholic, lepromatous and autonomic neuropathies). McLeod's interests extended to the neuromuscular junction and myasthenia gravis and its treatment, particular treatment by plasmapheresis or immunoglobulin therapy, measures that were to become part of routine clinical practice in due course.

John Pollard was involved in many of the studies and in time instigated his own program of investigation of the peripheral neuropathies, particularly those with an immunological basis. His work enhanced the understanding of some of the mechanisms involved in demyelination, particularly the complementary roles of antibody and T-cells in targeting the inflammatory processes involved. Nicholson, whose research orientation was more biochemical than many of his contemporaries, worked in particular on the genetic basis of the hereditary neuropathies, particularly Charcot-Marie-Tooth disease (Ouvrier and Nicholson 1995; Nicholson *et al.* 1998). Other paediatric neurologists also contributed to knowledge in the peripheral nerve area, e.g. Kathryn North and neurofibromatosis.

Muscle Disease

When skeletal muscle biopsy first began to come into common use, Byron Kakulas, in Perth, commenced a series of investigations into muscle disease in animals and humans which continued over several decades. The main thrust of the work was directed towards the muscle dystrophies and other myopathies. It began with morphological and electron microscopic studies, and later moved into genetic aspects. A clinical interface was maintained throughout the course of the investigations. Frank Mastaglia, an academic clinician in the same city, became involved in the investigations but expanded his interest into muscle disease more generally, including the inflammatory and drug-induced myopathies. Mastaglia produced, in collaboration with John Walton of Newcastle-upon-Tyne, a monograph upon the pathology of the subject, and other important writings.

In contrast to the predominantly morphological approach taken to muscle disease by this group of Western Australian collaborators, Edward Byrne at St Vincent's Hospital in Melbourne embarked on a series of studies on muscle disease in the 1980s, with emphasis on their biochemical aspects, particularly in relation to the mitochondrial disorders. His work extended to other neurological syndromes which involved disordered mitochondrial functioning, e.g. Leber's optic atrophy. Subsequently he moved into the area of their genetics, before making a new and very distinguished career in quite a different area, viz. academic administration, rising to the Vice-Chancellorship of Monash University and, later, that of the University of London, and to a British knighthood.

A younger generation of neurologists continued the Australian contribution into knowledge of skeletal muscle disorder, mainly from a biochemical and genetic standpoint, e.g. Carolyn Sue and her work on mitochondrial myopathies.

Neuropharmacology

In recent decades a number of Australian scientists have investigated various aspects of neuropharmacology. One, David Curtis, after a short period soon after graduation under the influence of Leonard Cox at the Alfred Hospital in Melbourne, made his whole career in research neuropharmacology, whilst continuing to maintain links with Australian clinical neurology from his base in Canberra. At the Australian National University, Curtis was for many years a member of the Physiology Department (then under J C Eccles), but subsequently was appointed to a Chair in Neuropharmacology, later changed in title to one in Pharmacology itself. Curtis's long series of painstaking studies into the pharmacology of synaptic neurotransmission, mainly within the spinal cord of experimental animals, brought him Fellowship of the Royal Society of London and the knowledge that he was one of the pioneers in the recognition of the role of amino acids, and particularly γ-aminobutyrate and glutamate, as central neurotransmitters.

Post-war clinical neuropharmacology in Australia began in Brisbane where, in 1968, an outbreak of intoxication from the antiseizure medication phenytoin was investigated. This outbreak occurred throughout Australia but did not occur simultaneously in the northern hemisphere. It was possible to show by circulating phenytoin concentration measurements that, for years prior to the time of the outbreak, calcium sulphate, the excipient in the marketed Australian phenytoin capsules, had caused some 25% of the oral phenytoin dose to fail to be absorbed and to be lost in the faeces. Replacement of the calcium sulphate by lactose (the excipient in the phenytoin capsules marketed in other countries) enabled the full drug dose to be absorbed. This change caused a significant number of patients taking the drug in already well-established nominal dosages to become overdosed (Bochner *et al.* 1972). From the pharmacologist's standpoint, this remains the best documented example existing of a clinically important interaction between a drug and an excipient in a drug preparation. As a by-product, the work also showed that a substantial number of patients taking phenytoin were not being adequately dosed with the drug, and that readjustment of their drug dosages, guided by pharmacokinetic principles, could produce improved control of their seizures, and also fewer adverse effects of the therapy. When this was realised, a program of systematic investigation of the pharmacokinetics and metabolism of the available antiseizure medications began in Brisbane. After a time, the approach was extended to other drugs used in neurology e.g. dexamethasone in the treatment of raised intracranial pressure, aspirin in migraine and stroke prophylaxis, and ergotamine in migraine attacks. The anticonvulsant clinical pharmacology work was also taken up in other Australian cities, notably by Vajda and Kilpatrick, separately, in Melbourne. During the last two decades of the 20th century several monographs on various aspects of clinical neuropharmacology were written or edited by Australian authors (see Appendix V). The effects of the phase of the menstrual cycle, and of pregnancy, on antiseizure medication pharmacokinetics were studied later.

Neuro-otology

In Sydney, in the Neurological Department of the Royal Prince Alfred Hospital, Michael Halmagyi, in collaboration with Ian Curthoys from the Department of Psychology of the University of Sydney, took up the study of vestibular mechanisms in animals and humans. In this case, the physiological work merged into the actual practice of clinical neuro-otology, with some of the earlier testing methods utilised by C S Hallpike gradually becoming replaced by simpler and more convenient methods, e.g. so-called 'head impulse testing'. Halmagyi, in conjunction with the American Robert Balogh, produced a book on the topic. Others have developed interests in the area, e.g. Waterson in Melbourne, while the clinic at the Royal Prince Alfred Hospital has increasingly passed into the hands of Halmagyi's disciples.

Dementia

At the time when the first generation of Australian neurologists was still practising, the problem of dementia and its management tended to fall into the hands of the psychiatrists, and to an extent this still happens. It was always realised over the years that dementia was the result of organic brain disease and that some varieties of such diseases were potentially treatable. With the increasing availability of neurologists, the decline in Freudian-type psychiatry, the recognition that fronto-temporal dementia takes in considerably more than the previously accepted entity of Pick's disease and awareness that modern brain imaging techniques plus biochemical investigations offer a reasonable chance of achieving a pathological diagnosis, dementia has increasingly moved into the domain of the neurologists, often ones working in conjunction with psychologists in clinics such as those in Sydney and Brisbane. John Hodges, in recent years in Sydney and before that in Cambridge, has made significant contributions to the area, and authored a standard text which over the years has appeared in three editions. The work of these clinics might not have so far yielded spectacular new knowledge, but their existence has certainly created wider and ongoing interest in what is an increasing community problem.

Neurophysiology

Patently, the most eminent figure in Australian neurophysiology since World War II has been the late Sir John Eccles, in his academic youth one of Sherrington's group at Oxford and later the first Professor of Physiology at the Australian National University in Canberra. Eccles' earlier work in Australia was on denervated voluntary muscle (1941) and subsequently extended to the study of the cerebellum and its connections and the functional organisation of the different types of neurons in the cerebellar cortex. Later, and during the years of his long retirement, his thought extended to wider topics e.g. neuronal plasticity, the physiological bases of consciousness, of memory, of motor control, of the emotions, before it finally spilled over into philosophy and the basis of the self.

Whilst of general relevance to the background of clinical neurology, the work of Eccles, and that of a number of other Australian neurophysiologists (e.g. McIntyre, Bishop, Pettigrew) was directed more towards obtaining basic knowledge than bettering the understanding of human disease mechanisms. Both psychiatry and psychology could have made claims on such work equal to those of neurology. However, particularly in Sydney in recent decades, neurophysiological investigations have also been carried out in which the basic knowledge obtained was almost incidental to the understanding of the disordered human nervous system function that was sought. This work also had a quite different motive from the purely diagnostic clinical neurophysiological studies which have increasingly become part of the day-to-day practice of clinical neurology. The more basic work began with James Lance, in parallel with his headache investigations. In patients, he studied the neurophysiological basis of spasticity, of Parkinsonian rigidity and tremor, of myoclonus and other involuntary movement disorders, and aspects of reflex activity. In collaboration with James McLeod, also of

Sydney, in 1981 he wrote a book relating to the subject (*A Physiological Approach to Clinical Neurology*) which appeared in more than one edition and was directed mainly towards the interests of postgraduate students in the area of clinical neurology. McLeod himself, early in his own career, had also done some experimental physiological work in Sydney.

Gradually Lance's own active participation in the area of neurophysiology, though not his interest in it, as judged from his publication record, began to lessen. Increasingly he bequeathed it to David Burke in his own Department. Burke, in earlier times often in association with Simon Gandevia, gradually seemed to transfer his interest from the basis of diseased to that of normal human neurophysiology. He involved himself in a very substantial series of continuing studies. These studies have investigated human fusimotor function and the afferent, cerebral and efferent components of the pathways involved in movement, and the effects of a number of factors, e.g. vibration, posture, cutaneous afferent input, on these various elements of the motor mechanism. However, clinical aspects have not been lost sight of in the investigations, and matters such as paraesthesiae and myotonia have been addressed.

Neuroanatomy

In the earlier and middle years of the 20th century there were Australian anatomists with a major interest in the nervous system e.g. Hunter, Wilkinson and Abbie, all referred to earlier, and in Melbourne Berry, Sydney Sunderland (also discussed above) and the anatomist-neurosurgeon Keith Bradley. Even earlier, there were the great cytoarchitectonic and comparative neuroanatomical studies of A W Campbell dating from more than a century ago. However, in the past 60 years which saw so much growth in Australian clinical neurology, the single major original neuroanatomical contribution has probably come from Nikolai Bogduk, another product of the Lance stable. Bogduk found for himself an interest in the applied anatomy of the spine, a hitherto relatively neglected area. Until recently holding the Chair of Anatomy in the University of Newcastle, Bogduk combined careful dissection studies of the spine and its ligaments and associated structures with nerve block studies in headache sufferers. In this way he tried to elucidate the contribution neck disorder may make to the production of headache. In so doing, he carried forward Lance's headache initiatives through a different line of approach to those adopted by the majority of those whose careers Lance influenced.

Another of Lance's disciples, Lambert, for a time also carried out anatomical studies relevant to headache mechanisms.

Neuropathology

In the pre-war British Queen Square tradition, neuropathology in a hospital was often the responsibility of the man earmarked for the next vacancy on the consultant staff of that institution. This pattern continued at Queen Square until JG Greenfield, having received the pathology appointment, chose to remain in it as pathologist to the Hospital until his formal retirement. In other places neuropathology was sometimes carried out by neurological clinicians with an interest in the area, or by pathologists who became increasingly interested in the nervous system as their careers progressed. From relatively early times, in Australia there have been pathologists with neurological or predominantly neurological interests, though they have collaborated with neurologists to obtain the material they subsequently studied.

The roles of men such as Flashman and Latham in Australian neuropathology prior to World War II have already been mentioned, and also the neuropathological studies of Alfred Walter Campbell, and the contribution in relation to glioma cytology and biology and to cryptococcal infection made by Leonard Cox.

The Nazi invasion of Poland in 1939 brought from Warsaw to Australia the 1911 Moscow medical graduate *Jacob Mackiewicz* (1887–1966) who, though a neurologist in his homeland, worked in Melbourne as a neuropathologist in the Mental Health Department. In Australia he studied the histological effects of antidepressant drugs and tranquillisers on the brain of the guinea pig, and investigated the pathology of the senile brain. He died before the latter work was published (Stoller 1966).

Brian Turner (1926–1974) took up the role in Sydney that was for so long occupied by Oliver Latham, working in the laboratory named in Latham's honour. Turner, a Sydney graduate who had been trained in Greenfield's department at Queen Square (Selby 1974), was initially interested in alcoholic cerebellar degeneration. Whilst never abandoning old-fashioned morphological neuropathology, before his untimely death he had moved progressively into early neurogenetic and neurometabolic work in relation to mental retardation in children.

Ross Anderson (1913–1988), a quiet, gentle man, was a medical graduate of Melbourne University, who subsequently trained in London with Godwin Greenfield and Dorothy Russell. He inherited the neuropathology mantle previously worn by Leonard Cox in Melbourne. Over many years, and continuing into his time of formal retirement, he not only provided a neuropathology service to the Alfred Hospital and to the city more generally, but investigated a number of matters, e.g. kuru, Murray Valley encephalitis, cerebral vascular disease.

In Perth, *Byron Kakulas* carried out the muscle investigative studies mentioned above, but also conducted investigations into other aspects of pathology, e.g. spinal cord trauma. Those whom he has trained over the years have come to occupy neuropathologist positions in most of the Australian State capital cities, Harper in Sydney in particular contributing to knowledge of the neuropathology of alcoholism, and Colin Masters, in Melbourne, to that of Alzheimer's disease.

Neurogenetics and Neuroimmunology

Some reference to aspects of these emerging areas has been made at several places in earlier parts of the present chapter, particularly in relation to epilepsy, and it seems that Australian neurologists in particular are developing an increasing interest in various autoimmune and other immune-mediated nervous system disorders, but it is rather early to attempt assessment of the history of the Australian contribution to knowledge in these areas.

PUBLICATIONS

Over the period of time being surveyed in this book, attitudes and practices in relation to the publication of medical work have changed considerably. In the middle of the last century, when Australian clinical neurology was beginning to become established, a record of a handful of papers, often single authored ones, over an individual's lifetime and published in medical journals after external review, would have been considered a highly meritorious contribution to knowledge and scholarship. Seventy years later, the names of a number of Australian clinical neurologists, some of whom are still involved in practice or academic activity, can be found amid the listed authorships of as many as several hundred individual papers. This proliferation of recorded scholarly activity over a comparatively short period of time probably reflects not only the increased activity and growth in neurologist numbers, but greater ease in preparing manuscripts, the availability of increased numbers of venues for publication, the advent of open access publication, and more papers having multiple (and sometimes quite numerous) authors. The proliferation of papers associated with the names of Australian neurologists also makes it almost prohibitively difficult to provide anything like a comprehensive list of Australian-authored journal publications, scattered as they are through the pages of numerous established and emerging medical journals and being increasingly available in electronic rather than hard copy form.

Book chapters written by Australian neurologists might provide a more easily assembled record, simply because the books that contain them often are easily visible on library shelves, but if they are to be found at all easily one would need to know beforehand in which books they are printed. But in the case of books themselves, authors' or editors' names nearly always appear on the book's covers or spines, or on both, so that identification is reasonably easy. Therefore, an attempt has been made to trace books written or edited by Australian neurologists to provide a measure of Australian neurology's scholarly activity over the years surveyed (Appendix V, Figure 1). As far as possible, a distinction has been made between works authored and works edited, but libraries do not appear to have always been scrupulous in making this distinction in their own catalogues.

In the Appendix the books have been listed chronologically in relation to the dates of appearance of their first editions, with indication given when further editions have been traced. It needs to be appreciated that a 'book' is defined as a collection of pages bound together and having front and back covers. The number of pages involved in being a book is not specified, though apparently Australian libraries take 20 as the minimum number. The contents of Appendix V need to be appreciated in the light of this knowledge, and an awareness that some books that would have been qualified for inclusion very probably have not been traced. It also needs to be appreciated that the table shows data for first editions only,

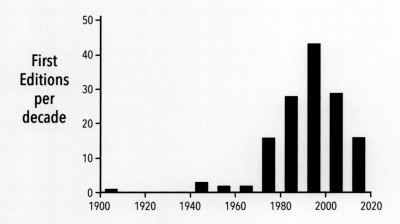

Figure 1. Numbers of first editions of medical books written or edited by Australian neurologists since 1900. Second and subsequent editions are not included in the graph.

and that the apparent book publication rate decline in the 21st century shown in Figure 1 is at least partly explained by the appearances of second and subsequent editions of books already listed. The neurologist-authored book publication scene today, as least numerically, certainly is a very different one from that of a century ago, when there was only that solitary volume, A W Campbell's great *Histological Studies on the Localisation of Cerebral Function,* with nothing to follow it for 40 years.

By the end of the 20th century it seemed not unreasonable to have concluded that Australian clinical neurology had come of age in its clinical, educational, scholarly and research capabilities and achievements. Subsequent events do not seem to necessitate any departure from that belief.

Chapter 7

SOME AUSTRALIAN NEUROLOGISTS FROM LATER GENERATIONS

With the passing of the years, death has overtaken increasing numbers of people from the generations of Australian neurologists that succeeded the foundation one, while even more who are still living have retired from neurological practice or have left it for other reasons. The previous edition of this book contained brief accounts of the careers of some of those who then were no longer living, but no attempt was made to define criteria that determined whose lives were included in the account. For the purposes of the present edition, it has seemed appropriate to continue to deal with those who are no longer living and for whom there exists accessible recorded evidence of their having made significant contributions to the advance of clinical neurology in Australia or internationally, dealing with them purely in order of seniority of their dates of birth. To do this has involved some nicety of judgement, and an awareness that some who practised clinically to the considerable benefit of those who were their patients, and whose illnesses they managed with devotion and skill, will appear to have gone unnoticed. Often this has been so simply because they made little contribution to the medical literature or did not find opportunity, or have time, to render forms of community service that attracted recording in documents that found their way into the public domain.

Ernest Beech (1908–1976)

To a generation accustomed to think of a medical life in specialist practice as involving a steady progression in a single area of medical activity with, at the most, only a single alteration in direction, the course of the career of Ernest Beech must seem something of an uncomfortable aberration. His obituary (Cohen 1994) described the course of his professional life. A graduate in Medicine from the University of Adelaide in 1932, Beech spent his first two postgraduate years in Perth, and then another two years in London. There he gained experience in neurology and respiratory disease and took the Membership of the Royal College of Physicians. From 1936 to 1945 he worked in general practice near the outskirts of Perth, where he became increasingly engaged in the practice of anaesthesia. In the latter capacity, he worked with the neurosurgeon James Ainslie, and also came to do Ainslie's medical neurological work. In 1938, Beech was appointed to the (Royal) Perth Hospital as Clinical Assistant to one of its senior physicians. Beech himself became a Physician to the Hospital in 1950, after having also been appointed in 1946 as Senior Physician to the Fremantle Hospital. During this period of simultaneous specialist practice as an anaesthetist, a physician and a neurologist, Beech was appointed President of the Australian Society of Anaesthetists in the immediate post-war years. He resigned his position as Anaesthetist to the Royal Perth Hospital in 1950 and in the following year replaced it with appointment as Neurologist to the Perth Children's Hospital. Soon after that, Gerald Moss resigned from the staff of the Royal Perth Hospital and was replaced as its Neurologist by Beech. As late as 1961 Beech sat for, and passed, the examination for Membership of the Royal Australasian College of Physicians, becoming a Fellow a decade later. After Beech retired as Senior Neurologist of the Royal Perth Hospital in 1968, he worked as co-ordinator of the Department of Radiology at that Hospital, and later as its Assistant Neuropathologist. He had become a Provisional Member of the Australian Association of Neurologists in 1957, but resigned from the Association in 1964, before his neurological appointment to the Royal Perth Hospital had expired.

Thus Beech's professional career comprised a most unconventional sequence and admixture of activities spanning a variety of medical specialties. His contribution to Australian neurology lay in his filling a potential vacuum by providing consultant neurological services to the major hospitals in Perth from the time Gerald Moss retired until the next generation of dedicated neurologists, Anthony Fisher and Mercy Sadka, had time to become established in practice in Western Australia. Beech does not seem to have become well-known to eastern state neurologists, or to have made significant original contributions to neurological knowledge, though he occupied an important place in the continuing development of the specialty in his own State.

WILLIAM J G BURKE (1913–1994)

A Sydney medical graduate (in 1946), Bill Burke's entire professional career was centred on St Vincent's Hospital in that city, except for the period 1950

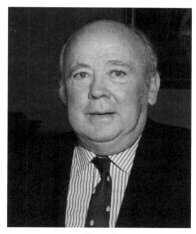

Bill Burke

and 1951 which he spent in London at the National Hospital at Queen Square and at the Maida Vale Hospital for Nervous Diseases. He became a Member of the Royal College of Physicians in 1950, having in the previous year taken the Membership of the Royal Australasian College of Physicians (of which he became a Fellow in 1961). By the time Burke returned to Sydney in 1952, Douglas Miller, later Sir Douglas, had established neurosurgery at St Vincent's Hospital in that city. Miller seems to have arranged for Burke to become Assistant Physician to the Hospital's Neurosurgical Department. Burke was also appointed Honorary Neurologist to the Mater Misericordiae and Lewisham Hospitals in Sydney and shared private consulting rooms with Miller. Burke's appointment at St Vincent's Hospital was converted to that of Neurologist to the Hospital and Head of its Department of Neurology when that Department was established in 1962. He continued to occupy this position until his retirement in 1988.

As a neurologist, Bill Burke was first and foremost a clinician and a teacher. He made little original contribution to neurological knowledge. Nor did he publish a great deal, though he delivered a memorable Graeme Robertson lecture in 1970 on the topic of myasthenia gravis, which testified to his extensive clinical experience with this particular disorder. Burke served his various hospitals in a number of leadership roles over the years. In 1954 he had become an Ordinary Member of the Australian Association of Neurologists and was a Council Member and the Association's Honorary Treasurer from 1963 to 1971. His memorial is the Neurology Department at St Vincent's

Hospital in Sydney, and the men he trained and who, over the years, came to be appointed to that Department, itself later named in Burke's honour.

John Vivian Gordon (1919–1999)

John Gordon graduated in Medicine from the University of Adelaide in 1942 and received a Doctorate in Medicine from that University in 1949. He became a Member of the Royal Australasian College of Physicians in 1947 and a Member of the Royal College of Physicians of London in 1950.

During a period of neurological training at the National Hospital at Queen Square in London, Gordon, like his friend George Selby, came under the influence of Sir Charles Symons. When Gordon returned to Adelaide in 1953, he was appointed as Clinical Assistant to the Neurosurgical Unit at the Royal Adelaide Hospital, the consultant physicians to that hospital at that time being reluctant to accept the desirability of a formal neurological appointment to the medical staff. In 1955 or 1956 Gordon became Assistant Physician to the Hospital, and in 1960 was appointed Honorary Neurologist to both the Royal Adelaide and the Adelaide Children's Hospitals and also to the Repatriation Department in South Australia (Rischbieth 1994).

John Gordon developed specialist neurological practice in Adelaide, both as a private consultant and at the various Adelaide hospitals to which he held appointments. He also induced younger men to take up the specialty, in particular Richard Burns. He did publish some clinical report type material, but he was not a researcher. In fact, as the years passed, his interest became increasingly directed towards music rather than medicine. In 1977 he left Adelaide and went to live in London where he pursued his cultural rather than his neurological interests. In 1994 he became an Honorary Member Emeritus of the Australian Association of Neurologists, to which he had been elected to Ordinary Membership in 1954. John Gordon had served on the Association's Council in its earlier days as its Honorary Treasurer (from 1974 to 1977).

Gordon was a rather large-framed, benign, genial and seemingly gentle man who established neurology on a secure basis in South Australia and inspired considerable affection in those he trained and in those with whom he was associated. His premature departure from the Australian neurological scene was a source of considerable regret to his colleagues in the national neurological community.

Arthur C Schwieger (1919–2010)

Many in his contemporary Australian neurological community may not have ever been aware that Arthur Schwieger, at least in his earlier life, had been a very promising musician and organist, and one who maintained strong musical interests throughout his days. He was Melbourne born, and seems to have settled on a medical rather than the musical career, graduating in Medicine from the University of Melbourne in 1942. After spending the following year at the Royal Melbourne Hospital, he enlisted in the Royal Australian Air Force during the war years. He returned to the Royal Melbourne Hospital from 1946 to 1948, taking the Membership of the Royal Australasian College of Physicians and obtaining a Melbourne MD degree. He then took himself off to London and Queen Square, taking the MRCP and beginning an enduring friendship with one John Walton, the future Newcastle-upon-Tyne neurologist who subsequently became Lord Walton. After Arthur Schwieger returned to Australia in 1953 he became assistant to Graeme Robertson at the Royal Melbourne Hospital, and also the first Honorary Neurologist to the Prince Henry Hospital. He also held a neurological appointment to the Repatriation General Hospital and engaged in private consulting practice.

To an outsider, his failure to be appointed as Graeme Robertson successor at the Royal Melbourne Hospital seemed a little surprising, but one does not know the circumstances and it may simply have been a matter of Schwieger's allegiance to, or preference for, Prince Henry Hospital, an institution to whose service he devoted much of his professional career.

Arthur Schwieger left behind no substantial corpus of publications, for he was not a researcher but a fine clinician and a gentle, kindly, courteous and likeable man.

John H W Tyrer (1920–2006)

Sydney-born John Tyrer, after an academically distinguished undergraduate career, graduated in Medicine from the University in his home city in 1941. After war service in a special research unit in the Royal Australian Air Force, he trained as a physician at the Royal Prince Alfred Hospital in Sydney, where he carried out animal experimental studies on cardiovascular dynamics which led in 1953 to the award of an MD from his alma mater. By this time, he had become a Member of the Royal Australasian College of Physicians and held appointment as an Honorary Assistant Physician to the Royal Prince Alfred Hospital. Late in the year of his MD award, he was appointed the first full-time Professor of Medicine in the University of Queensland. Before taking up that appointment, he spent a year as Travelling Fellow of the Australasian College of Physicians, increasing his neurological experience while working under the then Sir Russell Brain at the London Hospital.

When John Tyrer took up his Chair, and the permanent headship of the University of Queensland Department of Medicine, his empire consisted of himself and a half-time secretary. Over the next 31 years he built up his department into one of the largest and wealthiest ones in the University, one that spanned all the major teaching hospitals in Brisbane and the Queensland Gold Coast, his staff including four additional full-time university professors. Although John Tyrer held formal appointments as a Neurologist and a Physician at the Royal Brisbane Hospital, he never practised clinical neurology exclusively, believing that his appointment required him to remain involved in internal medicine more broadly. Indeed, with his intellectual, highly logical and rather perfectionistic qualities of mind, he probably was not entirely comfortable with the realities and improvisations sometimes required in clinical neurological practice. Even late in his academic career, he remained impervious to the temptations of academic preferments available to those who increasingly move into broader higher educational institutional administrative activity, for he realised that such a course would be inimical to what he preferred to do. He could be a little machiavellian at times, on one occasion defeating a request for more information from a newly appointed Dean of the Faculty of Medicine by flooding that Dean's office with copies of every single letter which left the Department of Medicine over a period of a fortnight. After that manifestation of efficiency and thoroughness, the Dean indicated that he now had the information that sufficed for his purposes.

John Tyrer's name appears on the authorship of a number of neurological papers in the literature, and on the title pages of several books on neurological and other medical topics. Although he never became an Ordinary Member of the Australian Association of Neurologists, remaining simply an Associate Member because of his continuing practice in general medicine, he did attend the Association's Scientific Meetings. For a dozen years after

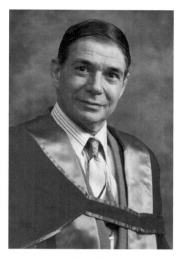

John Tryer

Graeme Robertson resigned from the Editorship of the *Proceedings of the Australian Association of Neurologists,* Tyrer edited the annual volumes of the *Proceedings'* successor, *Clinical and Experimental Neurology*. He also accommodated in his Department the library that Graeme Robertson left to the Australian Association of Neurologists when no other home could be found for it. Over many years he maintained a contact with French neurology and neurologists, visiting Paris annually for periods of several weeks, sometimes longer, over the Christmas weeks of Australian academic relative inactivity.

In retrospect, John Tyrer's main professional contribution to Australian medicine lay in his developing academic medicine in Queensland from a very small beginning into a substantial domain, but while doing this he also served Australian clinical neurology in a very significant way during its earlier years of growth.

John Mackay Sutherland (1920–1995)

John Sutherland was a Highlander, a Caithness man, educated at the Glasgow High School and the University of Glasgow, from which he graduated MB ChB in 1943. After naval service during World War II, he was awarded an MD from the University of Glasgow for investigations into multiple sclerosis and took the Membership of the Royal College of Physicians of Edinburgh while training in neurology under Douglas Kinchin Adams at the Western

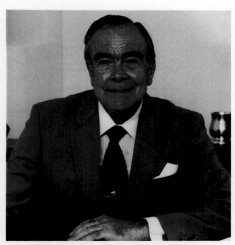

John Sutherland

Infirmary of Glasgow. Later, as a Senior Registrar based in Inverness, he provided a *de facto* neurological service to the north of Scotland and the Hebrides, while carrying out the major neuro-epidemiological study that demonstrated the role of genetic factors in multiple sclerosis. However, the queue of time-expired senior registrars that had developed in Britain by the end of his neurological training led to his accepting an academic appointment in Brisbane and emigrating to Australia. There, after a few years in the University of Queensland's Department of Medicine in the capacity of a Senior Lecturer, he became the first Senior Visiting Neurologist ever appointed to the Royal Brisbane Hospital, occupying that position from 1959 to 1977. He then retired, to practise in the quieter professional environment of the country city of Toowoomba, where he died in 1995.

Scientifically, John Sutherland's main achievements were the multiple sclerosis studies already outlined above, but he also obtained very considerable local fame in Brisbane as an expositor of clinical neurology. He took a major interest in medico-legal aspects of the specialty. He co-authored a set of educational case studies for medical students (*Exercises in Neurological Diagnosis*) with John Tyrer and later also with Eadie (Tyrer *et al.* 1981), and wrote a co-authored work *The Epilepsies – Modern Diagnosis and Treatment* (Sutherland and Eadie 1980) and, in passing, an autobiography intended for his grandchildren (*A Far-off Sunlit Place*). As well, in retirement, he produced a small textbook of neurology in note form (Sutherland: *Fundamentals of Neurology*) which appeared in 1981. He was the first man to practise in Queensland purely as a neurologist. He brought the Scottish neurological tradition, different in some ways from the Queen Square one, and at the time more therapeutically conscious, to Queensland soil, and he also made Australian neurology aware of the possibilities and dividends of neuro-epidemiological research.

(Lionel) Adrian Dawson (1921–1994)

Born in the Hunter region of New South Wales, Adrian Dawson (Dunlop 1996) was educated at Knox Grammar School, Sydney and became a Sydney medical graduate in 1944. After a year at Royal Prince Alfred Hospital, he spent almost his entire subsequent career in Newcastle. He went to Britain in the 1950s, where he became a Member of the Royal College of Physicians in 1954 (and a Fellow of that College in 1972) and took the Membership of the Royal Australasian College of Physicians. He was Senior Physician to the Newcastle Mater Hospital from 1955 to 1990, and in 1965 became Senior Consultant in Neurology at the Royal Newcastle Hospital. He retired from the latter position in 1991 and died three years later.

Dawson was the first neurologist to practise in Newcastle. He was a successful and admired consultant in that city, and a very pleasant and well-liked man. His interests within medicine were predominantly clinical. He did have some involvement in John Sutherland's epidemiological survey of the prevalence of multiple sclerosis in his home city (McCall *et al.* 1968), but otherwise seems to have had little record of research productivity.

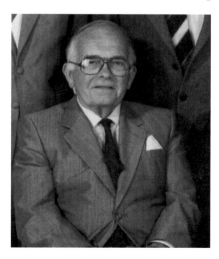

Adrian Dawson

JOHN D BERGIN (1921–1995)

Though a New Zealander, Jack Bergin was a long-standing Ordinary Member of the Australian Association of Neurologists and a fairly regular attendee at its Annual Scientific Meetings in Australian cities. The appropriateness of outlining his career in a history of Australian neurology, and not those of other significant New Zealand neurologists who have died subsequently e.g. Jock Caughey, Gavin Glasgow, Richard Hornabrook, is admittedly arguable, but it was included in the first edition of this book and it would seem ungracious to omit it now.

Bergin had graduated in Medicine from the University of Otago in 1943, and after war service held training positions in Wellington, becoming a Member of the Royal Australasian College of Physicians in 1947. Between 1950 and 1955 he worked in the United Kingdom, at the Hammersmith Hospital and the National Hospital at Queen Square, becoming a Member of the Royal College of Physicians in 1951. In 1955, soon after his return to Wellington, he succeeded Ivan Allen as Neurologist to the Wellington Hospital. He further developed the neurology service there, and trained a generation of New Zealand neurologists. He was elected to Fellowship of the Australasian (1957) and the London (1969) Colleges of Physicians. Bergin continued to work at the Wellington Hospital until his retirement from that institution, and then continued on in private consulting practice.

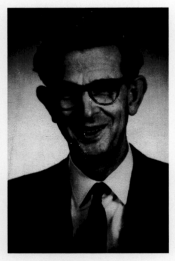

John Bergin

Jack Bergin was a clinical neurologist whose talents were thought of highly by his Australian contemporaries. He was a tall man with a quiet manner, who was capable of taking a firm line on matters which he considered important, but who otherwise did not seem to put himself forwards very often. He published occasionally in the medical literature, though more often on the topic of abortion than on any single neurological theme. As well as serving his profession, he served his community and his Church in a variety of ways and was appointed to a Papal Knighthood in the Order of St Gregory the Great in 1990.

KEITH S MILLINGEN (1922–1994)

Keith Millingen was a New South Welshman who made his professional career in Hobart. He was educated at the Sydney Church of England Grammar School and the University of Sydney, from which he graduated in Medicine. After spending the years 1945 and 1946 on the resident staff of Sydney Hospital, he moved to Hobart. He worked there for the remainder of his career, except for several periods of study overseas. He became a Member of the London, Edinburgh and Australasian Colleges of Physicians, and subsequently was elected to Fellowship of all of these bodies.

Millingen was appointed Honorary Physician to the Royal Hobart Hospital in 1952, and became Neurologist to that Hospital from 1977 to

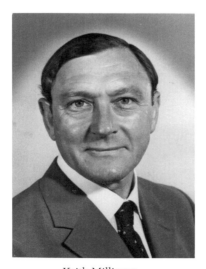

Keith Millingen

1987, when he retired with the title of Consultant Physician to the institution that he had served for more than a third of a century.

At first, Millingen worked in private consultative practice in Hobart, but later he became a member of the academic staff of the University of Tasmania, first as a Senior Lecturer and later as Reader in Medicine, while continuing to retain his consultant appointments to the Royal Hobart Hospital.

For many years, Keith Millingen was the only neurologist working in the whole of Tasmania and it fell to his lot to develop the neurology and clinical neurophysiology services of the State. His publication record indicates that his neurological interests ranged over several areas, e.g. multiple sclerosis, Parkinsonism, epilepsy. In addition, he formed collaborations with members of the Department of Pharmacy of the University of Tasmania which resulted in his co-authorship of papers on the clinical pharmacokinetics of several drugs used in neurology, and on the issue of compliance with prescribed medication in the management of epilepsy.

GEORGE M SELBY (1922–1997)

Vienna-born, George Selby emigrated to Australia with his parents in 1938, shortly before Nazi Germany annexed Austria. His secondary schooling was completed at Scotch College, Sydney. He then studied medicine at the University of Sydney, from which he graduated MB, BS in 1946. After spending a year on the resident staff of the Royal Prince Alfred Hospital and another year in neurological research in Sydney, he took himself off to Europe and the United Kingdom. There he worked for two years at the National Hospital at Queen Square, coming under the influence of, in particular, Sir Charles Symons. Selby returned to Sydney holding the Memberships of the Royal Colleges of Physicians of both London and Edinburgh, and soon afterwards took the Membership of the Royal Australasian College of Physicians.

At some stage around this time, if not earlier, he seems to have been taken under the wing of E L (Gus) Susman, despite their holding consultant appointments at different hospitals. As already mentioned, Susman later left George Selby the unusual Zeiss ophthalmoscope which he had owned, and also part of his library, including a volume of Gowers' *Manual* which George Selby much later passed on to the present writer.

In Sydney, Selby appears to have been the first man since A W Campbell half a century earlier to attempt to practise privately purely in clinical neurology. From 1951 to 1954 he was Neurologist-in-Charge of the new Northcott Neurological Centre, and in 1953 became Honorary Assistant Physician responsible for Neurology at the Royal North Shore Hospital of Sydney. In 1964, that appointment was converted to that of Honorary Neurologist to the Hospital, with charge of its Department of Neurology. After twenty-three years in that position George Selby became Consultant Neurologist to the Hospital, a position he held to the time of his death. Selby also was Neurologist to the Mater Misericordiae Hospital and the Hornsby Hospital in Sydney. In the fullness of time his Memberships of the various Royal College of Physicians became converted to Fellowships of those bodies, and in 1968 the University of Sydney conferred on him a Doctorate of Medicine for his thesis into research on Parkinson's disease.

George Selby was a great servant to the Australian Association of Neurologists. He became an Associate Member in 1951, when that category of membership was more or less tantamount to what became shortly afterwards its Provisional Membership. In 1954 he moved to Ordinary Membership of the Association and served as a Council Member from 1959 to 1969, and again from 1971 to 1978, being the Association's President between 1974 and 1978. In later years he was the Association's Honorary Archivist, and after his term of Presidency expired the Association conferred on him membership of its category of Honorary Member Emeritus. He was honoured by appointment as a Member of the Order of Australia in 1995, in recognition of his services to neurology.

The later years of George Selby's life were clouded by illness. Despite increasing handicaps, he remained active as long as he could, and bore with great dignity and courage the closing off of one after another of the aspects of life in which he had found fulfilment in better times. Over those long sad years, he was cared for devotedly by his wife Deirdre with the support of professional colleagues, notably Peter Williamson. He died on the 28 April 1997, on the day when the Australian Association of Neurologist was meeting with the Association of British Neurologists in his own home city.

George Selby was not only a fine clinical neurologist possessed of gracious European manners, but a man who was ever careful to preserve the feelings of other people. He was also an excellent clinical teacher and a

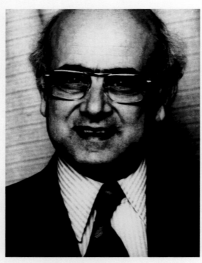

George Selby

lucid lecturer who created an active neurological department at the Royal
North Shore Hospital where he trained a succession of juniors. But he was
much more than that. He was an active clinical researcher throughout
much of his professional life who was well aware of research attitudes and
of statistical techniques and their place in collecting and analysing original
data. Parkinson's disease was his great intellectual hobby. His careful
longitudinal analysis of a large case series of patients with this disorder was
the basis of his MD degree. During his career he published over a wider
range of neurological topics e.g. parietal lobe syndromes (Selby 1956),
subacute myelo-optic neuropathy (Selby 1972). He also wrote a monograph
on *Migraine and its Variants* (Selby 1983) whose contents reflected his
extensive clinical experience.

George Selby played a number of very significant professional roles in
the evolution of Australian neurology. He was the pioneer of modern-day
exclusive neurological consultant practice in Australia's largest city, and
he made a long and influential contribution to advancing the affairs of the
Australian Association of Neurologists. But above all, he was an example
of that uncommon and important phenomenon, a clinical neurologist who
was also a clinical researcher, both in attitude and in achievement. His
career constitutes a notable bridge between clinical and academic neurology
in Australia. Had he lived at a slightly later date it seems highly probable that
his attainments would have received fitting academic titular recognition.

MARIE (MERCY) SADKA (1923–2001)

Mercy (as she seems to have always been known in neurological circles) Sadka was the first female practitioner of clinical neurology in Australia. Of Mesopotamian descent, her birth and earlier education took place in Singapore, and her education subsequently continued in England. She obtained her basic medical qualifications from the University of Oxford in 1947 and received postgraduate training in neurology at the National Hospital at Queen Square and later (1955 and 1956) at the Massachusetts General Hospital where she obtained experience in neuropathology. This overseas apprenticeship completed, she re-joined her family in Perth, becoming a Member of the Royal Australasian College of Physicians in 1955 (and a Fellow in 1967). She was appointed to the consultant neurology staff of the Royal Perth Hospital in 1959. There she instituted electroencephalography services, first in that hospital, and subsequently in other Perth hospitals. Later she developed an increasing interest in neurological rehabilitation. In the latter connection, over many years she was responsible for the Stroke Rehabilitation Unit associated with the Royal Perth Hospital, and in addition continued her clinical and clinical neurophysiological activities. She had a number of publications in the medical literature to her name and was responsible for the appearance of a booklet on *Stroke Disability, Whose Responsibility?* which became available in 1980.

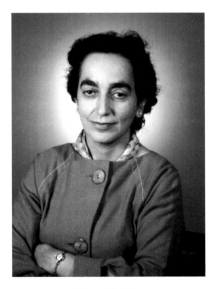

Mercy Sadka

Outsiders would probably have regarded Mercy Sadka as a rather private person who preferred to keep to herself, but she was also perceived as one who proved capable of persisting and effective advocacy for worthy causes, especially that of neurological rehabilitation. It was probably the latter activity that provided the major basis for her being created an Officer in the Order of Australia (in 1988, the year of her retirement).

PETER J B LANDY (1923–2006)

Peter Landy was the first man with formal neurological training to have practised in Brisbane, though he was not the first to have practised exclusively as a clinical neurologist in that city. He had been born in Toowoomba and graduated in Medicine from the University of Queensland in 1946. After two years in junior hospital appointments in that city, he travelled to London where he worked at the Central Middlesex Hospital and then at the Maida Vale Hospital under Russell Brain before returning to Brisbane in 1953, by then holding the qualification of MRCP (London). He was initially appointed as Neurologist to the Brisbane Mater Hospital, then a small institution where he had access to very few beds, but he also held appointment as an Assistant Visiting Physician to the Brisbane General Hospital (subsequently renamed the Royal Brisbane Hospital).

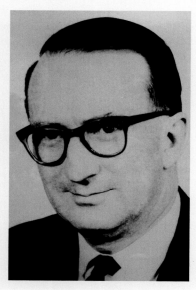

Peter Landy

When the new Princess Alexandra Hospital opened in Brisbane in 1956, Peter Landy transferred his allegiance to that institution, first in the capacity of a physician before being appointed as its first Visiting Neurologist in the early 1960s. After his formal retirement from that hospital long afterwards, he maintained contact with it while continuing in private consulting practice. Over the years, he had a substantial involvement with the Australian Medical Association and other medically related professional bodies, including various periods in chairmanship roles, and was awarded an OBE for his contributions to medicine in 1983. Clinically, his skills were in considerable demand as a neurologist throughout his long career. He was a quiet and slightly diffident man, though one who was greatly liked and respected by his colleagues. Throughout his career, he made some contributions to the neurological literature, but he was not primarily a researcher and his main enduring contribution to Australia neurology would be his initiating and sustaining roles in the earlier stages of the development of clinical neurology on the south side of the Brisbane River.

ANTHONY FISHER (1924–2007)

Adelaide-born Tony Fisher obtained his medical qualifications from the University of his home city in 1946, and two years later became Neurology Registrar to Leonard Cox at the Alfred Hospital in Melbourne. He took the MD of the University of Melbourne in 1954 and achieved Membership of the Royal Australasian College of Physicians. Between 1954 and 1957 he accumulated further neurological experience in London, at the West End Hospital for Neurological Disease and at the National Hospital at Queen Square. In the year after his return to Australia he was appointed Assistant Honorary Neurologist at the Royal Perth Hospital, where he became Senior Honorary Neurologist after Ernest Beech retired in 1968. For a time, Tony Fisher was also Neurologist to Fremantle Hospital, but in 1971 he transferred his activities in Perth from the Royal Perth Hospital to the Sir Charles Gairdner Hospital, where he served as Head of the Department of Neurology from 1977 to 1983. He continued to be an active member of that Department after he formally retired in 1988 and maintained links with it for another decade.

Tony Fisher had spent time in London at Queen Square with CS Hallpike, the pioneer English-language neuro-otologist, and this experience probably

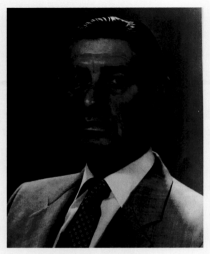

Tony Fisher

led him to set up neuro-otological investigative facilities at the Sir Charles Gairdner Hospital, where he employed them in studying external eye muscle movement disturbances, a particular interest of his.

Tony Fisher and Mercy Sadka had commenced consultant neurological practice at much the same time, in a city where neurological activity seems to have languished for some years before. Tony had a more outgoing and approachable personality than Mercy and to an outsider's probably superficial perception it was he who, more than anyone else, reactivated clinical neurology in Perth and set it on its continuing growth pathway.

PETER EBELING (1926–2013)

Peter Ebeling was the immediate successor to Graeme Robertson's role at the Royal Melbourne Hospital. Like Robertson, he was a Melbourne man, one educated at Scotch College in that city and then at the University of Melbourne from which he graduated with first class honours in Medicine. After postgraduate training in general medicine and neurology in his home city, where he took a Melbourne MD degree, Peter Ebeling went to Queen Square at a time when Roger Gilliatt was developing the methodology for clinical nerve conduction studies in that institution. At Queen Square, Ebeling used these techniques to study various ulnar nerve palsies, and subsequently brought the methodology back to Australia where he was the

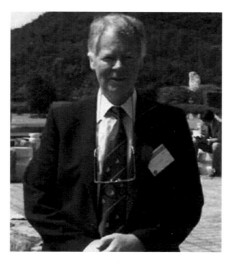

Peter Ebeling

first person to employ it in routine clinical practice. In this country, he was initially appointed as a Neurologist at the Royal Melbourne Hospital under Graeme Robertson and Arthur Schwieger, but in 1963 succeeded the former as Head of the Neurology Department at the Hospital, continuing in that role until 1991. Ebeling also held appointments at other Melbourne teaching hospitals and had a busy private consulting practice.

Peter Ebeling did a considerable amount of clinical teaching, played a substantial internal role in the politics of the Royal Melbourne Hospital and in the activities of the Royal Australasian College of Physicians, recruited capable and professionally successful and highly productive people to the consultant staff of the Royal Melbourne Neurology Department and encouraged their development of special areas of neurological knowledge and expertise. All this activity and his interests outside neurology left him little opportunity to take his own early clinical neurophysiological research further.

JAMES W LANCE (1927–2019)

A few of the younger members of the founding generation of Australian clinical neurologists, John Game in particular, used to speak of their hope that one day the importance of clinical neurology in the country would be recognised by the creation of an academic department and, as was the expectation of those times in relation to academic departments,

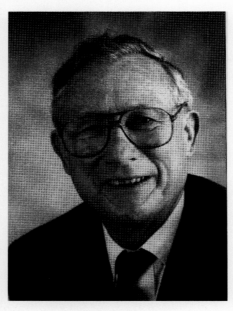

James Lance

of a professorship associated with it. John Game lived long enough to see that hope realised, in the form of James Waldo Lance, and fulfilled at the University of New South Wales.

James Lance had been born at Wollongong in New South Wales and graduated in Medicine from University of Sydney in 1950. After two years in resident positions at the Royal Prince Alfred Hospital in Sydney, he carried out research on pyramidal tract function under the guidance of the relatively recently arrived neurophysiologist Peter Bishop, an investigation resulting in the award of an MD from Sydney University. Lance then went to London to the Postgraduate Medical School at Hammersmith, followed by the National Hospital at Queen Square where he was allocated to look after the relatively few beds that the already retired Sir Francis Walsh had available to him.

On his return to Sydney, Lance took up various teaching and clinical appointments, including one at the Northcott Neurological Centre where the Director was George Selby. In those times, that directorship seems to have been the starting point for young neurologists or prospective neurologists beginning to make their careers in Sydney. Lance in turn became Director of the Centre for a time (1956–1957), but also held an appointment to the honorary staff of Sydney Hospital (1956–1961). In 1960, he spent time overseas again, in Boston with Raymond Adams at the Massachusetts General Hospital. After this, in 1961, he transferred his allegiance from University of Sydney-associated institutions to the newly opened Department of Medicine in the University of New South Wales where he held appointments to its associated Prince of Wales and Prince Henry Hospitals. He was initially appointed to the University in the capacity of a Senior Lecturer, becoming an Associate Professor in 1964 and a full Professor eleven years later, and holding Emeritus status after 1992. He continued his association with, and his teaching of neurology in, the Prince of Wales Hospital almost to the end of his life.

That sparse outline of James Lance's highly productive and distinguished neurological career omits mention of his roles in, and sometimes presidencies of, various international associations, particularly ones connected with headache, his long service to the Australian Association of Neurologists including a term as its fourth President, his Fellowships of the Royal Colleges of Physicians of London and Australasia, the honorary DSc conferred on him by the University of New South Wales around the time his formal retirement, and the national governmental recognition of his achievements in the awards of CBE in 1977 and an AO in 1991.

Throughout his career, Lance remained an active clinical neurologist, one alert to the existence of previously unrecognised phenomena, e.g. his description of the Harlequin syndrome and of neck-tongue pain, as well as his more famous account of post-anoxic myoclonus (the Lance-Adams syndrome). He interpreted neurological matters largely from an applied physiological standpoint, though also for a period from a chemical one when, in collaboration with the chemist Herta Hinterberger, he studied the behaviour of circulating serotonin concentrations in relation to migraine attacks. George Selby had earlier stimulated his interest into the then rather neglected topic of migraine, and together they had produced a major paper on its phenomena which marked the beginning of Lance's long series of major publications concerning headache, and particularly migraine. These works included several books, one of which, *The Mechanism and Management of Headache,* went through seven editions during his lifetime. James Lance's work was the origin of a school of headache research in Australia, initially preserved by people who worked with him such as Michael Anthony, Peter Goadsby and Andrew Zagami, but increasingly metastasised via his intellectual disciples into other Australian institutions.

But there was a second side to Lance's scientific publication record. The qualification 'scientific' is necessary in this connection as, during his career, he found relaxation in writing stories for children, one of which appeared in book form. This second scientific side reflected his physiological interpretation of neurological phenomena, taking the forms of an investigation into tendon reflex mechanisms in humans and of a book written in conjunction with his counterpart in the University of Sydney, James McLeod. That neurophysiological side of Lance's science also was developed further by people who he had trained, most notably by David Burke and Simon Gandevia.

If it was the presence on library bookshelves of Graeme Robertson's several volumes concerning the now superseded method of pneumoencephalography that first presented a more or less contemporary international medicine readership with enduring and easily observed evidence of the existence of Australian clinical neurology, it was surely the volumes bearing James Lance's name on their covers that next enhanced that international awareness.

RICHARD RISCHBIETH (1927–2007)

With the exception of a period of about five years obtaining postgraduate experience in Britain, Dick Rischbieth's life was spent in Adelaide. He was born there in 1927, educated at St Peter's College and the University of Adelaide, graduated in Medicine from the latter at the end of 1950. While in England he obtained Memberships of the London and Edinburgh Royal Colleges of Physicians and spent time at Queen Square. Back in Adelaide, he initially worked at the Royal Adelaide and the Adelaide Children's Hospitals, but in 1961 became involved in the establishment of the Neurology Unit at the Queen Elizabeth Hospital which was affiliated with the relatively new Flinders University. This was an institution which, at that time, was rather eagerly recruiting to its professorial staff bright young medical academics whose careers were clearly in growth phases. Rischbieth was appointed Head of the Queen Elizabeth Hospital's Neurology Unit from 1961 to 1992, during which time he saw it develop into a major Australian neurological facility.

Dick Rischbieth was neither a researcher nor by nature an academic. Rather, he was a well-liked practical clinical neurologist and clinical teacher who accumulated a few publications in the literature during his career. He will be remembered for his role in association with the early development

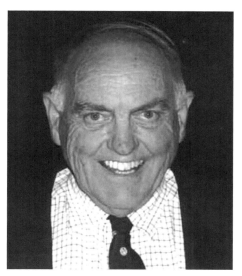

Dick Rischbieth

and long-continued oversight of the Neurological Unit at a major new Adelaide institution.

DAVID CURTIS (1927–2017)

David Curtis probably would generally be regarded as a great experimental neuropharmacologist whose original scientific achievements received considerable international recognition during his lifetime. In 2006 his autobiography appeared, providing an account of his career but with a very heavy emphasis on his scientific work. The autobiography was part of the series of volumes *The History of Neuroscience in Autobiography* and the Series Editor, in Volume 5, briefly summarised Curtis's scientific attainments thus:

> David Curtis pioneered the use of microelectrophoretic techniques to examine the effects of potential synaptic transmitters on single identified neurons in the mammalian central nervous system (CNS) in vivo. He similarly examined the effects of compounds that blocked or enhanced synaptic transmission at the synapses of particular excitatory or inhibitory pathways. He thus contributed to the identification of a number of central transmitters, particularly glycine, gamma-aminobutyric acid (GABA), and aspartic and glutamic acids.

One might therefore need to justify the inclusion of the name of David Curtis among the ranks of Australian clinical neurologists who are no longer

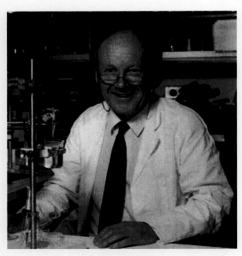

David Curtis

living. He had graduated in Medicine from the University of Melbourne in 1950 and spent his first two years after graduation at the Royal Melbourne Hospital where for a time he worked under the neurologist Graeme Robertson, and then in 1953 moved to the Alfred Hospital as Neurology Registrar to Leonard Cox and John Game. While occupying that position, he was greatly impressed by a visiting lecture from the future Nobel Laureate John Eccles, newly appointed to the John Curtin School of Medical Research in Canberra, and sought an opportunity to do research with him. David Curtis spent the remainder of his life in Canberra, first in the Department of Physiology and later in that of Pharmacology, achieving professorial status in 1973, and then the Chair of Pharmacology before, towards the end of his formal academic career, from 1989 to 1992, occupying the Howard Florey Chair of Medical Research at the National University and the Directorship of the John Curtin School. He had become an FAA in 1965, and President of that body from 1986 to 1990, a Fellow of the Royal Society of London in 1974 and was elected FRACP in 1987.

There is very little in that abbreviated formal career record that would justify Curtis being regarded as an Australian neurologist, but members of the post-founder generation of Australian clinical neurologists will perhaps recall that he was elected an Honorary Member of the AAN and served two terms on the Association's Council. Whenever the Association met in Canberra in earlier years, he facilitated its Scientific Meetings, attended them, and in the years afterwards was often present at these meetings when they were held in nearby Australian capital cities. At least some in the contemporary Australian neurological community had a sense that he continued to feel himself a part of that community over the years, and that he gained something from hearing about clinical matters and in return offered the clinical community insights and knowledge regarding advances in neuropharmacology, particularly advances for which he was at least partly responsible, which they otherwise might not have been aware of until long afterwards. In those now distant days, when many believed that the only neurotransmitters were acetylcholine and noradrenaline (and perhaps adrenaline) with dopamine beginning to find a place, it came as something of a surprise that he was alerting his clinical colleagues to evidence of a neurotransmitter role for excitatory and inhibitory amino acids, and in doing this preparing their thinking for the clinical use of newer pharmacological agents such as baclofen and, long afterwards, for certain antiseizure medications.

David Curtis may not have been so often present at AAN Scientific Meetings in his pre-retirement years, when he was more heavily involved in academic administration, but in his retirement, when he retained a connection with the National University, he did sometimes reappear at AAN meetings, giving the impression that he retained an interest in the thinking and welfare of his clinical colleagues. On one occasion I can remember his being asked how he was filling in his time when he no longer had his own laboratory, and his saying that he had taken to doing wood turning and was waiting for the moment when his wife would plead with him to stop making more wooden bowls.

While he did so much for neuroscience, David Curtis was a great friend to, and supporter of, Australian clinical neurology and clinical neurologists, and an example for their scientific aspirations to attempt to follow.

John Barrie Morley (1934–2019)

Although he was born at Maroubra in New South Wales, the earlier part of Barrie Morley's life occurred in Melbourne where he graduated in Medicine from its University in 1958. After three years at the Prince Henry Hospital in that city undertaking physician training, he spent the period 1962 to 1964 in Britain at the United Oxford Hospital's Neurology Unit, and at Queen Square and Guy's Hospital. After returning to Melbourne, he entered private

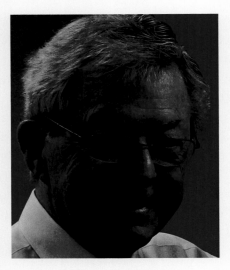

Barrie Morley

practice in neurology and resumed his relationship with Prince Henry Hospital and the Monash Medical School where, between 1978 and 1979, he was Dean of the Clinical School. He was also Head of Neurology and Chairman at the Monash Medical Centre between 1966 and 1989. During the earlier part of those years, he also devoted a great deal of time in serving as Honorary Secretary of the Australian Association of Neurologists, during the latter six years of John Game's long presidency.

The death of Barrie Morley's second wife, after his first wife had died relatively young, seemed to precipitate a change in the direction of his life. With a daughter, he moved to the rural city of Toowoomba in southern Queensland to enter into a new pattern of living, while practising privately in neurology. He continued in this activity until his last years, also providing consultations at nearby country towns such as Kingaroy. When the University of Queensland extended its medical student teaching to larger country towns, Barrie became involved in this activity, holding the status of Associate Clinical Professor.

Barrie Morley was a very sincere and likeable man, possessed of major musical interests and administratively gifted, not a researcher but a fine clinician. His greatest service to Australia neurology probably lay in his long period of secretaryship of the Australian Association during the early years of its development. One can hardly help wondering how his career might have developed had he not suffered the loss of his first wife so relatively early in his life, and again being bereaved a few years later.

Bernard Gilligan (1934–2006)

Victorian country born, Bernard Gilligan was educated at the University High School and then at Wesley College in Melbourne, matriculated into the Melbourne University Medical course from which he graduated with honours in 1957. He then commenced a career-long association with the Alfred Hospital in Melbourne, interrupted in 1959 by a year of doing paediatrics at the Princess Margaret Hospital in Perth. On return to the Alfred Hospital after that year, he began neurological training under John Game, becoming a Member of the Royal Australasian College of Physicians in 1961 (and a Fellow nine years later). Subsequently he went to Queen Square in London for further neurological experience, and on his return to Melbourne in early 1965 was appointed to the position of Neurologist to his old hospital and Head of the Neurology Unit there. This was a position which John Game had vacated in 1963 and to which Leonard Cox temporally returned in the interval before Gilligan became available. He continued to work at the Alfred Hospital until 1996 and continued in private consulting practice for the remainder of his life. He had also held a Neurology appointment at the Fairfield Hospital for a time. During the earlier part of those years at the Alfred he became a Fellow of the College of Rehabilitation Medicine.

For some years Bernard Gilligan was active in the affairs of the then Australian Association of Neurologists, serving as its Honorary Treasurer from 1978 to 1983 before becoming President from 1984 to1987. When Treasurer, he suffered the mild indignity of having almost the entire original consignment of Association neckties inundated by the overflow from a sink in his consulting rooms, beneath which he had stored the neckwear prior to its distribution. Although it not known for sure, Bernard Gilligan was such an efficient man that he almost certainly had the provision of a replacement consignment of ties covered by insurance. The incident is referred to again in Chapter 8.

As mentioned immediately above, and probably to an extent under John Game's tutelage, Bernard Gilligan was a careful and diligent man who looked after his responsibilities capably, and possibly with a more realistic awareness of practicality than his tutor. It seems very likely that,

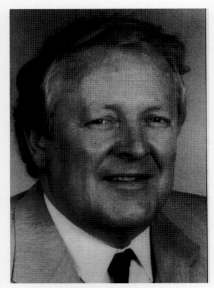

Bernard Gilligan

through John Game, he was able to approach the Van Cleef Foundation seeking funding for the establishment of a Chair in Neurology to be sited in the Alfred Hospital, which had become a teaching hospital of Monash University. After some years this approach came to fruition, and the Chair to occupation by Elsdon Storey.

Although Bernard Gilligan published some papers in the literature, by nature he was not a researcher but rather a capable and successful clinician who was an unusually good organiser and possessed of a will to expedite the progress of Australian clinical neurology. His capacities and his achievements led to his being awarded Membership of the Order of Australia in 2005.

IAN HOPKINS (1934–2019)

Ian Hopkins was the first person in Australia to practise exclusively as a full-time paediatric neurologist. He was a University of Melbourne medical graduate who subsequently took that university's MD degree in 1962 and the Membership of the Royal Australasian College of Physicians. He then travelled to Britain, in the 1963 and 1964 period holding a Nuffield Foundation Travelling Fellowship. In London, he worked at the Hammersmith Hospital, the Great Ormond Street Hospital for Sick

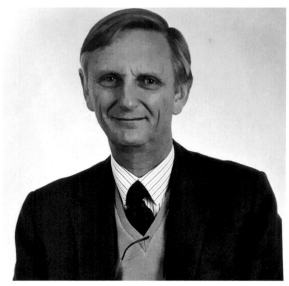

Ian Hopkins

Children and at the National Hospital, Queen Square. After that period in Britain, he obtained further neurological experience in the United States at the Johns Hopkins Hospital in Baltimore and the University of Kentucky.

After his return to Melbourne, he initially became First Assistant in the University of Melbourne's Department of Paediatrics and in 1968 was appointed Neurologist to the Royal Children's Hospital, becoming Director of its Department of Neurology from the beginning of that Department's existence (in 1977). He continued to practise neurology in the Hospital to the time of his retirement in 2001, by which stage he had allied himself to that small group of Australian neurologists who in later life were keener to talk about their wood turning activities than their medical ones.

During his career, Ian Hopkins' main interest probably was in childhood epilepsy. He was responsible for the authorship of a number of literature publications and his name has been attached to two different entities, the Hopkins syndrome and the Pitt-Hopkins syndrome.

JOHN BALLA (1934–2013)

Unusually for an Australian neurologist, the most complete account of John Balla's career is not to be found in places where one seeks information about Australian medical careers but in a newspaper, and not a newspaper

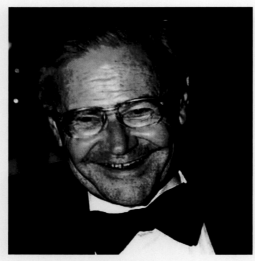

John Balla

from Balla's hometown, but the *Sydney Morning Herald* (Gibson 2013). Also unusual was that the thrust of the article, appropriately enough, concerned the analysis of clinical thinking and reasoning, particularly as it was connected with neurology and neurological education, rather than matters of conventional clinical neurological practice or clinical discovery.

Balla was born in Hungary and lived through the terrible stresses of the siege of Budapest that occurred near the end of World War II, events described by Balla's slightly younger contemporary Frank Vajda in his book *We Are Our Memories* (2021). In 1948, Balla's family left their homeland and made their way to Melbourne where John Balla was educated at the Melbourne High School and the University of Melbourne, from which he graduated in Medicine. After this, he worked overseas at several institutions in England before returning to Melbourne to Prince Henry Hospital where in due course he became Head of the Department of Neurology and Dean of the Clinical School. As he grew older, he became increasingly concerned with medical thinking more than clinical matters and spent various periods overseas engaged in activities related to these concerns, including a three-year period in a professorial appointment at Hong Kong.

John was a sincere and pleasant man. Whether his intellectual activities have had, or will have, any considerable continuing influence on Australian neurology remains to be seen, but Australia neurology is surely entitled to claim for itself John Balla both as a neurological clinician and for his role as an author of several medical books (see Appendix V).

Peter F Bladin (1929–2022)

Almost exactly a quarter of a century after those present at the 1997 Annual Scientific Meeting of the Australian Association of Neurologists in Sydney learned that a very distinguished figure in the clinical neurology of the country, George Selby, had died during the course of the Meeting, and in the city where the Meeting was held, this set of events was repeated in May 2022, but on this occasion in Melbourne, where Peter Bladin's life came to its end.

Peter Bladin had played a very influential part in re-enlivening Melbourne clinical neurology after the influences of the founding generation of Melbourne clinical neurologists began to wane as they grew older. Bladin's activities and achievements certainly became well enough recognised and appreciated within his home city, but one has the impression that his work may not have been as well known in the broader Australian neurological community as it deserved to have been, while such recognition as he received from his alma mater and the national government came rather belatedly.

After a distinguished undergraduate career in the Faculty of Medicine of the University of Melbourne, during which he took a BSc degree, Bladin graduated MB BS at the end of 1955. He spent the next 4 years in physician training positions at St Vincent's Hospital in Melbourne, becoming a MRACP in 1958. Fellowship of the College came a few years later, and subsequently Fellowship of the Edinburgh College of Physicians. Bladin also possessed a Melbourne MD degree taken by thesis in 1970.

Bladin spent two years in Britain, working at Queen Square, where from conversations later in life I gained the impression that he had developed a friendship with Willian Gooddy, a kindly man of less conventional attitudes and interests than many of his Queen Square colleagues. These were characteristics that I think Peter Bladin would have found congenial. In London Bladin also saw something of the surgical attempts to treat intractable seizure disorders at the Maudsley Hospital, an experience that may also have led to his developing a degree of empathy for organically oriented psychiatry and psychology.

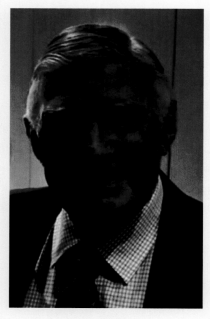

Peter Bladin

Bladin returned to Melbourne in 1961 to take up a Junior Consultant position at St Vincent's Hospital, where he worked under the Senior Neurologist John Billings. However, in 1965, with the resuscitation and expansion of the old Austin Hospital, and the arrival of Austin Doyle as its Professor of Medicine, Bladin transferred his allegiance to that institution as its founding Director of Neurology. The remainder of his professional career was spent there. In personality and strength of character he was able to cope with Austin Doyle and he progressively built up a large and vigorous neurological team and neurological facilities.

His personal neurological endeavours lay in three main directions. The first to make an impact on the wider Australian neurological community was stroke, which in those days was generally regarded as the territory of the general physician, who tended to pursue masterly investigative inactivity during the acute phase of the illness. Bladin and the junior colleagues whom he increasingly attracted adopted more active roles in the situation. With the aid of the then contemporary imaging techniques, certain clinical stroke syndromes were defined, and more active management policies adopted. Gradually his interest in this area seemed to wane and it increasingly became the territory of his disciple Geoffrey Donnan, and largely moved with the latter to the Florey Institute.

Over the years in the late 1960s and 1970s it became increasingly apparent to the outsider that epilepsy had become Bladin's principal professional interest, though if one reads his account of his *Career in Epilepsy* (Bladin 2017) it seems that, even before he went to Queen Square, epilepsy began to hold intellectual appeal for him. Peter Bladin was not a man to contemplate or investigate aspects of epileptogenesis in the laboratory. He was suited to rapid action, intellectually and physically. He was also sensitive to the psychological issues arising from experiencing the threat of, or the actual occurrence of, epileptic seizures, and the limitations of their current drug therapy. When he proceeded to set up Australia's first comprehensive Epilepsy Service at the Austin Hospital, he catered for both the psychological and physical aspects of epilepsy management. There had certainly been sporadic attempts at neurosurgical treatment of refractory epilepsy in Australia before the Austin service was instigated, but once it was underway, until similar facilities were set up elsewhere, the Austin provided the only satisfactory site in Australia for the evaluation and surgical management of drug treatment-resistant seizure disorders. Peter Bladin is deservedly regarded as the founding influence on epilepsy surgery in Australia, as well as being the instigator (and inaugural President) of the Epilepsy Society of Australia, where his achievements are honoured by those who deliver its annual Bladin Lecture.

Over the years, Peter Bladin's Epilepsy Service attracted many medical graduates who went on to make distinguished careers in epileptology, none more so than his successor at the Austin Hospital Samuel Berkovic whose distinguished genetic investigations led to Fellowship of the Royal Society of London.

Bladin's third field of professional endeavour was a less outwardly noticeable one professionally. In the years of his formal retirement his interest in the history of neurological illness, particularly epilepsy, flourished in a series of publications. He traced the record of epilepsy as it had occurred in his home State of Victoria from the earliest times of European settlement, and set down the outcome in a handsome privately produced but undated 250-page volume. There are also single-author historical publications in the medical literature associated with his name, together with some historical chapters in books and co-authorship of a monograph *A Disease Once Sacred*.

In 1993, the year of his retirement from the Austin Hospital, Bladin was honoured by the Australian Government with the award of an AO. He continued his medical interests and maintained his connection with the Austin Hospital Epilepsy Service and his old friendships, particularly that with Frank Vajda, during his post-retirement years. He lost his wife and life's companion Dawn in 2018, though in his last years he was consoled by knowing that their son Christopher was already well established in his own neurological career.

JAMES GRAHAM MCLEOD (1932–2022)

The death of James McLeod in June 2022 brought to its end the long and distinguished career of a man who played a very great role in the development of scientific clinical neurology in his home city of Sydney.

Jim McLeod's early career in medicine took a slightly unusual course compared with that which was customary in Australia in the 1950s. He interrupted his undergraduate medical studies at the University of Sydney for a year to acquire the qualification of BSc (Med) in Physiology, and then, as a Rhodes scholar, spent three years in Oxford doing research on the physiology of pain that led to the award of a D.Phil. Following this, he returned to Australia to graduate from the University of Sydney with an MB BS qualification in 1959. After doing early post-qualification clinical work at the Royal Prince Alfred Hospital in Sydney he returned overseas to spend a year at Queen Square followed by another year at Harvard. In 1967, after his second return to his home city, he took up an appointment as Senior Lecturer in Medicine at the University of Sydney, becoming an Associate Professor there three years later. In 1978 he was appointed to the Bosch Chair of Medicine in the University of Sydney and, in addition, though later in that same year, as Bushell Professor of Neurology. These were appointments that he retained until the time of his retirement. Academic, professional and governmental honours came his way as the years passed – a DSc from Sydney University, an honorary doctorate from the University of Aix-Marseille, Fellowship of the Australian Academy, Fellowships of the London and Australasian Colleges of Physicians and appointment as an Officer in the Order of Australia (in 1986).

His clinical activities throughout his postgraduate career were largely confined to the Royal Prince Alfred Hospital where he was Head of that institution's Department of Neurology and, from 1990 onwards, Chairman of its Institute of Neuroscience.

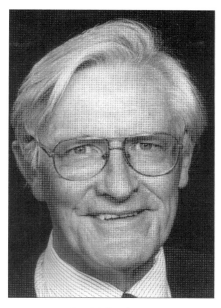

Jim McLeod

Jim's influence on the development of Australian neurology began well before he became President of the then Australian Association of Neurologists from 1981 to 1984, and continues at the time of writing. James Lance had initiated a program of clinical neuroscience research at the University of New South Wales and its teaching hospitals in the early 1960s, and Jim McLeod, from his position in the University of Sydney, proceeded to likewise before the end of that decade. At least from the perspective of an outsider, there was no sense of any tension or unhealthy rivalry between the two men or their respective research programs going on in the same city, and they collaborated in the writing of a book published in 1984 by Blackwells of Oxford (*Introductory Neurology*) that went to a second edition. A decade later Jim McLeod authored a second book dealing with his main area of professional interest, *Inflammatory Neuropathies,* published by Elsevier.

Jim McLeod's own research interests lay in two main directions. Initially his studies appeared to be concerned chiefly with disorders of peripheral nerves and the neuromuscular junction, and the application of clinical neurophysiological investigations in their elucidation. These were matters both of clinical interest and of practical importance to the then younger generation of neurologists, several of whom joined his research program (John Pollard, John Walsh, Pamela McCombe and Garth Nicholson, among others) while Michael Halmagyi's concerns became focused on vertigo and disorders of balance. As time passes, the Australian neurological community will increasingly and enduringly associate McLeod's name with his work on the chronic inflammatory demyelinating peripheral neuropathies, even if details of the extension of his peripheral nerve interests into related disorders through the activities of his intellectual disciples fades from collective neurological memory.

Soon after the Australian neurological community began to become aware of Jim McLeod's interest in the peripheral nervous system it became apparent that he was also concerned with primary demyelinating disease of the central nervous system and, in particular, in the epidemiology of multiple sclerosis in his homeland. John Sutherland had pioneered work in this latter area overseas and later in Australia, and with co-investigators had published on it. But I am reasonably sure that Jim McLeod moved into the area quite independently of Sutherland's interests and came to dominate it over a couple of decades after Sutherland ceased active research. In essence, McLeod's work brought up to date the earlier data on the Australian regional distribution of the disease, and also involved participation in clinical trial studies of measures designed to retard or reverse the process of primary demyelination.

Through his work and his research achievements, and with his unostentatious, persevering and helpful ways, James McLeod played a very major and successful role in introducing and then sustaining a scientific background to the practice of clinical neurology in his home city. It is not only those whom he trained who are now nearing or at the ends of their professional careers, but a whole younger generation of Australian neurologists who have reason to be grateful for his endeavours.

Byron Kakulas (1932–2023)

Though Byron Kakulas in the earlier years of his professional life was engaged to a degree in clinical neurological activities, and in the 1970s was a member of the Council of the Australian Association of Neurologists, his dominant role throughout the greater part his career was that of a neuropathologist with a particular interest in muscle and spinal cord disease. A Western Australian, he had been a medical student in Adelaide and graduated from that University in 1956 before the Perth medical course was ready to produce its own graduates. After early clinical training in neurology at

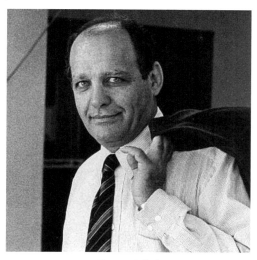

Byron Kakulas

the Royal Perth Hospital he became involved in an investigation into the weakness that developed in the small marsupial, the Quokka, that was found on Rottnest Island off the Western Australian coast. This work led to the award of an MD from the University of Western Australia and, later, to an expanding program of research on neuromuscular disorders back in Perth after Byron had undertaken neuropathology training at Harvard with Raymond Adams and his colleagues.

The neuromuscular investigative work continued to occupy Byron over the remainder of his long life. It led to recognition of the entity inclusion body myositis, to a substantial publication record including several books and monographs (see Appendix V), an international reputation in his chosen field, the award of an AO by the Australian Government and an MD from the University of Athens, the foundation and initial directorship of a Neuromuscular Research Institute in Perth (later the Perron Institute) and to the existence of a Perth school of neuromuscular disorder scholars, including among others Frank Mastaglia. In a way, Byron's professional career followed the opposite course to the typical one for a late 19th and first-half 20th century neurologist, viz. some neuropathology first while waiting for the opportunity for clinical work, but that certainly did not prevent it enhancing the reputation of Australian clinical neuroscience.

Chapter 8

THE AUSTRALIAN ASSOCIATION OF NEUROLOGISTS – IN MORE RECENT TIMES

The last four decades of the 20th century and the first two of the 21st have seen the Australian neurologists' professional association grow in financial strength, in organisational maturity, and in influence within the local medical profession, the wider community and at a governmental level. At the same time the Association has continued to serve the needs of Australian neurologists, particularly in relation to education, and to provide them with a national voice and a forum. The various aspects of this growth may be more easily traced if dealt with individually.

Organisational Matters

The Association's Constitution

Over the latter half of the 20th century there were a number of revisions in aspects of the Australian Association of Neurologists' Constitution. The initial revision, occurring some 10 years after the founding of the organisation, was discussed in Chapter 4. The principal purposes of that revision were to define the Association's membership categories more precisely, and to set a timetable for members to retire from the Australian Association of Neurologists' Council as the years passed and the pool of persons available to serve on that body increased in size. Subsequent revisions of the Constitution arose from a need to refine the membership categories still further as professional and other circumstances changed with the passage of time, or because of the desirability of otherwise advancing the interests of the Association or those of its members. Each change in the Constitution usually had a gestation period of one to three years. This allowed time for the alteration to be approved at an Annual General Meeting following the one at which it was first mooted, and for the subsequent necessary legal drafting to be done to allow the Constitutional change to be put into effect. None of the alterations changed the basic organisational structure or the philosophy of the Association, though one change opened the way for the Association to include all New Zealand neurologists, with the Association then becoming the Australian and New Zealand Association of Neurologists. The changes were intended to serve what were seen to be desirable purposes at the times they were made. None caused the Association to deviate from the directions envisaged, and legislated for, by its founders.

The Constitutional changes described in Chapter 4, more clearly defining the various membership categories, came into effect in 1961. In 1966, the Constitution was modified again to allow the Association's fiscal year to coincide with the community financial year, and the possibility of termination of membership for non-payment of the annual subscription was stated explicitly.

In 1968, a mechanism was sought to honour the Association's first and second Presidents, Leonard Cox and E Graeme Robertson, respectively. Council, without referring the matter to an Ordinary General Meeting of the Association, created a new category of Honorary Member Emeritus to accommodate these men. The name of K B Noad was added to the category at the time it was first utilised. Later the names of Gerald Moss, John Game, David Curtis, George Selby, John Gordon and John Sutherland were added, and later still, those of J W Lance and M J Eadie.

During a period of prolonged and delicate negotiation to set up the Australian Neurological Foundation, and to seek governmental acceptance of a differential fee for a neurological consultation, the Australian Association of Neurologists in 1971 suspended Article 45 of the Constitution. This made it possible for the then President, John Game, to serve an additional two-year term in office, which permitted him to progress the negotiations in which he was already heavily involved. At the same time provision was made for an additional member to be added to the Council, or, if the Honorary Secretary and Honorary Treasurer happened to be the one person, for two extra members to be added. It was specified that no Associate, Honorary or Provisional Member could be elected to the Council, though an Honorary Member Emeritus could be.

During the latter part of John Game's eight-year term as President, a detailed general revision of the Association's Constitution was carried out. This culminated in 1976 in a series of Constitutional changes which specified that a Council Member could serve no more than two consecutive three-year terms in that office, that after an initial three-year term the President could be re-elected annually for up to a maximum of a further three consecutive years, so long as he or she had not already spent a total time on Council in excess of nine consecutive years. Honorary Secretaries or Honorary Treasurers could occupy these offices for up to six consecutive years. Provision was made for the position of an Honorary Assistant Secretary who would attend Council meetings but not have voting rights there. There would also be an Executive of the Council comprising the President, Honorary Secretary and Honorary Treasurer. In the same revision it was specified that non-medically qualified persons could become Associate Members, and that the Australian Association of Neurologists' Constitution could not be modified without the approval of an Ordinary General Meeting of the Association.

In 1975 the Constitution was again altered to create a new membership category of Affiliate-in-Training, intended to accommodate medical practitioners, generally ones possessing an appropriate postgraduate level of qualification, who were undergoing training as neurologists.

In the following year Provisional Members were accorded voting rights at Ordinary General Meetings of the Association, and also the right to nominate Association members for positions on the Council. In 1977 Associate Membership was made open to consultant physicians who had an interest in neurology but were not practising on a full-time basis in that specialty.

After this, there were no changes in the Constitution for almost a decade. The possibility of incorporating the Australian Association of Neurologists as a company limited by guarantee was raised in 1977, as it offered certain advantages. The necessary Constitutional changes were put in place a year later. At the same time a new category of Retired Member was created, and the quorum for an Ordinary General Meeting of the Association was set at 30 members instead of 30% of the membership. The term in office for the Honorary Treasurer and Honorary Secretary was set at three years, following which they could serve one further three-year term if re-elected.

In 1991 a new category of Overseas Membership was created for neurologists living overseas who wished to have a relationship with the Association. It was determined that such Overseas Membership would terminate if the holder commenced residence in Australia. The annual subscription to the Association for Overseas Members was to be the same as that for Ordinary Members of the Association who resided overseas. Five years later, in 1996, the Constitution was altered again, to allow for creation of the position of President-elect of the Association. This appointment was to be made in the penultimate year of the term of office of the current President, to ensure a smooth transition to the next Presidency. Categories of Corresponding Member and Corresponding Affiliate Member were created in 1997, the latter category to take in overseas graduates who were undertaking neurological training in Australia but who intended to return to practise neurology in their home countries on completion of their training.

Subsequently, the Constitution was revised to convert its language to a gender-neutral form. The category of Provisional Member was extinguished, with those who would previously have been appointed to that category becoming entitled to Ordinary Membership of the Association immediately they were considered qualified to practise as neurologists. The last conversions from Provisional to Ordinary Membership occurred in 2000. Ordinary Membership itself became known as Full Membership of the Association from 2003 on. A category of Junior Affiliate was created to accommodate younger persons interested in neurology, but who were not undergoing neurological training at the time. They were not accorded voting rights at Association meetings.

In late 2005, the Council of the Australian Association received an approach from the corresponding New Zealand Association (founded in 1955) suggesting a merger of the two bodies. In general, this largely formalised an existing *de facto* situation, for a number of New Zealand neurologists in their individual capacities were already members of the Australian Association. Some details had to be organised, but apparently these were dealt with swiftly and satisfactorily, for by July 2006 the Australian and New Zealand Association of Neurologists (ANZAN) was in formal existence. The ANZAN Council's membership was enlarged to ensure it always contained at least one Member from New Zealand.

As one looks at the Constitutional changes made between when the Australian Association's inauguration and ANZAN's coming into being, it can be seen that their effect was to broaden the range of persons with neurological or neuroscience interests who could become members of the Association , and to include trainees in neurology within its embrace.

Nevertheless, the alterations still preserved the ability of dedicated clinical neurologists to have the major influence within the Association. Consequently, the Association remained the voice of, and the meeting point for, Australian clinical neurology. The Association would continue to serve as a *de facto* register of Australian clinical neurologists – one which could rapidly assume a *de jure* status if such a register became necessary at some future time. Any other changes made in the Constitution were to facilitate the Association's workings and to enhance its security and stability.

In 2019, a decision was taken to create a Fellowship of the Association, available to persons of good standing who had been Full Members for at least 7 years. The category was to be recognised by use of the post-nominal FANZAN, though at the time of writing it is unclear whether this will be accepted as a registerable medical qualification in Australia or New Zealand. Creation of this category seems akin to the long-standing practice whereby Membership of overseas Royal Colleges of Physicians may in appropriate instances be converted into Fellowship, a practice that was also followed by the Royal Australasian College of Physicians prior to 1970.

Membership Growth

Over the period of almost 75 years since the Australian Association of Neurologists was founded, its membership had grown from the 8 Originating Members, who could be regarded as equivalent to present-day Full Members, to, in 1999, a total of 323 Ordinary Members, 57 Provisional Members, 69 Associate Members, 28 Honorary Members, 3 Honorary Members Emeritus, 29 Affiliates-in-Training and several Overseas Members and Corresponding Members. The subsequent growth in the Association's membership has resulted in there being, at the time of writing of this edition, 677 Full Members (equivalent to the former Ordinary plus Provisional Members), some 45 of them in New Zealand, 22 Associate Members, 198 Members-in-Training, 32 Honorary Members (4 of them Emeritus) and 94 Retired Members (Figure 2). An additional 22 Full Members were based overseas. Over the years of the Association's existence, a number of those in various categories of Membership have left the Association, mainly by reason of death, but sometimes resignation. Therefore, the total number of persons who have held membership of the Association is rather greater than the total of the contemporary existing membership. Although in 1964 the Ordinary General Meeting of the Association had rejected a proposal to include mention of New Zealand in the Association's name, as mentioned above individual New Zealand neurologists had been elected to its Ordinary or Provisional Membership of the Australian Association over the years before ANZAN came into formal being.

The main interest in these membership statistics probably lies in the growth of the numbers of Ordinary and Provisional Members, and subsequently Full Members, with the passage of time. These two classes of member, plus the occasional Honorary Member Emeritus who continued in practice, provide a reasonable measure of the total Australian neurological consultant workforce at a given time. The growth since 1950 in the numbers of Australian-based Full (and previously equivalent) Members, and other main classes of Members, is plotted against time in Figure 2. Figure 3 shows the growth in numbers of Full (or equivalent) Members on a state-by-state basis, for the major Australian States, the numbers in that Figure reflecting neurologist numbers per million head of population. While the numbers expressed on this basis have grown with time, it is noticeable that, in the past two decades, the growth in New South Wales has tended to slow, and that in Victoria to accelerate. This may correlate with the activity of neurological research that occurred in Sydney in the 1970 to 1990 period, and the subsequent acceleration in Melbourne neurological research. Keen neurological trainees have tended to move to research-active training centres, and then made their careers there. The consistently fewer neurologists per head of population in Queensland over the past quarter of a century is noticeable.

Office-bearers

Following the six-year terms of each of the first two Presidents, Leonard Cox and E Graeme Robertson, the eight-year term of John Game, and the subsequent four-year term of George Selby (cut short by health considerations), it became the norm for the President of the Association to remain in office for a single term of three years' duration. Simply as a matter of convenience, the Honorary Secretary was always based in the same city as the President, since this expedited the day-to-day management of the Association. The terms of office of the Honorary Secretaries tended to coincide with those of the Presidents. In contrast, it proved quite practicable for the Honorary Treasurers to work in different cities from those where the President and the Honorary Secretary resided. No disadvantage seemed to follow from the Treasurer's term of office not coinciding with that of the other two members of the Council's Executive.

The Association's Council adopted the practice of meeting just before each annual Ordinary General Meeting of the Association, and over many years also meeting at one or two reasonably evenly spaced intervals during the intervening months. In recent years, the Council has found it desirable to meet four times a year. For a time in the early 1970s, an Honorary Assistant Secretary attended Council Meetings and undertook the responsibility for compiling the Council's Minutes and those of the Ordinary General Meetings. After a few years the position was allowed to lapse when the Association's Secretary became available to record the Minutes of the Meeting.

In 2003, the size of the Association's Council was increased. It had been virtually unchanged from the time of the Association's inception more than half a century before, and over the intervening years the size of the Association's membership had increased manyfold. The Council's expanded size was set at a maximum of 7 persons plus the Executive, with Chairpersons of certain Council Committees also attending Council Meetings. After the Association became an Australian and New Zealand one, the Council's size increased further to ensure that at least one Council Member's position was occupied by a New Zealander, even if someone from that country was also a member of the Council's Executive.

The names of the members of the Association's Councils over the years of the Association's existence (Presidents, Presidents-elect, Honorary Secretaries, Honorary Treasurers, and other Council Members) are set out in Appendix VI. The names of the Presidents of the Association, and the dates of their terms of office, are shown in the table opposite. Photographs of the Presidents of the Association whose photographs do not appear elsewhere appear on the pages following Table 1.

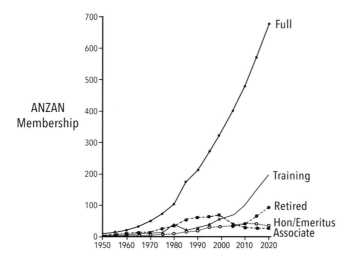

Figure 2. Growth in numbers of Australian members in the current various classes of ANZAN membership.

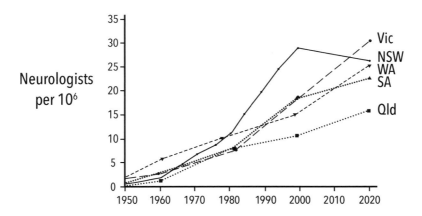

Figure 3. Growth in neurologist numbers per million head of population in each Australian State since 1950.

Table 1

Presidents of the Australian / Australian and New Zealand Association of Neurologists

Year	President
1950–1957	Leonard Cox
1957–1965	Graeme Robertson
1965–1974	John Game
1974–1978	George Selby
1978–1981	James Lance
1981–1984	James McLeod
1985–1987	Bernard Gilligan
1987–1990	Peter Rice
1990–1993	John King
1993–1996	John Morris
1996–1998	Richard Burns
1998–2001	William Carroll
2001–2003	Geoffrey Donnan
2003–2007	David Burke
2007–2010	Stephen Davis
2011–2013	Richard Frith
2014–2016	Richard Macdonnell
2017–2019	Michael Kiernan
2020–2022	Pamela McCombe
2023–	Alan Barber

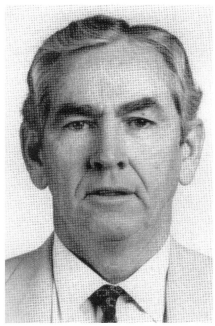

Peter Rice

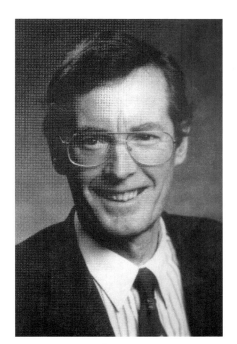

John King

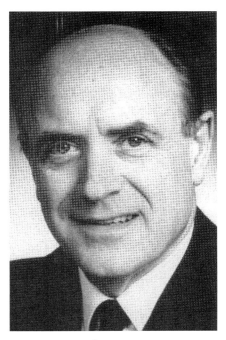

John Morris

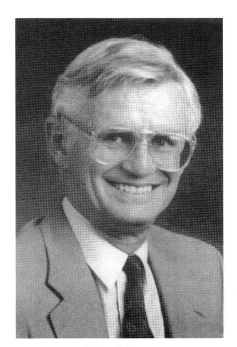

Richard Burns

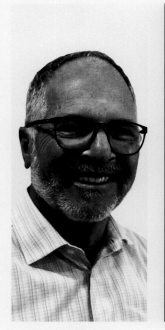

Richard Frith

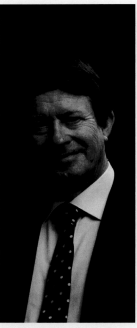

Richard Macdonnell

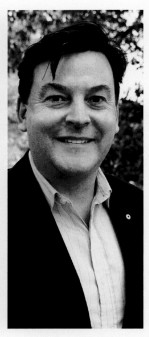

Matthew Kiernan

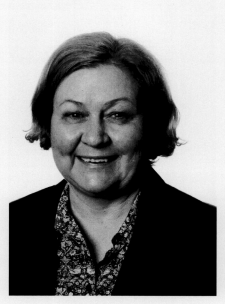

Pamela McCombe

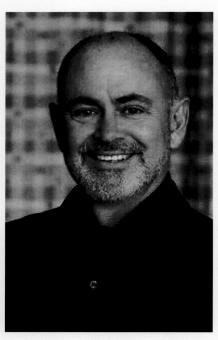

Alan Barber

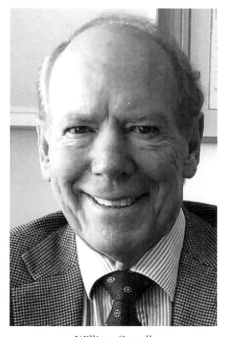

William Carroll

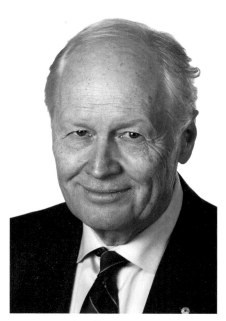

Geoffrey Donnan

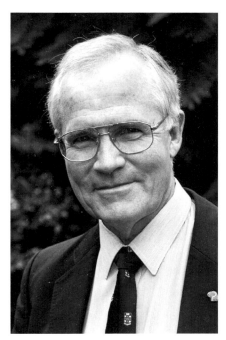

David Burke

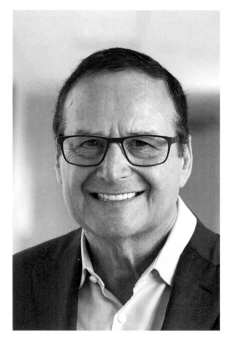

Stephen Davis

The Secretariat

The first three Presidents of the Australian Association of Neurologists, whose combined term of office spanned some twenty years, lived and worked in Melbourne. Initially, the President and the Honorary Secretary provided the secretarial support for the Association from their own consultant practices. However, in the latter part of Graeme Robertson's term of office, and throughout that of John Game, a part-time secretary was employed by the Association and worked in an office in the building of the Royal Australasian Colleges of Surgeons in Spring Street, Melbourne. When the Presidency move to Sydney in 1974, a part-time secretary was employed and based in the then President's consulting rooms at the North Shore Medical Centre. Thereafter a pattern of shifting Presidents and shifting part-time secretariats every few years began, with its inevitable inefficiencies and discontinuities, and went on for some years. Where possible, accommodation was found for the part-time secretary in the institution at which the President held his institutional appointment. By the mid-1990s the Australian Association of Neurologists had grown too large, and its activities too complex, for such essentially makeshift arrangements to continue to be practicable. In 1997 it became possible for the Association to obtain space in the Royal Australasian College of Physicians building in Macquarie Street, Sydney as a permanent base for the secretariat. A continuing rather more senior part-time secretary was employed to work there, almost in the role of an executive officer. Additional part-time secretarial help was provided in the home city of the President and Honorary Secretary. Thus by the latter half of the 1990s the Association had achieved a situation in which it at last possessed a stable and continuing secretariat, and a home for it. For some years, until 2001, Ms Alice Boyce was the Association's Sydney-based Secretary. On her resignation, she was replaced by Mrs Mandy Jones who, now designated Executive Director, and with an expanded office staff, has continued to serve the Association's needs with very considerable efficiency.

Financial Matters

The Australian Association of Neurologists began its financial existence in 1950 with an anonymous donation of £5.0.0 and a decision to set the annual subscription for each Ordinary and Associate Member at £1.1.0 (it was still a time when professional fees were expressed in terms of guineas). Almost half a century later, the Association had accumulated assets of $285,652, and had an annual subscription rate of $320 for each Ordinary Member, $ 270 for each Provisional and Associate Member and $210 for each Affiliate-in-Training. By 2020 the Association's total assets were recorded in its Treasurer's report as $ 3,550,090, while the annual subscription for a Full Member had risen to $677 (Figure 4). It should be appreciated that the subscription rates for a number of years included the cost of each member receiving the six issues each year of the *Journal of Clinical Neuroscience* (at a value of $208 per annum in 1999). No adjustment of values for the effects of inflation has been included in the *Journal's* pre-2020 subscription rates, but £1.10 in 1950 would have been more or less equivalent in value to $ 62.00 in 2020.

Details of the changes in the inflation-adjusted annual subscription rates for Full Members, converted into 2020 Australian dollars, over the years of the Association's existence, are shown in Figure 4. It will be noted that, after the early years when the Association was finding its way and some costs were probably absorbed into the expenses of the private practices of members of the Executive of the Association Council, the value of the annual subscription for Full Members was reasonably stable over a third of a century, but has subsequently risen, probably reflecting the Association's growing role in neurological education and in professional medico-political negotiation and associated activity.

The Association's finances did not progress smoothly to their apparently satisfactory situation at the close of the 20th century, and thereafter. In the 1960s and early 1970s the financial state of the Association was sometimes rather precarious, mainly because of the cost of producing the annual volume which recorded the proceedings of its Scientific Meetings. The history of that publication and of its financing will be dealt with shortly. Once a mechanism was finally organised to relieve the Australian Association of Neurologists from having to provide full financial support for its publication, and when after 1973 a registration fee was charged for attendance at the Association's annual Scientific Meetings, the Association's financial surplus began to grow, particularly as the Annual Scientific Meetings nearly always proved profitable. During the period of high interest rates in Australia in the latter part of the 1980s, the Association's financial reserves were able to accumulate fairly rapidly. After that time the Association conducted its various operations so that they continued to produce a substantial profit each year. As well, at a time in the early 1980s when the annual subscription was raised, there was an unanticipated fall in the cost of producing the Association's publication over a few years, and this boosted the assets of the Association.

Considered overall, and if allowance is made for the effects of the costs of the Association's publications, the data suggest continuing responsible and prudent financial management of the Association in the hands of the various Honorary Treasurers, and also relatively inexpensive day-to-day operation of the Association's secretariat.

The Insigne of the Association

At the 1961 meeting of the Council of the Australian Association of Neurologists there was discussion concerning some form of insigne for the Association. At the next Annual General Meeting the possibility was raised of an insigne comprising a picture of the head of John Hughlings Jackson ringed by a representation of the circle of Willis, but the matter was left in the hands of the President to progress further. In the following year, Graeme Robertson returned to Council with the concept of using an illustration of a waratah (that reproduced as the frontispiece of the present book) as the insigne. This illustration had been published in 1793. It was based on a specimen sent to London by John White, the first Surgeon-General to the newly founded colony at Sydney Cove. It could be regarded as an Australian parallel to the emblem (a rose, a thistle, a daffodil and a shamrock) of the National Hospital for Nervous Diseases at Queen Square in London, the institution to which Australian neurology has had such a close and continuing relationship. Moreover, this particular illustration of the waratah had a historical association with some of the earliest medical activities in Australia.

Graeme Robertson's suggestion was accepted by the Council and by the Annual General Meeting of the Association, and the insigne has been used by the Association since that time, and subsequently registered.

The E Graeme Robertson Book Collection

Near the end of his life, the second President of the Association, E Graeme Robertson, presented his collection of neurology books to the Australian Association of Neurologists. At the time of the bequest, the Association possessed no property where the collection could be kept on

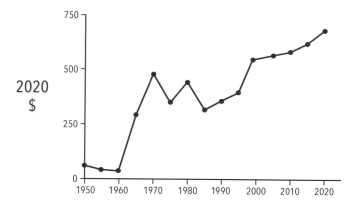

Figure 4. Annual subscription rates, converted to 2020 Australian dollars, for ANZAN full members (or equivalent) between 1950 and the present time

a long-term basis. In 1974, Professor J H Tyrer offered to accommodate it in the Department of Medicine of the University of Queensland. There it remained until 2009, when arrangements were put into place for it to be accommodated in a special bookcase in the Library of the Royal Australasian College of Physicians, in Sydney. The collection comprises a considerable number of texts from the classical era of clinical neurology in the latter part of the 19th century, and some more recent works. It would probably be fair to say that the material in the collection would be of interest to neurologists, and would be of modest monetary value, but it contains no really old or very rare and valuable works.

SCIENTIFIC AND EDUCATIONAL ACTIVITIES

The Research and Education Foundation

By the time the Association was celebrating a half-century of existence, and its financial situation was reasonably secure, the idea of setting up an Education and Research Foundation began to be mentioned in the Council Minutes. The gestation period proved to be a rather long one, probably largely explained by issues with regards to tax deductibility. It seems that these issues were finally bypassed by some sort of conjoint arrangement with the Royal Australasian College of Physicians so that, by 2007, the Association in conjunction with the College of Physicians was supporting various educational initiatives. Later, aided by profits from the 2005 World

Congress of Neurology held in Sydney, the Foundation moved to set up research funding for the support of two National Health and Medical Research Council scholarships annually, one devoted to dementia-related investigations, each potentially to be held for three years. These scholarships were first advertised in 2014 and began to be occupied in the following year and have continued to be available since.

Scientific Meetings

The annual scientific meetings have been the main focus of the Association of Neurologists' scientific activities. These meetings have been rotated around the Australian State capital cities and the national capital, and the larger New Zealand cities. Occasional meetings have been held outside Australasia (Singapore, Hong Kong, Vancouver) and in later years sometimes in easily accessible resort sites within Australia which possessed suitable conference facilities (e.g. Broome, Alice Springs). Some of the earlier meetings were held in conjunction with those of other scientific bodies e.g. the Royal Australasian College of Physicians and the Neurosurgical Society of Australasia, whilst the Association's meeting for 1967 was replaced by the Second Asian and Oceanian Congress of Neurology held in Melbourne. The World Congress of Neurology, organised in conjunction with the Australian and New Zealand Association of Neurologists, took place in Sydney in November 2005, with some 5200 delegates registered. There was another meeting in conjunction with the Asian and Oceanian Congress of Neurology that was held in Melbourne in 2012.

As the membership of the Australian Association of Neurologists grew and increasing amounts of material for presentation at its meetings became available from within its own membership, the scientific meetings more and more came to involve the Association alone, and not in conjunction with other professional bodies. As well, the meetings became longer, because of the amount of material offered and because special interest groups within the Association began to meet immediately before or after the meeting of the whole Association. The sites where the Annual Scientific Meetings have been held are listed in Appendix VII.

The scientific meetings at first were one-day affairs, with a presentation scheduled each half hour. As time passed, and the numbers of papers on offer increased, spoken presentations were shortened to 20 minutes each (including 5 minutes for discussion), and in 1979 to 15 minutes each (the time again including 5 minutes for discussion). An increasing proportion of the scientific material on offer came to be presented in the form of posters, with the main thrust of the scientific content of these posters being delivered to the audience in a series of two-minute spoken presentations in particular designated sessions during the course of the Scientific Meeting. Moreover, increasing proportions of the 15-minute presentations were given not to the meeting audience as a whole but in one or other of two (or later more) concurrent sessions. In these concurrent sessions, as far as feasible, papers on related tropics were brought together in the same individual session. The necessity for such concurrent sessions had been recognised by 1986. A little earlier, poster presentations had been introduced to permit more research to be reported to the meetings. Despite these devices permitting a greater amount of scientific material to be accommodated within the program of the meetings, the durations of the meetings themselves had to be increased from one day to one and a half days by 1960, to two days by1962, then to three days and finally, by 1997, to four days. The realities and logistics of clinical neurological practice in Australia made further prolongation of the meetings impracticable. Even as early as 1970, it sometimes proved necessary to reject papers that were offered, simply because of lack of time to permit their presentation.

As time passed, the contents of the Annual Scientific Meetings ceased to involve predominantly reports of original observations and experimental studies on neurological topics. Sessions of a more didactic nature on recent progress in areas of basic or applied neuroscience were commissioned by those arranging the program of the Annual Scientific Meetings. As well, from 1980, guest lecturers from overseas or from within Australia were invited to present formal lectures on topics relating to their areas of expertise. Once it was inaugurated in 1978, the E Graeme Robertson Memorial Lecture became a focal point of the meeting program and, in time, other named lectures were added to the programs (see below).

The topics of the papers presented at the various Annual Scientific Meetings of the Association in its earlier days provide some indication of the types of case material that passed through the hands of Australian neurologists over the course of almost three-quarters of a century, and of the scientific matters that proved of interest to them. A complete listing of the titles of all the papers and posters presented at the meetings would now be too extensive to include in this book. However, for interest, the titles of the papers presented at the first 12 Annual Scientific Meetings, when the program was much shorter than it later became, are listed in Appendix II. After the 12th meeting it was possible for papers presented at the Annual Scientific Meetings of the Association to be published in the *Proceedings of the Australian Association of Neurologists,* and later in its successor *Clinical and Experimental Neurology,* and many such papers were included in the volumes. The contents of the various issues of those earlier publications are set down in Appendix VIII. They provide a record, though an incomplete one, of the material presented to Annual Scientific Meetings of the Association in earlier times. The contents of the various volumes have now become available on the ANZAN website, but it may be convenient for prospective readers to have available the listing of paper titles to locate articles of interest.

The Annual Scientific Meetings of the Association have served a number of purposes which collectively have advanced the practice of neurology in Australia. They have provided the mechanism and the stimulus for Australian neurologists once a year to discuss their problems, compare their experiences, express their views on various matters of concern to them, and to plan together for the future. They have exposed Australian neurologists to educational opportunities relevant to their professional activities, made them aware of neurological research going on in the country and overseas at an early stage, and given them a forum at which they could describe and discuss their own original work and afford their younger colleagues an initiation into the techniques of presenting research material to an audience.

The E Graeme Robertson Memorial and Other Named Lectures

In 1976, following the death of the second President of the Association, Edward Graeme Robertson, the Council of the Australian Association of Neurologists determined to fund an invited annual lecture in honour of his memory at each Annual Scientific Meeting of the Association. The first E Graeme Robertson Lecture was given in Hobart in 1978. There was a lecture given in each subsequent year with the exception of 1998 when circumstances prevented the lecturer from doing so, and in 2020, when no meeting was held because of the Covid outbreak. The contents of many, but not all, of the earlier such lectures appeared in the pages of *Proceedings of the Australian Association of Neurologists* or those of the publications which have succeeded it. The names of the Graeme Robertson Lecturers, and the titles of their lectures, are shown in Appendix IX. The annual Graeme Robertson Lecturer is now intended to be a member of ANZAN who has made both a substantial contribution to the Association and to Australasian neurology and neuroscience. In earlier times, the lecturers sometimes were overseas neurologists invited to the Australian Association's Annual Scientific Meetings, with the initial lecture being given by Graeme Robertson's cousin, the Melbourne neurosurgeon Mr Reginald Hooper.

Subsequently, the Australian Association created an annual Mervyn Eadie Lecture (beginning in 2001) and, after the Association became the Australian and New Zealand one, the Ian McDonald Lecture (beginning in 2009). These lectures were to be delivered, respectively, in recognition of the recipient's career achievements and international recognition of excellence in neuroscience research, and by distinguished neurologists, particularly in the field of multiple sclerosis. In 2019, a James Lance Oration was created. The names of those who delivered the above-named lectures/orations, and their lecture/oration titles, are also set down in Appendix X.

The name of Leonard Cox was earlier perpetuated in an annual award and, beginning in 2009, in the L J Cox Lecture given in recognition of the quality of the scientific work of an early career stage neurologist within 10 years of obtaining Fellowship of the Royal Australasian College of Physicians.

In 2010 an annual ANZAN Medal was first awarded, acknowledging services to Australasian neurology (Appendix XI).

There also are a Jim McLeod Award for an Advanced Trainee in Neurology whose work is presented at each Annual Scientific Meeting of the Association, and a Jim Lance Award for work done for a Higher Degree and presented at an Annual Scientific Meeting of the Association.

THE PUBLICATIONS OF THE ASSOCIATION

The Journals

As already mentioned (Chapter 4), within a few years of the foundation of the Australian Association of Neurologists, the Minutes of its Council and of its Ordinary General Meetings began to mention the possibility of preserving the contents of the presentations given at its Annual Scientific Meetings. The first venue considered for their publication (in 1954) was the Royal Australasian College of Physicians' journal, the then *Australasian Annals of Medicine*. Later (1960) the possibility of having a stenographer record the presentations as they were delivered was mentioned. There was also some speculation about the possibility of founding a local neurology journal. Such ideas seem to have smouldered on for a few years. Then the decision was taken to publish the papers given at the Association's Scientific Meetings in the form of an annual volume to be called *The Proceedings of the Australian Association of Neurologists,* under the editorship of E Graeme Robertson. The first volume appeared a year later, in 1963. It comprised the papers from the 1962 meeting, contained in a 74-page volume with a light grey cardboard cover with the title of the publication in red lettering (see next page). In the following year the cover took on the form it retained throughout the remaining 30 years of the publication's existence, white card (and after 1976 white hard cover) featuring the Association's insigne, a waratah flower (in colour), with black lettering for the title and the other details.

Almost from the outset, the publication encountered difficulties. Potential authors sometimes proved reluctant to provide their manuscripts to the Editor, or provided them only after substantial delays. The editorial work, done in Graeme Robertson's private time, and the subsequent printing delays, often meant that the *Proceedings* from one meeting had not appeared by the time of the subsequent Annual Scientific Meeting. Such delays discouraged the publication of original work in the *Proceedings.* As well, though the *Proceedings'* contents were not copyrighted, editors of overseas journals were sometimes reluctant to accept work which had appeared in the *Proceedings,* or which was in press in it. Even though a paper had been accepted by the *Proceedings* earlier than by an overseas journal, if it first appeared in the public domain in a copyrighted overseas journal there were potential legal problems when it later appeared in the *Proceedings.* Such matters always remained potential rather than actual issues, but they tended to deter prospective authors from having their work appear in the *Proceedings* if they thought it might be accepted by an overseas journal with a higher profile and wider readership. Nevertheless, at least some researchers were still prepared to present the material at the Association's Annual Scientific Meetings. For a time, attempts were made to prevent presentation of material at Annual Scientific Meetings unless it was guaranteed by the presenter that the material would be submitted to the *Proceedings,* and at one stage the Association's Council determined that this would become the Association's policy. Unfortunately, it was never practicable to implement

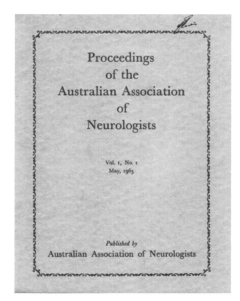
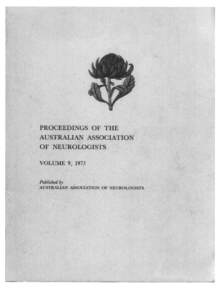

Proceedings of the Australian Association of Neurologists. Front covers of Volumes 1 & 9.

that policy without denying the audience at Annual Scientific Meetings the opportunity to hear about the best recent neurological research occurring in the country. Inevitably, the problems in publishing such material militated against the success and wider dissemination of the *Proceedings*. In addition, the unavailability of the best Australian neurological research in its pages, and the comparatively limited circulation of the publication, denied the *Proceedings* the opportunity to publish the very work which might have allowed it to be more successful.

After almost a decade in the editorial role Graeme Robertson resigned from his office, to be replaced in 1974 by Professor John Tyrer, of Brisbane, with MJ Eadie becoming Assistant Editor a year later.

In the mid-1970s the *Proceedings* faced problems resulting from several factors, viz. increasing annual printing costs, termination of the Commonwealth book bounty that had previously helped finance publication costs, a failure to find a cheaper source of printing, the impracticality of scaling back the length of individual publications too radically and thus reducing the size of each volume, and the possible reduction in the drug companies' contributions to the cost of the printing at a time of growing inflation. At that time, it seemed that the *Proceedings* faced progressive financial strangulation.

However, by 1977 the then President of the Association, George Selby, was able to inform the Ordinary General Meeting of the Association that Adis Press, of Sydney, had agreed to undertake responsibility for the publication of the *Proceedings,* and for its distribution. Adis were willing to promote the publication internationally. Copies for Australian Association of Neurologists' members were to be provided from their annual subscription to the Association. However, Adis Press considered that the title of *Proceedings of the Australian Association of Neurologists* was too limiting to encourage a wider readership. In response to this, the publication's title was changed to that of *Clinical and Experimental Neurology.*

For several years the arrangement with Adis Press, and later with its successors Williams and Wilkins-Adis and then MacLennan and Petty, appeared to work well, though the anticipated growth in circulation did not occur. The publication of each issue became slower as the publishers seemingly lost interest in the volume as their attempts to enhance its circulation faltered and failed. It became increasingly, indeed embarrassingly, apparent that the growing mass of academic neurological research in Australia was not being offered for publication in the volume.

John Tyrer resigned his editorship in 1984, while Eadie took on that role with C M Lander, later joined by M P Pender, as the Assistant Editors. The publication arrangement with MacLennan and Petty was terminated in 1990. After that time, the Australian Association of Neurologists reverted to its earlier role of publisher. The printing was carried out by the University of Queensland for the next two years. For the 1993 and 1994 volumes, the entire material was prepared by desk-top publishing within the Department of Medicine of the University of Queensland, with the final printing being done by Merino Lithographics in Brisbane. These changes considerably reduced costs for the Association, but nothing redressed the declining proportion of papers presented to Annual Scientific Meetings of the Association that was offered for publication in its journal. Some years earlier, in 1969, the Association's Council had authorised the Editor to accept papers dealing with neurological topics which had not been presented to Annual Scientific Meetings of the Association. This policy change led to the submission of some such papers, often from Asian countries, but publishing these involved an increased effort in organising refereeing and often considerable editorial correction. Unfortunately, no papers of outstanding scientific merit became available as a result of the process. The issue of refereeing papers submitted to the journal had arisen at a much earlier stage, when the Australian National Health and Medical Research Council, the main source of medical research funding in the country, decreed that it would not take into account publications in non-refereed journals when determining the research track record of applicants for its grants. In relation to the available facilities, it would not have been logistically possible to send out for formal refereeing all the papers which would have been submitted to the journal in a single batch over a period of a few weeks in each year following the Annual Scientific Meeting of the Association. To have then engaged in further correspondence with authors about referees' criticisms, would have further delayed the already almost unacceptably slow production process of the journal. Rather than adopting such a practice, it was argued that the discussion occurring after the presentation of papers at the Annual Scientific Meetings of the Association provided a form of refereeing. Formal refereeing by outside advisers was organised only for papers about which reservations were expressed at the time of their discussion, when doubts arose after the papers were subsequently read by the Editor, or when papers which had never been presented at Annual Scientific Meetings of the Association were on offer. In 1980 the National Health and Medical Research Council accepted that appearance of a paper in the Australian Association of Neurologists' journal was to be considered an instance of publication in a refereed journal.

At intervals over the years, at meetings of the Association, the possibility of an Australian neurological journal, not merely the publication of the contents of the Association's Scientific Meetings, continued to be mentioned. In 1987 and again in 1988, at the Ordinary General Meetings the matter was discussed at some length. By this time the shortcomings of *Clinical and Experimental Neurology* and its inability to meet the growing scientific aspirations of an increasingly academic and research orientated body had become obvious. However, at that stage the majority of members present felt the time was not ripe, nor were the mechanisms available, for *Clinical and Experimental Neurology* to become a journal which would appear at regular intervals throughout the year.

In 1994 the situation changed. After making the Australian Association of Neurologists aware of its initiative, the Neurosurgical Society of Australasia launched the quarterly *Journal of Clinical Neuroscience,* with Professor Andrew

Kaye of Melbourne as its editor, and with its publisher the old Edinburgh firm of Churchill-Livingstone. The Australian Association of Neurologists was invited to make this new journal its own official publication. Realising that *Clinical and Experimental Neurology* was withering away, the Association accepted the opportunity. It was decided that the existence of *Clinical and Experimental Neurology* would terminate after 31 years of production, with the appearance of the 1994 volume. Eadie became the Co-Editor of the *Journal of Clinical Neuroscience* in 1995, and neurologists joined its editorial board. The *Journal of Clinical Neuroscience* subsequently expanded in bulk, grew to six issues per year, and finally to eight, and increased substantially in cost to subscribers. Unfortunately, there was no major increase in the number of papers from Australian neurologists which were offered to it, and the journal's contents increasingly became dominated by papers from overseas sources and material of predominantly surgical interest.

Eadie remained as Co-Editor until 2000, being succeeded in the role by Stephen Davis (till 2006), then Elsdon Storey (till 2012), and finally by Richard Gerraty, who continued until 2015 when the publisher, by then Elsevier, imposed a new Editor and shifted the editorial facilities overseas. Following this, the Australian and New Zealand Association ceased to regard the publication as its journal.

After a period of negotiation, the Association in 2019 adopted a new open-access journal, the *British Medical Journal's Neurology Open,* as its publication, with Gerraty resuming the editorship. It is rather early to know how successful this particular endeavour will prove, occurring at a time when new open-access medical journals are appearing with considerable rapidity, and some are almost pleading for papers to be submitted to them, and with the financial costs being borne by the authors of accepted papers.

Financial Aspects of the Journals

The *Proceedings of the Australian Association of Neurologists* encountered financial problems from its beginning. Some of these have already been alluded to in relation to the financial affairs of the Australian Association of Neurologists. Some have been touched on immediately above in relation to the history of the Association's journals. The costs of printing each annual volume could not be anticipated, and at times came to imperil the solvency of the Association in the late 1960s and early 1970s. In some of the early years of the *Proceedings'* existence, its cost per member exceeded that member's annual subscription to the Association. For several years in earlier times, the Australian Association of Neurologists' finances were extricated from embarrassment only by virtue of grants to support publication of the *Proceedings* which were received from the three major Swiss drug companies of the time, and by the receipt of the book bounty that the Commonwealth Government of the day provided over a number of years to encourage the printing of books in Australia. As well, on at least one occasion, an injection of funds from the Van Cleef Foundation was needed to rescue the Association financially. However, receiving the book bounty precluded having the printing of the *Proceedings* done more cheaply but outside Australia. In the late 1960s the cost of the *Proceedings* drove up the annual membership subscription. In the later 1970s, another financial crisis for the Association was impending before the arrangement with Adis Press referred to above came into operation. This relieved the situation for a time, but Adis clearly overestimated their prospects of generating income from selling *Clinical and Experimental Neurology* outside the membership of the Australian Association of Neurologists. When this became apparent to their successor, it resulted in rapidly mounting costs to the Association in the later 1980s. As already mentioned, the Association then reduced its costs by reverting to the role of publisher and using a University-based printing mechanism, and later by making use of desk-top publishing and a commercial printing firm for the final stages of production. With the advent of the *Journal of Clinical Neuroscience* the Association finally reached a position in which it knew in advance the likely annual costs of the publication, and could adjust its annual subscription accordingly, making its whole financial operation more predictable. That situation continued while the journal remained the official publication of the Australian and New Zealand Association of Neurologists.

Other Association Publications

In 1994 John Morris, during his term as President of the Australian Association of Neurologists, brought out two small books under the aegis of the Association. One was *A Directory of Neurology in Australia*. It comprised a systematic listing of the various neurological units in institutions around the country, with details of their staffing, special interests and expertise and included an outline of their histories and philosophies. The second book,

Neurology in Australia, comprised a collection of previously published and specially written accounts of events and persons significant in the development of Australian neurology. Overall, it provided a reasonably wide-ranging though not totally systematic brief account of the history of neurology in the country.

The Significance of the Association's Journals

As an outcome of a seemingly fortuitous though happy circumstance, and in the face of mounting evidence of failure, by the end of the 20th century *The Proceedings of the Australian Association of Neurologists* and its successor *Clinical and Experimental Neurology* had arrived at the main final purpose for which they had been intended. They were transmuted into an Australian-based neurological journal which had the potential to be commercially viable. Nonetheless, it can hardly be denied that the two earlier publications of the Australian Association of Neurologists fell short of achieving most of their more immediately intended purposes. Despite the editorial efforts, they never published the complete array of papers presented to any Annual Scientific Meeting of the Australian Association of Neurologists. They never became increasingly used by Australian neurologists as the venue for publication of their research. Rather, the reverse was the case. As Australian neurological research became increasingly competitive internationally, researchers ensured that their work was published overseas and not locally. The Association's journal was forced into an inconsistent policy about the acceptance of papers from authors outside the Association's membership. As well, it always needed some financial subsidy to survive.

Yet the Association's two publications should not be considered total failures, even before their unexpected final and seemingly successful transformation. They were able to appear annually over a span of 31 years. Their very existence over this period proved a source of pride for Australian neurology. No other Australian medical specialist group of similar size, and relatively few neurological associations in overseas countries, were able to boast of possessing a publication which could be found on the shelves of medical libraries in many countries throughout the world. The publications yielded another dividend which could have been apparent only to those who had attended Scientific Meetings of the Australian Association of Neurologists before, and in the first few years after, the *Proceedings* began to appear. The discipline of having to prepare papers for presentation in a form suitable for publication, and the lessons to be learned from seeing the editorial corrections of submitted text, had a salutary effect on the standard of verbal presentation of material at the Association's Scientific Meetings. Over a few years the old discursive ways and evidences of lax thinking largely gave way to crisper, clearer, more direct and better reasoned and better delivered accounts. Those who could learn the more rigorous and better structured ways of presentation prospered; those who could not ceased to offer material at the Scientific Meetings of the Association as the deficiencies in their presentations became more obvious. A standard of scientific presentation was achieved, and remains in force, which has contributed to training more than two generations of Australian neurologists in the writing of scientific papers and in the public presentation of scientific material. It may be difficult to provide documentary evidence to support that assessment, but this training and discipline, as much as pioneering the way to a new national clinical neuroscience journal, appear to have been the great contributions that *The Proceedings of the Australian Association of Neurologists* and *Clinical and Experimental Neurology* have made to the development of the specialty of clinical neurology in Australia.

THE TRAINING OF AUSTRALIAN NEUROLOGISTS

At no stage of its existence did the Australian Association of Neurologists or its successor the Australian and New Zealand Association have formal control of, or direct responsibility for, the training of prospective neurologists in the country, or for assessing their fitness to practise the specialty, although progress seems to have been made towards these possibly desirable ends. However, members of the Association were involved in both of these activities in their individual capacities as consultants in various teaching hospitals throughout the country, and on occasions by virtue of the offices they held within the mechanisms of the Royal Australasian College of Physicians. The latter was the body which, throughout the latter half of the twentieth century, and since, granted the relevant specialist diploma which opened the door to recognition as a neurologist.

Nonetheless, the Australian and New Zealand Association of Neurologists has become the acknowledged professional body which speaks for Australian neurology. Because of its carefully defined membership categories, and their qualifying criteria, the Association has become, in effect, though not de jure, a second body whose standard needed to be met before acceptance as a specialist neurologist was likely to be achieved. This is a situation unlike that which has applied for many of the other specialties of internal medicine where the relevant sub-specialty body's membership is neither so exclusive professionally, nor so tightly defined. The Association of Neurologists had been positioned, almost certainly by the foresight of its founders, so that in time it could relatively easily function as an examining body for assessing the matter of fitness to practice as a neurologist in Australia. The possibility of its taking on that role was broached within the confines of the Association as early as 1964, and continued to be raised on later occasions. This was a serious possibility when, in the period around 1968 to1970, the Royal Australasian College of Physicians revealed that it was in the process of altering its training programmes for all areas of internal medicine, converting them into a two-stage process. The first stage of the training was to be in general internal medicine and to culminate in an examination. Success in this examination would open the way to two or three years of further apprenticeship style training either in general medicine or in one of its sub-specialties. Following this, and subject to satisfactory reports being received from the training supervisors, Fellowship of the College was to be granted, permitting specialist registration to occur. There was some disagreement between the Australian Association of Neurologists and the Royal Australasian College of Physicians over certain of the details of the second stage of training. In these circumstances a degree of tension arose within the Association between those who took the broader College view of training, and those more concerned with the advancement of neurology per se. It was a partial recrudescence of what had gradually become the dwindling argument between those who expected the physician to be omni-competent in all areas of medicine, and those who believed that the growing bulk of medical knowledge had made that no longer a reasonable expectation. It was at this time that the foundation of a College of Neurologists, with its potential for becoming an examining body, was mooted (Minutes of Council 1976). In 1974, the Council had already sought legal advice about its becoming a diploma-granting body. However, over the subsequent few years the Royal Australasian College of Physicians gradually found itself increasingly in agreement with the Australian Association of

Neurologists' views about the second stage of the College Fellowship. The issue of a separate College of Neurologists faded as the current pattern of Australian neurological training gained general acceptance in 1977, and then settled into place. Nonetheless, with the increasing numerical strength of the Association of Neurologists as the years have passed, the increasing volume of neurological and basic neuroscience knowledge that must be mastered, and the tendency of neurology to become further separated from psychiatry, psychology, and areas such as speech pathology, it continued to seem likely that the issue of a College of Neurologists would be resurrected at some point in the future.

In 1977, the Australian Association of Neurologists negotiated the availability of a training position for one of its advanced trainees at the National Hospital, Queen Square, London and for an analogous position at the Mayo Clinic in the United States. From that time, these posts have continued to be occupied by Australian trainees. After 1989, a similar arrangement was entered into at the United Oxford Hospitals and, later, one at the Royal Free Hospital in London.

In 2006, a type of reciprocal arrangement was mooted between English and Australian neurology, but negotiations must have been protracted, as final agreement does not seem to have been reached until 2011, with the arrangement first being implemented in 2014 resulting in one of the initial English appointees, after his period in Sydney was completed, moving successfully into a consultant neurological appointment in Brisbane.

Within Australia, the Association has increasingly undertaken the provision of facilities for the training of clinical neurologists, and the continuing education of its full members. Many such activities have been on-going once they have proved their worth. Thus, among others, there have been, for instance, annual clinical neurophysiology and registrar training workshops and annual registrar training weekends, EEG and neuropathology courses, a regular monthly so-called 'Brain school' and various competitive intellectual activities with an underlying educational motive at Scientific meetings.

The Australian Neurological (Brain) Foundation

It could be argued that the story of the Australian Neurological Foundation is not a proper topic for discussion in relation to the affairs of the Australian and New Zealand Association of Neurologists. However, the Foundation was the brainchild of John Game and he became its first President. He conceived it, and he devoted years of his life to planning its organisation and its welfare and continued to promote its purposes until, by 1980, his health made that no longer possible. The Foundation had a long and painful gestation during John Game's years as President of the Australian Association of Neurologists. There was much negotiation with the neurosurgeons, with lawyers, and with the Taxation Department before the Foundation became a tax-exempt charity, a pre-requisite to successful fundraising in Australia. The news of the granting of that tax exemption became available during a meeting of the Australian Association of Neurologists, and the restrained and dignified satisfaction with which John Game announced it to his colleagues on that occasion, remains a pleasurable memory.

Sadly, the Foundation did not prosper to the extent that John Game had hoped. The main, though certainly not the sole original purpose of the Foundation in Game's mind, if not in the minds of the other main protagonists, was to obtain funds to set up one or more chairs of neurology in Australia. Game believed that this would do more than anything else to advance the cause of neurology in the country, and subsequent events suggested that he was right in his assessment. However, to obtain the tax exemption, it was necessary to make the Foundation's priorities those of patient care, education and research, so that the chairs had to accept a lower publicly avowed precedence. When the Foundation was inaugurated, the late Henry Miller, that formidable and ebullient Northumbrian neurologist who had, by then, become Vice-Chancellor of the University of Newcastle-upon-Tyne, despite being in fading health, travelled around the Australian State capitals attempting to make the Foundation's existence known. A selective appeal for support, rather than one directed to the wider community, was decided on, and met with some success. However, as time passed, the impetus died away and problems arose. The chief one centred on the argument that moneys raised within one State should be spent within that State and not be redistributed for national purposes. The issue came into the open in 1979. John Game had envisaged the Foundation as a national body which would have a national vision and not be dominated by more parochial concerns and influence. One can appreciate the force of the State argument, and in the end the Foundation had to be partly reconstituted to give it effect. Unfortunately, doing this added to the difficulties of the States which had less potential for fundraising. In general, in these States the Foundation, later renamed the Australian Brain Foundation to enhance its popular appeal, tended not to prosper, whereas it has been rather more successful in the more populous and wealthier States.

At one time, over a period of several years, the affairs of the Australian Neurological Foundation occupied some half of the contents of the Minutes of the Ordinary General Meetings of the Australian Association of Neurologists. However, after the Foundation was established that proportion declined and, whilst members of the Association of Neurologists may have continued to be members of the Foundation, the two bodies themselves reached a stage where they followed their own rather separate paths, though retaining some degree of contact. John Game almost inevitably was the initial President of the Foundation, and was followed in that role by Bernard Gilligan and, later, by Michael Halmagyi.

The story of the Australian Brain (Neurological) Foundation comprises a chapter in the history of the Australian Association of Neurologists. The Foundation was the product of a splendid vision. The initial high hopes which were held for it were not realised in full, but the Foundation continues to exist and, indeed, to grow, funding neurology research so that it appears to be playing something of the role that John Game envisaged for it half a century ago, though in the meanwhile his vision of Chairs in Neurology became reality through other means.

SPECIAL FOCUS GROUPS WITHIN THE ASSOCIATION

The Australian and New Zealand Association of Neurologists emerged from the membership of the Royal Australasian College of Physicians because of the perceived need for a venue and mechanism to cater for the special interests of a sufficiently sized group of practitioners who worked solely, or chiefly, within the particular area of neurological medicine, and who still wished to retain links to the parent body. In like manner, as the Australian Association of Neurologists' membership grew, special focus groupings with that body developed and have, at the time of writing, remained within the purview of the Association. The first groupings to appear (in 1980) were those of the Child Neurologists, who had grown in number to some 21 persons by 1994, and the Neuropathologists, many of whom were Associate rather than Ordinary Members of the Association of Neurologists. A number of subsequently formed special focus groups have done likewise e.g. the Women in Neurology, the Movement Disorder group and the groupings of those focused on Neurological Rehabilitation and in Electroencephalography. The memberships of these groupings are not necessarily limited to, or even dominated by, neurologists, so they are usually offshoots rather than branches of the Association of Neurologists.

At least four special focus groupings – the Epilepsy Society of Australia, the Stroke Society (both originally centred on the neurologists of the Austin Hospital in Melbourne), the Australian Headache Society (originally based on the Department of Neurology of the University of New South Wales) and the Neuro-ophthalmology group – commenced holding their meetings at separate times and at different sites to the one where the Annual Association of Neurologists met in the same year. These various arrangements seem to have worked harmoniously enough, and the Epilepsy Society and Stroke Society Meetings, both held roughly six months from the time of the Annual Australian Association of Neurologists' Meetings, in effect have provided a second opportunity for Australian neurologists to come together during each year. The Epilepsy Society has already attained sufficient size and duration of existence to warrant publication of its history, written by Frank Vajda.

As well, in more recent times, further highly focused special groups have appeared within the Association, e.g. ones for Asian-Pacific affairs, neuro-otology, neuromuscular disorders. There is also a long-standing subcommittee that deals with fitness to drive (motor vehicles), which has often been called on to advise the Commonwealth Governmental body concerned with this matter (Austroads), though the final decisions in relation to this matter seem to be made at individual State level.

At the time of writing, the proliferation of such special focus groups, and the natures of their formal and informal affiliations with the Association, are being studied by the ANZAN Council, presumably in the hope of further rationalisation and coordination.

RELATIONSHIPS WITH OUTSIDE BODIES
The Australian Medical Association

Over the years, particularly in the earlier ones of the Association's existence, there were ongoing interactions between the Australian Association of

Neurologists and the Australian Medical Association. The main issue dealt with was that of fees for the various professional activities provided by neurologists. At one stage (1973) the situation was reached at which the Australian Medical Association agreed to negotiate the listing of a fee for a neurological consultation which was 25% greater than that which it recommended for a physician's consultation. However, the Australian Medical Association fairly rapidly reversed its position on the matter (in 1974), to the considerable disappointment of at least some Australian Association of Neurologists' members. There have also been interactions between the two bodies concerning the principles of specialist recognition, and about the changed basis of the composition of the representation of special interest groupings within the Australian Medical Association's structure. As time has passed, interactions between the Australian Medical Association and the Association of Neurologists appear to have become less frequent.

The Royal Australasian College of Physicians

The major and continuing interaction between the Royal Australasian College of Physicians and the Australian and New Zealand Association of Neurologists has occurred in relation to neurological training, as discussed earlier in this chapter. Underlying the contacts and relationships between the two bodies, though to a lessening extent as the years have passed, has been the long-standing territorial tension between the claims of the self-acknowledged pluri-competent physician and those of the dedicated and focused specialised professional neurologist. Relationships between the College and the Association have become increasingly close and harmonious, particularly in relation to neurological training, as time has passed. In a way, the Association has reached a stage in its growth and membership size similar to that reached by the College of Physicians several decades ago, and this may have encouraged a degree of mutual sympathy between them, particularly in relation to the matter of splintering into sub-specialised fragments.

Australian Government

A number of sections within the Australian Commonwealth Government have approached the Australian Association of Neurologists on different occasions to seek advice and comment on various matters. This has been particularly the case in relation to the variously named Commonwealth Department responsible for Health matters. There has also been ongoing interaction over the quantum of fees for certain professional services provided solely, or predominantly, by neurologists, including the appropriate costing for certain neurophysiological investigations. The matter has tended to keep recurring in new guises as new technologies become available. The issues concerning neurologists' fees have often involved the Australian Medical Association as a third party, and on the whole usually have not led to a satisfactory outcome from the standpoint of the Australian members of the Association, when any outcome at all has emerged. Nevertheless, the fact that the Commonwealth has chosen to consult, and to listen to the Australian and New Zealand Association on such matters is some recognition of the status that Association enjoys in the medical community.

By 1970 the Australian Association of Neurologists had found it desirable to set up a Drug Advice Committee to deal with the enquiries made by Government and other instrumentalities concerning the use of therapeutic drugs in neurological disorders. This Committee remained active over a number of years whilst its brief gradually broadened to take in a wider range of matters e.g. the issue of vehicle driving and epilepsy. At one stage. the Committee was re-designated the General Advisory Committee of the Association, but later reverted to a Therapeutics Advisory title. In later years this Committee expanded its initial, largely reactive, role and began to initiate correspondence with Government bodies, in response to requests from Australian members of the Association of Neurologists, and sometimes from the Australian pharmaceutical industry. Members of the Association, in roles as individual persons and not as Association members. have also been positioned at times to be able to convey neurologists' attitudes and advice to relevant Commonwealth Governmental bodies, e.g. Eadie and Herkes to the Australian Drug Evaluation Committee, Eadie to the Pharmaceutical Benefits Advisory Committee and the Therapeutics Goods Standards Committee.

International Societies

The Australian Association of Neurologists has been affiliated with the World Federation for Neurology since the inception of the latter, and pays it a relatively nominal contribution on behalf of each Association member. The tangible dividend emanating from the linkage between the two bodies appears to have been relatively small, though an ANZAN member, William Carroll, after occupying the Vice-Presidency for some years, became President of the Federation in 2017. Richard Stark, of Melbourne, served as Treasurer of the Foundation for a time

A reasonably similar affiliation has existed in relation to the International EEG Society.

Other Australian Professional Societies

Throughout its existence, the Australian Association of Neurologists has maintained links with the Neurosurgical Society of Australasia and at least once, in earlier times, met in conjunction with that Society in Canberra. The existence of the *Journal of Clinical Neuroscience* depended on the linkage between the two societies. Once the Editorship of the journal was changed by the publisher without prior agreement, and ANZAN ceased to acknowledge it as its official publication, that aspect of the linkage lapsed.

The Australian and New Zealand Society of Neuropathologists, which began its existence as a club and became a society in 1980, was an offshoot of the Australian Association of Neurologists, as mentioned earlier. For several years, the abstracts of the Neuropathologists Society were printed in *Clinical and Experimental Neurology,* and the Society usually met in conjunction with the Australian Association of Neurologists. However, some members of Neuropathologists Society did not become members of the Australian Association of Neurologists, and the relationship between the two bodies appears to have atrophied.

There has been a long-standing relationship between the Society of EEG Technicians and the group of Australian Association of Neurologists members interested in this aspect of technology. The Australian Association of Neurologists for a time advised the EEG Technicians Society on a variety of matters of common interest, including aspects of technician training. However, as time has passed the EEG Technicians seem to have found a closer alliance with, and potentially membership in, the Epilepsy Society of Australia.

The Australian Council for Rehabilitation of the Disabled has also interacted with the Association of Neurologists over many years, though the relationship seems to have tended to be a rather distant one.

Social Activities

From the time of the foundation of the Australian Association of Neurologists, it was the custom for its Members to attend a formal dinner on one evening during each Annual Meeting. In 1969 the decision was taken to invite members' spouses to the dinner, and three years after that it became accepted that lounge suits rather than dinner jackets would be a suitable form of male attire for the occasion.

The Association also arranged for a necktie bearing its insigne to be produced in 1978. After only three such ties had been purchased by members, the entire stock was ruined by a minor flood in the rooms of the then Honorary Treasurer. There was some delay before another batch of ties could be procured. About this time, through the generosity of a pharmaceutical firm, members were provided with a set of cuff links bearing the Association's insigne. More recent male fashion has rendered these items almost historical relics.

From small beginnings, over the space of almost 75 years, guided by wise foresight and a dedicated sense of purpose, and with prudent organisational and financial management, the Australian and, later, Australian and New Zealand Association of Neurologists has grown into a very significant professional body which provides a recognised public voice for Australasian neurology. Its views are nationally based ones, and parochialism has been almost non-existent within it. The Association has reached a stage where it appears to be stable and well established professionally and in the eyes of government and outside bodies. It is positioned by virtue of its size, cohesiveness and Constitution to take on a more influential role and an enhanced formal qualification-awarding status quite quickly, if that is seen as desirable at some stage in the future.

Chapter 9

WHY and HOW?

When one considers what can be gleaned from the record of events described in the previous chapters, one obvious question that arises is why neurology in Australia developed as it did, roughly half a century after it appeared in Britain as a recognised specialist area of medical endeavour, when British medicine has always been the main source of Australian medicine. Why was there the delay? And how, over the passage of the better part of a century after its delayed beginning, did Australian neurology then manage to achieve a status of clinical practice and research largely comparable with that of the neurology of British and other Western societies?

The development of clinical neurology in Britain and Western Europe in the latter half of the 19th century seems to have been the outcome of three major circumstances. Firstly, medicine had achieved a sufficient knowledge of bodily function and disease to be able to understand and apply the knowledge of nervous system structure and function which was becoming available. Secondly, in enough places there was a sufficient accumulation of sufferers from nervous system disease, and sufficient community wealth, to permit medically trained individuals to restrict their clinical practices, and in some cases devote their research, to such disease. Thirdly, in some of these places there was a sufficient aggregation of men of some genius who were able to derive new knowledge from the study of the disorders that they were attempting to manage, and then to propagate that knowledge more widely. By the 1860s or soon afterwards, the two leading sites of such constellations of circumstances had appeared, the National Hospital for Nervous Diseases at Queen Square, London, and the Salpêtrière in Paris. In the former, John Hughlings Jackson and William Gowers and, to some extent David Ferrier, were the major figures, with Jean-Martin Charcot at the latter. But they were not alone, and London and Paris were not the only places for long, before additional sites and men devoted to neurology began to emerge. Accounts of the history of the development of British neurology sometimes give the impression that everything happened in London, and in that city at Queen Square. However, quite soon after the Queen Square Hospital opened, neurology was springing up in independent growth in some larger British provincial cities such as Manchester, with James Ross, in Edinburgh with Laycock and Byrom Bramwell, and in Glasgow with Alexander Robertson.

In the same later decades of the 19th century, the Australian situation was rather different. Those practising medicine in the country, even if Australian born, had nearly always received their medical educations in Britain or Western Europe. They therefore might be expected to have possessed a general level of medical knowledge comparable to that of their northern hemisphere counterparts. However, they may have been disadvantaged to an extent by a delay of weeks, at the most months, before new relevant information originating in the northern hemisphere became available in a group of British colonies half the globe away. In Australia in those times there was no single centre of population large enough or wealthy enough to provide the amount of clinical material and the facilities that would have permitted an individual, however talented, to practise purely in clinical neurology. George Rennie became the first in the country whose activities began to approach what was predominantly neurological practice. In some ways his situation was akin to that of the London physicians Robert Bentley Todd and John Russell Reynolds who, just before the Queen Square Hospital opened, were carrying out and describing important neurological investigations but who continued throughout their professional lives to practise as general physicians. One can scarcely equate the activities of A W Campbell, the first Australian to practise purely as a clinical neurologist, with those of John Hughlings Jackson, the 'father of English neurology'. Relative to the circumstances of his time, Campbell may have been a great, though often not appropriately appreciated, neuroscientist, but he does not appear to have been an outstanding or especially influential clinician. Jackson, older than Campbell, was possessed of a philosophical cast of mind and his main limitation, that of an inability to express himself in writing that was clear and direct and non-repetitive, was largely compensated for by the ability of his slightly younger colleague William Gowers to convey Jackson's ideas, and also the results of Gowers' own analysis of data and synthesis of concepts, in clear direct English. Australian clinical neurology did not really get underway until Leonard Cox, largely self-educated neurologically, came on the scene in the 1920s. Within Australia, the greatness of his achievements has probably never been adequately appreciated, the general feeling, at least until recently, having been that Edward Graeme Robertson, bearing the imprimatur of Queen Square training and the holding of a consultant neurological appointment in London, was the most influential founding figure in Australian neurology. Robertson's influence began just before the onset of World War II, considerably more than half a century after Jackson, Gowers and Charcot had made their marks.

How from that comparatively small and protracted emergence did Australian clinical neurology, over a period of about half a century from its beginning, more or less manage to catch up with the contemporary performance of clinical neurology in Britain and other Western countries?

Two factors come to mind. Firstly, the tempo of the advances in international neurological knowledge after World War II tended to slow. The major early clinical neurological problems had already been investigated by then with the tools available and, as far as they could be at the time, had been solved. The issues that remained were on the whole of lesser magnitude and also were more difficult to study, even with advances in investigational technology. Also, Australian life and intellectual activity had been disrupted by World War II to a lesser extent than that in Europe and Britain, so the development of Australian clinical neurology was able to proceed from a less disturbed base in the immediate post-war years, expediting its ability to reach standards comparable to those of other Western countries. There probably was a second factor that operated, at least in relation to British neurology. Britain was very slow to make academic appointments in clinical neurology; Australia made them relatively sooner and then made more of them, proportionately. Such appointments offer greater opportunities for research, and at the present time, with its ease of communication, it is research more than anything else that tends to determine the perceived standard of clinical neurology in medically trained eyes.

Others will almost certainly interpret differently the events discussed immediately above. Even so, at the time of writing one hopes that they will not disagree that Australian clinical neurology seems to have found its way to a worthwhile place in the international clinical neurological community.

REFERENCES

Abbie AA (1937) 'The anatomy of capsular vascular disease'. *Medical Journal of Australia* 2:564-567.

Abbie AA (1941) 'The anatomy of the cerebellum'. *Medical Journal of Australia* 1:159–163.

Abbie AA (1969) *The original Australians*. Wellington: Reed.

Abercrombie J (1828) *Pathological and practical researches on diseases of the brain and the spinal cord*. Edinburgh: Waugh & Innes.

Allen IM (1938) 'Results of the investigation of reflex epilepsy'. *Medical Journal of Australia* 1:1052–1055.

Allen IM (1939) 'On compulsive grasping, the grasp reflex, tonic innervation and associated phenomena'. *Medical Journal of Australia* 1:717-727.

Allen IM, Spencer FM (1935) 'Acute aseptic meningitis'. *Medical Journal of Australia* 2:275-281.

Allsop JL (1954) 'Thallium poisoning'. *Australasian Annals of Medicine* 3:144–160.

Allsop J (1994) 'A history of neurology in New South Wales'. In: Morris J, ed. *Neurology in Australia*. Sydney: Australian Association of Neurologists: pp. 35-45.

Anderson AG (1917) 'Some remarks on the occurrence of the "Mysterious Disease" in Southern Queensland'. *Medical Journal of Australia* 2:270-272.

Anderson C, English JC (1938) 'Streptococcal meningitis treated with sulphanilamide'. *Medical Journal of Australia* 2:287-288.

Anderson D (1933) 'John White: Surgeon-General to the first fleet'. *Medical Journal of Australia* 1:183–187.

Anderson N (2016) *Dusty Allen rediscovered: a neurologists life*. Auckland, Mary Egan Publishing.

Anderson SG (1952) 'Murray Valley encephalitis: epidemiological aspects'. *Medical Journal of Australia* 1: 97–100.

Anderson SG, Donnelly M, Stevenson WJ, Caldwell NJ, Eagle M (1952) 'Murray Valley encephalitis: surveys of human and animal sera'. *Medical Journal of Australia* 1:110–114.

Anderson SG, Price AVG, Nanadai-Koia, Slater K (1960) 'Murray Valley encephalitis in Papua and New Guinea'. *Medical Journal of Australia* 2:410-413.

Anonymous (1917) 'Obituary: James Froude Flashman'. *Medical Journal of Australia* 1:174–176.

Anonymous (1922) 'An historical account of the occurrence and causation of lead poisoning among Queensland children'. *Medical Journal of Australia* 9:148–152.

Anonymous (1923) 'Obituary: George Edward Rennie'. *Medical Journal of Australia* 2:211-213.

Anonymous (1924) 'Obituary. John Irvine Hunter'. *Medical Journal of Australia* 2:669-671.

Anonymous (1926) 'Current comment. Sympathetic innervation and skeletal muscle tonus'. *Medical Journal of Australia* 2:390-391.

Anonymous (1960) *Queen Square and the National Hospital 1860–1960*. London: Edward Arnold.

Baldwin AH, Heydon GM (1925) 'X disease in Townsville'. *Medical Journal of Australia* 2:394-396.

Balls-Headley W (1896) 'Demonstration'. *Intercolonial Medical Journal of Australasia* 1:380.

Bancroft J (1884) 'Queensland ticks and tick blindness'. *Australasian Medical Gazette* 4:37, cited by Cleland JB (1912) *loc cit*.

Bancroft J (1892) 'Leprosy in Queensland'. *Australasian Medical Gazette* 1:427-430.

Basten A, McLeod JG, Pollard JD, *et al.* (1980) 'Transfer factor in treatment of multiple sclerosis'. *Lancet* ii:931-934.

Bell G, Latham O (1928) 'Tumour of the brain: spongioblastoma multiforme'. *Medical Journal of Australia* 2:757-761.

Bentley BJ (1912) 'Some further points in the treatment of epilepsy with chloretone'. *Medical Journal of Australia* 32:599-601.

Bentley J (1911) 'Epilepsy'. *Australasian Medical Gazette* 30:121–126.

Bertrand S, Weiland S, Berkovic SF, Steinlein OK, Bertrand D (1998) 'Properties of neuronal nicotinic acetylcholine receptor mutants from humans suffering from autosomal dominant frontal lobe epilepsy'. *British Journal of Pharmacology* 125:751-760.

Billings J, Robertson P (1955) 'Paraplegia following chest surgery'. *Australasian Annals of Medicine* 4:141–144.

Birkett AN (1944) 'Norman Dawson Royle'. *Medical Journal of Australia* I:570-571.

Black GHB (1934) 'Migraine'. *Medical Journal of Australia* 2:37-46.

Bladin P, Eadie M, Wehener V (2004) 'Leonard Bell Cox (1894–1976) – pioneer of Australian clinical neurology'. *Journal of Clinical Neuroscience* 11:819-824.

Bladin PF (2017) 'Reflections on a life in epilepsy. Evolution of epileptology in Australia. Early days'. *Epilepsy and Behavior* 71:108–115.

Blackburn CB, Latham O (1922) 'Pernicious anaemia with early spinal symptoms'. *Medical Journal of Australia* 2:735-737.

Blunt M (1955) *John Irvine Hunter of the Sydney Medical School 1898–1924*. Sydney. Sydney University Press.

Bochner F, Hooper WD, Tyrer JH, Eadie MJ (1972) 'Factors involved in an outbreak of phenytoin intoxication'. *Journal of the Neurological Sciences* 16:481-487.

Bostock J (1926) 'Diabetic tabes so-called'. *Medical Journal of Australia* 2:82-83.

Braak H, Del Tredici K, Rub U, de Vos RAI, Steur ENHJ, Braak E (2003) 'Staging of brain pathology related to sporadic Parkinson's disease'. *Neurobiology of Aging* 24:197-211.

Breinl A (1917) 'The mysterious disease'. *Medical Journal of Australia* 1:454.

Breinl A (1918) 'Clinical, pathological and experimental observations on the 'mysterious disease', a clinically aberrant form of acute poliomyelitis'. *Medical Journal of Australia* 5:209-213 & 229-234.

Breinl A, Young WJ (1914) 'The occurrence of lead poisoning amongst Queensland children'. *Annals of Tropical Medicine and Parasitology*:575.

Brothers CRD (1964) 'Huntington's chorea in Victoria and Tasmania'. *Journal of the Neurological Sciences* 1:405-420.

Brown-Sequard CE (1860) *On the etiology, nature, and treatment of epilepsy, with a few remarks on several other affections of the nervous centres. In: Course of lectures on the physiology and pathology of the central nervous system.* Philadelphia: Lippincott & Co: pp. 178-186.

Buchanan AL (1929) 'Experiences with encephalography'. *Medical Journal of Australia* 2:812-817.

Buchanan AR (1937) 'The Lange colloidal gold reaction as a routine test: a preliminary note on the results'. *Medical Journal of Australia* 2:175-178.

Burkitt N (1944) 'Obituary. Norman Gilmore Royle'. *Medical Journal of Australia* 1:570-571.

Burnell GH (1917) 'The Broken Hill epidemic'. *Medical Journal of Australia* 2:157-163.

Burnell GH (1918) 'The Broken Hill epidemic'. *Medical Journal of Australia* 1:278-280.

Burnell GH (1922) 'X disease'. *Medical Journal of Australia* 1:126.

Burnet FM (1934) 'Louping ill virus as a possible cause of the X disease epidemics of 1917–1918'. *Medical Journal of Australia* 1:679-681.

Burnet FM (1952a) 'Murray Valley encephalitis'. *American Journal of Public Health* 42:1519–1521.

Burnet FM (1952b) 'Poliomyelitis and Murray Valley encephalitis: a comparison of two neurotropic virus diseases'. *Medical Journal of Australia* 1:169–175.

Burns C (1963) 'Ivan Macdonald Allen'. *New Zealand Medical Journal* 62:244-245.

Burns R, 'Thomas DW, Barron VJ (1974) 'Reversible encephalopathy possibly associated with bismuth subgallate ingestion'. *British Medical Journal* 1:220-223.

Burrow JNC, Whelan PI, Kilburn CJ, Fisher DA, Currie BJ, Smith DW (1998) 'Australian encephalitis in the Northern Territory: clinical and epidemiological features, 1987–1996'. *Australian and New Zealand Journal of Medicine* 28:590-596.

Burston RA (1988) 'Fry, Henry Kenneth'. In: McDonald GL, ed. *Roll of the Royal Australasian College of Physicians. Volume 1.* Sydney: Royal Australasian College of Physicians: pp. 100–101.

Burt T, Blumbergs P, Currie B (1993) 'A dominant hereditary ataxia resembling Machado-Joseph disease in Arnhem Land, Australia'. *Neurology* 43:1750–1752.

Burt T, Currie B, Kilburn C, *et al.* (1996) 'Machado-Joseph disease in east Arnhem Land, Australia: chromosome 14q32.1 expanded repeat confirmed in four families'. *Neurology* 46:1118–1122.

Cade JF (1947) The anticonvulsant properties of creatinine. *Medical Journal of Australia* 2:621-623.

Calov WL (1940) 'Cerebro-spinal meningitis'. *Medical Journal of Australia* 2:51-64.

Cameron J, Capra MF (1993) 'The basis of paradoxical disturbance of temperature perception in ciguatera poisoning'. *Journal of Toxicology and Clinical Toxicology* 31:571-579.

Cameron J, Flowers AE, Capra MF (1991) 'Effects of ciguatoxin on nerve excitability in rats'. *Journal of the Neurological Sciences* 101:87-92.

Campbell AW (1894a) 'A contribution to the morbid anatomy and pathology of the neuro-muscular changes in general paresis of the insane'. *Journal of Mental Science* 40:177–195.

Campbell AW (1894b) 'Degenerations consequent on experimental lesions of the cerebellum'. *British Medical Journal* 2:641-642.

Campbell AW (1894c) 'On vacuolation of the nerve cell of the human cerebral cortex'. *Journal of Pathology and Bacteriology* 2:380-393.

Campbell AW (1897) 'On the tracts of the spinal cord and their degenerations'. *Brain* 20:488-535.

Campbell AW (1903) Communicated by Sherrington, CS. 'Histological studies on cerebral localisation'. *Proceedings of the Royal Society of London* 488-492.

Campbell AW (1905) *Histological studies on the localisation of cerebral function.* Cambridge: Cambridge University Press.

Campbell AW (1910) 'The treatment of trigeminal neuralgia by injections of alcohol'. *Australasian Medical Gazette* 29:66-75.

Campbell AW (1911) 'On the localisation of function in the cerebellum'. *Transactions of the Ninth Australasian Medical Congress*, Sydney 847-852.

Campbell AW (1913) 'A case of syringomyelia'. *Australasian Medical Gazette* 34:478-479.

Campbell AW (1916) 'Remarks on some neuroses and psychoses in war'. *Medical Journal of Australia* 1:319-323.

Campbell AW (1919) 'A case for diagnosis (Thomsen's disease)'. *Medical Journal of Australia* 2:506-508.

Campbell AW (1924a) 'The evolution and functions of the labyrinth'. *Medical Journal of Australia* Suppl:428-429.

Campbell AW (1924b) 'Infantile paralysis of cerebral origin'. *Medical Journal of Australia* 1:512-515.

Campbell AW (1927a) 'The epilepsies of childhood'. *Medical Journal of Australia* 1:774-775.

Campbell AW (1927b) 'Some modifications of nervous disease in childhood'. *Medical Journal of Australia* 1:697-699.

Campbell AW (1928a) 'The sympathetic innervation of skeletal muscle'. *Medical Journal of Australia* 1:258.

Campbell AW (1928b) 'The value of ocular signs in neurological diagnosis'. *Transactions of the Australasian Medical Congress* 125–126.

Campbell AW (1930) 'Cerebrospinal syphilis'. *Medical Journal of Australia* ii: 26-27.

Campbell AW (1931) 'Affections of peripheral nerves'. *Medical Journal of Australia* 2:544-546.

Campbell AW (1933a) 'The nervous child'. *Medical Journal of Australia* 2:535-538.

Campbell AW (1933b) 'The treatment of migraine'. *Medical Journal of Australia* 1:36-37.

Campbell AW (1935) 'Dr John Hughlings Jackson'. *Medical Journal of Australia* 2:344-347.

Campbell AW, Cleland JB, Bradley B (1918) 'A contribution to the experimental pathology of acute poliomyelitis (infantile paralysis)'. *Medical Journal of Australia* 5:123–128.

Campbell AW, Dowling N (1920) 'A case of nervous or hysterical fever'. *Medical Journal of Australia* 1:171–172.

Cheek DB (1950) 'Pink disease: an investigation of its cause and treatment (preliminary report)'. *Medical Journal of Australia* 1:101–107.

Cheek DB, Hicks CS (1950) 'Pink disease or infantile acrodynia: its nature, prevention and cure'. *Medical Journal of Australia* 1:107–121.

Chinner ME (1940) 'A clinical survey of nine cases of encephalomyelitis in association with measles'. *Medical Journal of Australia* 2:526-529.

Clark FJ (1937) 'The treatment of trigeminal neuralgia'. *Medical Journal of Australia* 2:784-785.

Clayton HJ (1923) 'Obituary. George Edward Rennie'. *Medical Journal of Australia* 2:213-214.

Cleland JB (1912) 'Injuries and diseases of man in Australia attributable to animals (except insects)'. *Australasian Medical Gazette* 32:269-274; 295-299.

Cleland JB (1916) 'Some aspects of the aetiology and epidemiology of cerebrospinal fever'. *Medical Journal of Australia* 2:496-499 & 516-518.

Cleland JB (1917) 'Mysterious disease'. *Medical Journal of Australia* 2:171–172.

Cleland JB (1923) 'Epidemic encephalitis'. *Medical Journal of Australia* 2:594.

Cleland JB (1937) 'Small aneurysms at the base of the brain and subarachnoid haemorrhage'. *Medical Journal of Australia* 1:141–142.

Cleland JB (1942) 'Injuries and diseases in Australia attributable to animals (insects excepted)'. *Medical Journal of Australia* 2:313-320.

Cleland JB, Campbell AW (1919) 'The nature of the recent Australian epidemics of acute encephalo-myelitis. Successful conveyance of the virus to sheep, a calf, and a horse'. *Medical Journal of Australia* 1:232-236.

Cleland JB, Campbell AW (1920a) 'The epidemiology of acute encephalomyelitis ('X disease') in Australia'. *Proceedings of the Royal Society of Medicine* 13:185-205.

Cleland JB, Campbell AW (1920b) 'An experimental investigation of an Australian epidemic of acute encephalomyelitis'. *Journal of Hygiene* 18:272-316.

Clements FW (1940) 'Pink disease: a consideration of three aetiological possibilities'. *Medical Journal of Australia* 2:430-432.

Clements FW (1960) 'The rise and decline of pink disease'. *Medical Journal of Australia* 1:922-925.

Clendinnen FJ (1897) 'Skiagrams of the skull and intra-cranial blood-vessels'. *Intercolonial Medical Journal of Australasia* 2:819.

Clubbe CPB (1925) 'Some aspects of infantile paralysis'. *Medical Journal of Australia* 1:527-533.

Cohen A (1994) 'Beech, Ernest Robert'. In: Wiseman JC, Mulhearn RJ, eds. *Roll of the Royal Australasian College of Physicians. Volume 2*. Sydney: Royal Australasian College of Physicians: pp. 14–16.

Collins AJ (1928) 'Epidemic encephalitis'. *Medical Journal of Australia* 2:72-74.

Cook RD (1981) 'Multiple sclerosis: is the domestic cat involved?' *Medical Hypotheses* 7:147–154.

Cook RD, Flower RL, Dutton NS (1986) 'Light and electron microscopical studies of the immunoperoxidase staining of multiple sclerosis plaques using antisera to a feline derived agent and to galactocerebroside'. *Neuropathology and Applied Neurobiology* 12:63-79.

Corkill AB, Ennor AH (1937) 'Choline esterase in myasthenia gravis'. *Medical Journal of Australia* 2:1121–1123.

Covernton JS, Draper MH (1947) 'A study of myotonia, with special reference to paramyotonia'. *Medical Journal of Australia* 2:161–175.

Cox LB (1931) 'The origin of Sluder's or spheno-palatine neuralgia'. *Medical Journal of Australia* 1:435-441.

Cox LB (1932a) 'Ganglioneuroma of the cerebrum, with an additional case'. *Medical Journal of Australia* 1:347-351.

Cox LB (1932b) 'On the relation of Sluder's neuralgia to the trigeminal nerve, and other facial neuralgias'. *Medical Journal of Australia* 1:292-298.

Cox LB (1933) 'The cytology of the glioma group: with special reference to inclusion of cells derived from invaded tissue'. *American Journal of Pathology* 9:839-898.

Cox LB (1934) 'Observations upon the nature, rate of growth, and operability of the intracranial tumours derived from 135 patients'. *Medical Journal of Australia* 1:182–196.

Cox LB (1935) 'Tumour of the brain as met with in general practice'. *Medical Journal of Australia* 1:425-541.

Cox LB (1937) 'Tumours of the base of the brain: their relation to pathological sleep and other changes in the conscious state'. *Medical Journal of Australia* 1:742-752.

Cox LB (1938a) 'The relation of myasthenia gravis and allied conditions to "Prostigmin" therapy'. *Medical Journal of Australia* 1:344-348.

Cox LB (1938b) 'On the origin and treatment of syringomyelic cavities'. *Medical Journal of Australia* 1:481-483.

Cox LB (1939a) 'Haemorrhage of the brain stem as a significant complication of intracranial tumours'. *Medical Journal of Australia* 1:259-262.

Cox LB (1939b) 'Trauma and intracranial tumours'. *Medical Journal of Australia* 1:256-259.

Cox LB (1949a) 'The treatment of neurosyphilis'. *Medical Journal of Australia* 1:449-451.

Cox LB (1949b) 'Medical sequelae of brain injury'. *Medical Journal of Australia* 1:519-521

Cox LB, Fantl P, Fitzpatrick M (1949) 'The treatment of disseminated sclerosis by prolonged lowering of the blood prothrombin level'. *Medical Journal of Australia* 1:577-579.

Cox LB, Tolhurst JC (1946) *Human torulosis*. Melbourne: Melbourne University Press.

Cox LB, Trumble HC (1939) 'Tumours and malformations of the blood vessels of the brain and spinal cord'. *Medical Journal of Australia* 2:308-319.

Crago WH (1890) 'Notes on a case of ascending paralysis of Landry'. *Australasian Medical Gazette* 10:19-21.

Crago WH (1923) 'Obituary: George Edward Rennie'. *Medical Journal of Australia* 2:213.

Creed JM (1889) 'Leprosy: in its relation to the European population of Australia'. Intercolonial Medical Congress of Australasia:499-503.

Critchley M (1990) *The ventricle of memory. Personal recollections of some neurologists*. New York: Raven Press.

Crowther WELH (1946) 'A case of so-called hydrophobia: a matter of diagnosis'. *Medical Journal of Australia* 1:69-72.

Cullen W (1805 (originally 1789)) *First lines of the practice of physic. Volumes 1 & 2*. New York: Duyckinck, Swords, Falconer *et al*.

Curtis JB, Miller D, Simpson D (1980) 'The neurosurgical society of Australasia: the first forty years'. *Australian and New Zealand Journal of Surgery* 50:434-437.

Dandy WE (1918) 'Ventriculography following the injection of air into the cerebral ventricles'. *Annals of Surgery* 68:5–11.

Dawson WS (1928) 'The treatment of general paralysis by malaria'. *Medical Journal of Australia* 1:10–13.

Dawson WS (1937) 'Cerebral arteriosclerosis: a review'. *Medical Journal of Australia* 2:499-506.

Dawson WS (1938) 'Obituary. Alfred Walter Campbell'. *Medical Journal of Australia* 1:183–185.

Dawson WS, Latham O (1931) 'A case of encephalomyelitis'. *Medical Journal of Australia* 2:236-238.

Dawson WS, Latham O (1943) 'Pathological states in dementia praecox as revealed in a fatal case of picrotoxin medication'. *Medical Journal of Australia* 1:245-248.

De Crespigny CT (1938) 'Cerebral vascular accidents and their treatment'. *Medical Journal of Australia* 1:1077–1081.

De Crespigny CTC (1944) 'G E Rennie Memorial Lecture. Torula infection of the central nervous system'. *Medical Journal of Australia* 2:605-615.

De Crespigny CTC, Hurst EW (1942) 'A demyelinating condition apparently localized in the brain stem'. *Medical Journal of Australia* 1:408-410.

De Crespigny CTC, Woollard HH (1929) 'A case of Schilder's disease'. *Lancet* ii: 684.

Delasiauve LJF (1854) *Traite de l'epilepsie*. Paris.

Denny-Brown D, Robertson EG (1933a) 'On the physiology of micturition'. *Brain* 56:149–190.

Denny-Brown D, Robertson EG (1933b) 'The state of the bladder and its sphincters in complete transverse lesions of the spinal cord and cauda equina'. *Brain* 56:397- 463.

Denny-Brown D, Robertson EG (1935) 'An investigation of the nervous control of defaecation'. *Brain* 58:256-310.

Dew HR (1922) 'Tumours of the brain: their pathology and treatment'. *Medical Journal of Australia* 1:515-521.

Dew HR (1936) 'Some aspects of intracranial surgery, with special reference to the meningiomata'. *Medical Journal of Australia* 2:69-76.

Donnan GA, Bladin PF, Berkovic SF, Longley WA, Saling MM (1991) 'The stroke syndrome of striato-capsular infarction'. *Brain* 114:57-70.

Donnan GA, McNeill JJ, Adena MA, Doyle AE, O'Malley HM, Neill GC (1989) 'Smoking as a risk factor for cerebral ischaemia'. *Lancet* ii:643-647.

Donnan GA, O'Malley HM, Quang L, Hurley S, Bladin P (1993) 'The capsular warning syndrome: pathogenesis and clinical features'. *Neurology* 43:957-962.

Douglas RA (1977) 'Dr Anton Breinl and the Australian Institute of Tropical Medicine'. *Medical Journal of Australia* 1:713-716; 748-751; 784-790.

Downing JH (1919) 'Coma following influenza'. *Medical Journal of Australia* 2:69.

Duhig JV (1922) 'Polio-encephalitis'. *Medical Journal of Australia* 2:261-263.

Dunlop DB (1996) 'Obituary. Adrian Dawson'. *Medical Journal of Australia* 164:182.

Eadie M J (1963) 'The pathology of certain medullary nuclei in Parkinsonism'. *Brain* 86:781-792.

Eadie MJ (1981) 'A W Campbell-Australia's first neurologist'. *Clinical and Experimental Neurology* 17:27-35.

Eadie MJ ed (1992) *Drug therapy in neurology*. Edinburgh: Churchill-Livingstone.

Eadie MJ (1994) 'Epileptic seizures in 1902 patients: a perspective from a consultant neurological practice (1961–1991)'. *Epilepsy Research* 17:55-79.

Eadie MJ, Sutherland JM, Doherty RL (1965) 'Encephalitis in the aetiology of Parkinsonism in Australia'. *Archives of Neurology* 12:240-245.

Eadie MJ, Tyrer JH (1980) *Neurological clinical pharmacology*. Auckland: Adis Press.

Eadie MJ, Tyrer JH (1985) *The biochemistry of migraine*. Lancaster: MTP Press.

Eadie MJ, Tyrer JH (1989) *Anticonvulsant therapy: pharmacological basis and practice*. 3rd ed. Edinburgh: Churchill-Livingstone.

Eadie MJ, Vajda FJE eds (1999) *Antiepileptic drugs: pharmacology and therapeutics*. Berlin: Springer.

Eadie MJ, Vajda FJE (2015) *Antiepileptic drugs in pregnancy*. Heidelberg. Adis

Eaton EM (1913) 'A case of tick-bite followed by wide-spread transitory muscular paralysis'. *Australasian Medical Gazette* 33:391-394.

Eccles JC (1941) 'Changes in muscle produced by nerve degeneration'. *Medical Journal of Australia* 1:573-575.

Editorial (1892) 'Leprosy in New South Wales'. *Australasian Medical Gazette* 11:165–166.

Editorial Comment (1926) 'Sympathetic innervation and skeletal muscle tonus'. *Medical Journal of Australia* 2:390-391.

Editorial (1927) 'Tick paralysis'. *Medical Journal of Australia* 1:548-549.

Edwards AT, Latham O (1943) 'Alzheimer's disease'. *Medical Journal of Australia* 1:251-253.

Edye BT (1926) 'The technique of cisternal puncture and its application in the treatment of general paralysis of the insane by arsenicalized serum'. *Medical Journal of Australia* 1:272-273.

Elkin AP (1935) 'Primitive medicine men'. *Medical Journal of Australia* 2:750-757.

Ellery RS (1926) 'On the treatment of general paralysis of the insane by malaria'. *Medical Journal of Australia* 1:401-404.

Evans W (1925) 'Preanaemic combined degeneration of the cord'. *Medical Journal of Australia* 2:508-509.

Evans W (1931) 'Pink disease or erythroedema polyneuritis'. *Medical Journal of Australia* 2:86-87.

Fairley NH, Guest JV (1915) 'Cerebro-spinal fever: an analysis of fifty cases'. *Medical Journal of Australia* 2:383-389.

Farquhar J, Gajdusek DC eds (1981) *Kuru. Early letters and field notes from the collection of D Carleton Gajdusek.* New York: Raven Press.

Ferguson EW (1924) 'Deaths from tick paralysis in human beings'. *Medical Journal of Australia* 2:346-348.

Ferrier TM, Eadie MJ (1973) 'Clioquinol encephalopathy'. *Medical Journal of Australia* 2:1008-1009.

Ferrier TM, Schwieger AC, Eadie MJ (1986) 'Delayed onset of partial epilepsy of temporal lobe origin following acute clioquinol encephalopathy'. *Journal of Neurology, Neurosurgery and Psychiatry* 50:93-95.

Findlay JP (1933) 'Facial paralysis due to toxic inflammation of the geniculate ganglion'. *Medical Journal of Australia* 1:251-253.

Flashman JF, Latham O (1915) 'A contribution to the study of the aetiology of disseminated sclerosis'. *Medical Journal of Australia* 2:265-269.

Flecker H (1944) 'Sudden blindness after eating "finger cherry" (Rhodomyrtus macrocarpa)'. *Medical Journal of Australia* 2:183-185.

Fleetwood TF (1889) 'A case of Thomsen's disease'. *Australian Medical Journal New Series* 11:393-394.

Flynn J, Greenaway TM (1935) 'Diffuse "encephalitis", presumably Schilder's disease'. *Medical Journal of Australia* 2:120.

Ford E (1979) 'Campbell, Alfred Walter (1868–1937)', *Australian Dictionary of Biography*, National Centre of Biography, Australian National University.

Frayne J (undated). Gilligan, Bernard Sutcliffe (1934-2006) *Roll of the Royal Australasian College of Physicians.* <https://www.racp.edu.au/about/our-heritage/college-roll/college-roll-bio/gilligan-bernard-sutcliffe>.

French EL (1952) 'Murray Valley encephalitis: isolation and characterization of the aetiological agent'. *Medical Journal of Australia* 1:100-107.

Frith JA (1988) 'History of multiple sclerosis. An Australian perspective'. *Clinical and Experimental Neurology* 25:7-16.

Frith JA, McLeod JG, Basten A, *et al.* (1986) 'Transfer factor as a therapy for multiple sclerosis: a follow-up study'. *Clinical and Experimental Neurology* 22:149-154.

Fulton (1879) 'On a case of chorea, treated by subcutaneous injection, in progressive doses, of curara'. *Australian Medical Journal New Series* 1:273-278.

Fulton JF (1938) 'Obituaries: Alfred Walter Campbell MD ChM 1868-1937'. *Archives of Neurology and Psychiatry* 40:566-568.

Gajdusek DC (1981) 'Introduction'. In: Farquhar J, Gadjusek DC, eds. *Kuru. Early letters and field notes from the collection of D Carleton Gadjusek.* New York: Raven Press: pp xv-xx.

Game J (1946) 'A case of periarteritis (polyarteritis) nodosa'. *Medical Journal of Australia* 1:295-298.

Game J (1951) 'Cerebral tumour: early symptoms and methods of investigation'. *Medical Journal of Australia* 1:367-373.

Game JA (1975) 'The Australian Association of Neurologists – a review of twenty-five years'. *Proceedings of the Australian Association of Neurologists* 12:1-6.

Game J (1976) 'Obituaries. Edward Graeme Robertson'. *Archives of Neurology and Psychiatry* 13:1-3.

Gandevia B, Cobley J (1974) 'Mortality at Sydney Cove, 1788-1782'. *Australian and New Zealand Journal of Medicine* 4:111-125.

Gibson JL (1896) 'Traumatic rupture of carotid into cavernous sinus – pulsating exophthalmos'. *Australasian Medical Gazette* 5:147-149.

Gibson JL (1904) 'A plea for painted railings and painted walls of rooms as the source of lead poisoning amongst Queensland children'. *Australasian Medical Gazette* 23:149.

Gibson JL (1905) 'Pulsating exophthalmos – post-mortem'. *Australasian Medical Gazette* 24:107-108.

Gibson JL (1912) 'The importance of lumbar puncture in the plumbic ocular neuritis of children'. *Australasian Medical Gazette* 31:25-27.

Gibson JL, Love W, Hardie D, Bancroft P, Turner AJ (1892) 'Notes on lead-poisoning as observed among children in Brisbane'. *Transactions of the Intercolonial Medical Congress of Australasia* 3rd Session:76-83.

Gibson S (2013) 'Researcher and educator whose desire to learn never waned'. *Sydney Morning Herald.* https://www.smh.com.au/national/researcher-and-educator-whose-desire-to-learn-never-waned-20131007-2v4bw.html

Gillespie NC, Lewis RJ, Pearn JH, *et al.* (1986) 'Ciguatera in Australia. Occurrence, clinical features, pathophysiology and management'. *Medical Journal of Australia* 145:584-590.

Gillett BStP, Farmer F, Anderson M, Sadka M (1973) 'Obituary: Gerald Carew Moss'. *Medical Journal of Australia* 59:44-45.

Gilligan BS (1996) 'John Aylward Game'. *Medical Journal of Australia* 164:497.
Goadsby PJ, Lipton RB (1997) 'A review of paroxysmal hemicranias, SUNCT syndrome and other short-lasting headaches with autonomic features, including new cases'. *Brain* 120: 193-209.

Goulston DL (1930) 'The action of radiation from radium needles on nerves'. *Medical Journal of Australia* 2:651-661.

Gowers WR (1886 & 1888) *A manual of diseases of the nervous system. 1st ed. Volumes 1 & 2.* London: Churchill.

Graham J (1893) 'Multiple neuritis among Chinamen in Sydney'. *Australasian Medical Gazette* 12:357-360.

Gray DF (1948) 'Human botulism in Australia'. *Medical Journal of Australia* 2:37-42.

Greenfield JG (1956) *The spino-cerebellar degenerations.* Oxford: Blackwell

Scientific Publications.

Greenfield JG, Robertson EG (1933) 'Cystic oligodendrogliomas of the cerebral hemispheres and ventricular oligodendrogliomas'. *Brain* 56:247-264.

Greenwood B (1967) 'The origins of sympathectomy'. *Medical History* 11:165-169.

Griffiths (1922) 'Insular sclerosis'. *Medical Journal of Australia* 2:658-659.

Guillain G (1959) *J-M Charcot 1825-1893. His life – his work*. London: Pitman.

Hagen PB, Noad KB, Latham O (1951) 'The syndrome of lamellar cerebellar degeneration associated with retinitis pigmentosa, hypertopias, and mental deficiency, with report of a case'. *Medical Journal of Australia* 1:217-223.

Hall B, Noad KB, Latham O (1945) 'Familial cortical cerebellar atrophy: a contribution to the study of heredo-familial cerebellar disease in Australia'. *Medical Journal of Australia* 1:101-108.

Ham BB (1905) 'The recent epidemic of infantile paralysis'. *Australasian Medical Gazette* 24:193-199.

Hamilton DG (1940a) 'The treatment of meningitis due to the meningococcus, haemophilus influenzae and streptococcus'. *Medical Journal of Australia* 2:342-346.

Hamilton DG (1940b) 'Tick paralysis: a dangerous disease in children'. *Medical Journal of Australia* 1:759-765.

Hammond SR, de Wytt C, Maxwell IC, *et al.* (1987) 'The epidemiology of multiple sclerosis in Queensland, Australia'. *Journal of the Neurological Sciences* 80:185-204.

Hammond SR, English DR, de Wytt C, *et al.* (1989) 'The contribution of mortality statistics to the study of multiple sclerosis in Australia'. *Journal of Neurology, Neurosurgery and Psychiatry* 52:1-7.

Hammond SR, English D, de Wytt C, *et al.* (1988a) 'The clinical profile of MS in Australia: a comparison between medium- and high-frequency prevalence zones'. *Neurology* 38:980-986.

Hammond SR, McLeod JG, Millingen KS, *et al.* (1988b) 'The epidemiology of multiple sclerosis in three Australian cities: Perth, Newcastle and Hobart'. *Brain* 111:1-25.

Hammond WA (1871) *A treatise on diseases of the nervous system*. New York and London: Appleton & Co. and Trubner & Co.

Hare F (1903) 'Mechanism of the paroxysmal neuroses'. *Australasian Medical Gazette* 22:283-291; 333-340; 387-394.

Hawkes CS (1903) 'The mechanism of trigeminal neuralgia'. *Australasian Medical Gazette* 22:497-501.

Hawkes CS (1905) 'The treatment of epilepsy'. *Australasian Medical Gazette* 24:644-650.

Haymaker W, Schiller F eds (1970) *The founders of neurology*. 2nd ed. Springfield: Thomas.

Head H, Campbell AW (1900) 'On the pathology of herpes zoster and its bearing on sensory localisation'. *Brain* 24:353-523.

Henderson JK, Henderson MA (2021) *Arthur Schüller: founder of neuroradiology – a life on two continents.* Ormond, Victoria. Hybrid Publishers.

Hickey MF (1963) 'Obituary: Herbert John Wilkinson'. *Medical Journal of Australia* 1:869.

Himmeloch E, Latham O, McDonald CG (1947) 'Alzheimer's disease complicated by a terminal salmonella infection'. *Medical Journal of Australia* 1:701-703.

Hogg CA, Latham O (1923) 'Encephalitis lethargica'. *Medical Journal of Australia* 2:90-95.

Hogg GH (1902) 'On the medicine of the Tasmanian aboriginals'. Transactions of the Sixth Session, Australasian Medical Congress, Hobart:176-177.

Hogg GH (1906) 'A case of myasthenia gravis in special relation to eye and throat conditions'. *Australasian Medical Gazette* 25:184-186.

Hogg GH (1915) 'Leber's disease'. *Medical Journal of Australia* 1:253.

Hogg GH (1928) 'Hereditary optic atrophy'. *Medical Journal of Australia* 1:372-374.

Holmes G (1904) 'On certain tremors in organic cerebral lesions'. *Brain* 27: 327–375.

Holmes G (1954) *The National Hospital Queen Square.* Edinburgh: E & S Livingstone.

Holmes GM (1956) 'The Croonian lectures on the clinical symptoms of cerebellar disease and their interpretation'. In: Walshe FMR, ed. *Selected papers of Sir Gordon Holmes.* London: MacMillan & Co: pp 49-111.

Holmes a Court AW (1923) 'Discussion on encephalitis'. *Medical Journal of Australia* Suppl:38.

Holmes a Court A, Latham O (1935) 'Schilder's disease'. *Medical Journal of Australia* 2:117-120.

Hood J (1902) 'Epidemic cerebro-spinal meningitis'. Proceedings of the Sixth Session, Australasian Medical Congress:158-164.

Hooper R (1978) 'Graeme Robertson and the golden age of neurology'. *Clinical and Experimental Neurology* 15:1-10.

Hopkins WF (1898) 'Case of gunshot wound of brain'. *Intercolonial Medical Journal of Australasia* 3:486-489.

Howson F (1918) 'A case of muscular atrophy'. *Medical Journal of Australia* 2:305.

Hughes JF (1940) 'Parkinsonism: an account of the disorder and its treatment, with special reference to high atropine dosage therapy'. *Medical Journal of Australia* 2:174-176.

Hughes TD (1927) 'Arsenical neuritis treated by the intravenous injection of sodium thiosulphate'. *Medical Journal of Australia* 1:543.

Hunter JI (1924a) 'The postural influence of the sympathetic innervation of voluntary muscle'. *Medical Journal of Australia* 11:86-89.

Hunter JI (1924b) 'The significance of the double innervation of voluntary muscle illustrated by reference to the maintenance of the posture of the wing'. *Medical Journal of Australia* 11(1):581-587.

Hunter JI (1924c) 'On the choice of procedure adopted in the operation of ramisection for spastic paralysis'. *Medical Journal of Australia* 11:590-591.

Hunter JI, Latham O (1925) 'A contribution to the discussion of the histological problems involved in the conception of a somatic and sympathetic innervation of voluntary muscles'. *Medical Journal of Australia* 1:27-36.

Hurley LE (1926) 'Disseminated sclerosis'. *Medical Journal of Australia* 1:25.

Hurst EW (1941a) 'Acute haemorrhagic leucoencephalitis: a previously undefined entity'. *Medical Journal of Australia* 2:1-6.

Hurst EW (1941b) 'G E Rennie Memorial Lecture. Demyelination: a clinicopathological and experimental study'. *Medical Journal of Australia* 2:661-666.

Huxtable LR (1892a) 'Records of clinical cases. Case VI – paralysis agitans'. *Australasian Medical Gazette* 11:211-213.

Huxtable LR (1892b) 'Records of clinical cases. Case VII – insular sclerosis'. *Australasian Medical Gazette* 11:213-215.

Jackson ES (1924) 'Historical notes: a comparison of two annual lists, those of 1827 and 1832, from Brisbane Hospital records'. *Medical Journal of Australia* 11:381-385.

Jackson JH (1870) 'A study of convulsions'. St Andrews Medical Graduates' Association Transactions 162-204.

Jamieson J (1873) 'On a case of chorea of unusual severity'. *Australian Medical Journal* 18:47-48.

Jamieson J (1883) 'Diphtheritic paralysis'. *Australian Medical Journal New Series* 5:386-387.

Jamieson J (1886) 'Cases of multiple neuritis'. *Australian Medical Journal New Series* 8:295-302.

Jamieson S (1894) 'Case of pseudo-hypertrophic paralysis'. *Australasian Medical Gazette* 13:294-295.

Jamieson S (1895-6) 'Record of cases illustrating some of the effects of syphilis upon the central nervous system'. *Intercolonial Quarterly Journal of Medicine and Surgery* 2:207-222.

Johnston WWS (1927) 'Disseminated sclerosis'. *Medical Journal of Australia* 2:417.

Jones SE (1917) 'Huntington's chorea'. *Medical Journal of Australia* 1:376-377.

Kelly M (1942) 'Headaches, traumatic and rheumatic: the cervical somatic lesion'. *Medical Journal of Australia* 2:479-483.

Kennedy J (1944) 'Obituary. John Fullarton Mackeddie'. *Medical Journal of Australia* 2:601-602.

Kenny G (1988) 'HJ Wilkinson – the travail of a pioneer with muscle'. In: Pearn J, ed. *Pioneer medicine in Australia*. Brisbane: Amphion Press: pp 269-279.

Kneebone J le M, Cleland JB (1926) 'Acute encephalitis (X disease) at Broken Hill: probable successful transmission to a sheep'. *Australian Journal of Experimental Biology and Medial Science* 3:119-127.

Lalor P, Haddow G (1920) 'Toxaemia in epilepsy'. *Medical Journal of Australia* 1:251-260.

Lambie CG, Latham O, McDonald GL (1947) 'Olivo-ponto-cerebellar atrophy (Marie's ataxia)'. *Medical Journal of Australia* 2:626-632.

Lance JW (1969) *Mechanism and management of headache*. 1st ed. Oxford: Butterworth-Heinemann.

Lance JW ed (1987) *Mind, movement and migraine*. Sydney: University of New South Wales.

Lance JW (1988) 'Robertson, Edward Graeme'. In: McDonald GL, ed. *Roll of the Royal Australasian College of Physicians. Volume 1*. Sydney: Royal Australasian College of Physicians: pp. 247-248.

Lance JW, Goadsby PJ (1998) *Mechanism and management of headache*. 6th ed. Oxford: Butterworth-Heinemann.

Lance JW, McLeod JG (1981) *A physiological approach to clinical neurology*. London: Butterworth.

Larkins N (1959) 'Obituary. Eric Leo Susman'. *Medical Journal of Australia* 2:339-340.

Latham LS (1922) 'Report of a case of encephalitis lethargica'. *Medical Journal of Australia* 2:426.

Latham O (1926) 'Trophic glial states in spinal cord lesions'. *Medical Journal of Australia* 1:507-510.

Latham O (1927) 'The pathology of two cases of sudden death'. *Medical Journal of Australia* 1:121-123.

Latham O (1930) 'Some difficulties met with in the pathological diagnosis of encephalitis'. *Medical Journal of Australia* 1:376-382.

Latham O (1931) 'Some thoughts on the term acute disseminated encephalomyelitis and its affinities'. *Medical Journal of Australia* 2:677-681.

Latham O (1934) 'Some activities of a mental hospital laboratory during thirty years'. *Medical Journal of Australia* 1:739-746; 767-776; 797-804.

Latham O (1938) 'The role of the small intracranial blood vessels in the pathology of brain conditions'. *Medical Journal of Australia* 1:292-295.

Latham O (1939) 'Haematomyelia'. *Medical Journal of Australia* 1:529-534.

Latham O (1941) 'Some notes on the pathology of the cerebellar system'. *Medical Journal of Australia* 1:164-167.

Layton W, Sutherland JM (1975)' Geochemistry and multiple sclerosis: a hypothesis'. *Medical Journal of Australia* 1:73-77.

Lind WAT (1924) 'Epiloia'. *Medical Journal of Australia* 2:290-294.

Lindon LCE (1936) 'Cerebral arteriography'. *Medical Journal of Australia* 1:849-853.

Litchfield WF (1917) 'The mysterious disease'. *Medical Journal of Australia* 1:384.

Litchfield WF, Latham O, Campbell AW (1917) 'A clinical and anatomical report of a case of Freidreich's disease'. *Medical Journal of Australia* 1:135-140.

Littlejohn ES (1923) 'Pink disease – erythroedema'. *Medical Journal of Australia* 1:689-692.

Lockwood L (1931) 'Post-vaccinal encephalomyelitis'. *Medical Journal of Australia* 1:662-663.

Lowe RF (1940) 'Pneumococcal meningitis treated with sulphapyridine'. *Medical Journal of Australia* 2:536-538.

Macdonald WL (1927) 'A case of chronic lenticular degeneration'. *Medical Journal of Australia* 2:718.

Macewen W (1879) 'Tumour of the dura mater removed during life in a person affected with epilepsy'. *Glasgow Medical Journal* 12:210.

Mackeddie JF (1926) 'Cisterna magna puncture'. *Medical Journal of Australia* 2:447-449.

MacKeddie JF (1927) 'Localization of spinal tumours'. *Medical Journal of Australia* 1:511.

Mackeddie JF (1929) 'Encephalography and the use of "lipiodol"'. *Medical Journal of Australia* 2:511.

Mackeddie JF (1931) 'Lipiodol; in neurological diagnosis'. *Medical Journal of Australia* 2:221-227.

MacLaurin C (1917) 'Obituary. James Froude Flashman'. *Medical Journal of Australia* 1:176.

MacLeod RA (1920) 'Congenital word blindness'. *Medical Journal of Australia* 1:593-596.

MacMillan M (2016) *Snowy Campbell, Australian pioneer investigator of the brain.* Melbourne. Australian Scholarly Publishing.

Macnamara J (1929) 'The treatment of acute poliomyelitis by means of human immune serum'. *Medical Journal of Australia* 2:838-850.

Macnamara J (1953) 'Elizabeth Kenny'. *Medical Journal of Australia* 1:85.

Maddox K (1959) 'Obituary: Eric Leo Susman'. *Medical Journal of Australia* 91:338-340.

Marten RH (1897) 'Notes on cases of post-herpetic neuralgia'. *Intercolonial Medical Journal of Australasia* 2:195-196.

Mathewson THR (1921) 'A rare type of intra-cranial tumour'. *Medical Journal of Australia* 2:400-402.

Mathewson THR (1922) 'Discussion following papers on epidemic encephalitis'. *Medical Journal of Australia* 2:283.

Mathewson THR, Latham O (1917) 'Acute encephalitis of unknown origin'. *Medical Journal of Australia* 2:352-356.

Maudsley HC (1906) 'Brachioplegia of cerebellar type, and rhythmical tremor, with an attempt to explain the symptoms and to localise the lesion'. *Intercolonial Medical Journal of Australasia* 11:302-319.

Maudsley HF (1925) 'Disseminated sclerosis'. *Medical Journal of Australia* 1:326.

Maudsley HF (1926) 'The sequelae of lethargic encephalitis'. *Medical Journal of Australia* 1:696-703.

Maudsley HF (1926) 'Disseminated sclerosis'. *Medical Journal of Australia* 1:836-837.

Maudsley HF (1928) Ocular signs in neurological diagnosis. Transactions of the Australasian Medical Congress 126-127.

Maund J (1856) 'Epilepsy produced by pressure on the brain'. *Australian Medical Journal* 1:20-27.

McAdam RL (1895) 'Notes of a case of intractable epilepsy much relieved by borax'. *Australasian Medical Gazette* 14:492-493.

McCall MG, Brereton TL, Dawson A, Millingen K, Sutherland JM, Acheson ED (1968) 'Frequency of multiple sclerosis in three Australian cities – Perth, Newcastle and Hobart'. *Journal of Neurology, Neurosurgery and Psychiatry* 31:1-9.

McCall MG, Sutherland JM, Acheson ED (1969) 'The frequency of multiple sclerosis in Western Australia'. *Acta Neurologica Scandinavica* 45:151-165.

McDonald JEF (1906) 'The treatment of cerebral haemorrhage'. *Australasian Medical Gazette* 25:186-188.

McDonald SF (1933) 'Swift's or pink disease: recent work on pathology and treatment'. *Medical Journal of Australia* 2:276-280.

McLean DM, Stevenson WJ (1954) 'Between Australian X disease and the virus of Murray Valley encephalitis'. *Medical Journal of Australia* 1:636-638.

McLeod JG, Hammond SR, Hallpike JF (1994) 'Epidemiology of multiple sclerosis in Australia. With NSW and SA survey results'. *Medical Journal of Australia* 160:117-122.

McWhae (1924) 'Headache'. *Medical Journal of Australia* 2:78-81.

Miles JAR, Howes DW (1953) 'Observations on viral encephalitis in South Australia'. *Medical Journal of Australia* 1:7-12.

Mills AE (1917) 'Obituary. James Froude Flashman'. *Medical Journal of Australia* 1:176-177.

Mills AE (1919) 'Multiple peripheral neuritis due to toxaemia of pregnancy'. *Medical Journal of Australia* 2:331-332.

Mills AE (1922) 'Encephalitis'. *Medical Journal of Australia* 2:197-198.

Milroy WH, Hughes BL (1945) 'A case of pneumococcal meningitis successfully treated with penicillin'. *Medical Journal of Australia* 2:434.

Minogue SJ (1926) 'The differential diagnosis of cerebral syphilis'. *Medical Journal of Australia* 2:444-447.

Minogue SJ (1927) 'Progressive lenticular degeneration'. *Medical Journal of Australia* 2:695-696.

Minogue SJ, Latham O (1945) 'Cerebellar degeneration with epilepsy'. *Medical Journal of Australia* 1:430-433.

Molesworth EH (1926) 'The leprosy problem'. *Medical Journal of Australia* 2:365-381.

Money A (1896) 'Epilepsies – cerebral paroxysms'. *Intercolonial Medical Journal of Australasia* 1:578-581.

Monson RBP (1926) 'The surgical technique of pneumoventriculography with an illustrative case'. *Medical Journal of Australia* 1:271-272.

Morgan F (1958) 'Obituary: Arthur Schuller'. *Medical Journal of Australia* 2:241-242.

Morgan I (1920) 'A review of four cases of syphilis of the nervous system'. *Medical Journal of Australia* 1:477-481.

Morlet C (1921) 'Hereditary optic atrophy as a possible menace to the community'. *Medical Journal of Australia* 2:499-502.

Morris J (1994a) *A directory of neurology in Australia*. Brisbane: Australian Association of Neurologists.

Morris J (1994b) *Neurology in Australia*. Brisbane: Australian Association of Neurologists.

Morris JN (1908) 'Hereditary cerebellar ataxia'. *Intercolonial Medical Journal of Australasia* 13:185-188.

Moss GC (1941) 'Meningococcal infections with special reference to meningococcal septicaemia'. *Medical Journal of Australia* 1:548-552.

Moss GC (1949) 'Encephalitis and encephalomyelitis'. *Medical Journal of Australia* 1:414-416.

Moss GC (1963) 'The mentality and personality of the Julio-Claudian emperors'. *Medical History* 7:165-175.

Murphy E (1924) 'Amyotrophic lateral sclerosis'. *Medical Journal of Australia* 1:10-11.

Newland H (1937) 'Obituary: Harry Swift'. *Medical Journal of Australia* 2:976.

Newman AK (1875) 'On insular sclerosis of the brain and spinal cord'. *Australian Medical Journal* 20:369-374.

Nicholson GA, Yeung L, Corbett A (1998) 'Efficient neurophysiologic selection of X-linked Charcot-Marie-Tooth families: ten novel mutations'. *Neurology* 51:1412-1416.

Noad KB (1933) 'Simulation of vascular disease of the geniculo-calcarine pathway by cerebral tumour'. *Medical Journal of Australia* 2:400-404.

Noad KB (1943) 'Head injuries'. *Medical Journal of Australia* 2:141-144.

Noad KB (1944) 'Uncinate epilepsy: the subjective symptoms of an attack'. *Medical Journal of Australia* 2:641.

Noad K (1975) 'Obituary: Oliver Latham'. *Medical Journal of Australia* 2:492.

Noad KB, Haymaker W (1953) 'Neurological features of tsutsugamushi fever, with special reference to deafness'. *Brain* 76:113-131.

Noble R (1926) 'The value of the ventriculogram in the localization of cerebral tumours'. *Medical Journal of Australia* 1:268-271.

Nowland HH, Hunter JI, Latham O (1924) 'Supra-pituitary tumour with Frohlich's syndrome'. *Medical Journal of Australia* 2:194-196.

Nye LJJ (1933) *Chronic nephritis and lead poisoning*. Sydney: Angus & Robertson.

Officer DM (1903) 'Case of disseminated sclerosis in a child'. *Intercolonial Medical Journal of Australasia* 8:347-349.

O'Hara HM (1893) 'A case of trigeminal neuralgia of five years' duration – curetting of Gasserian ganglion from cavum Meckelii'. *Australian Medical Journal* New Series 15:513-517.

Ouvrier RA, Nicholson GA (1995) 'Advances in the genetics of hereditary hypertrophic neuropathy in childhood'. *Brain Development* 17 (Suppl):31-38.

Parker LR (1938) 'Obituary. Alfred Walter Campbell'. *Medical Journal of Australia* 1:181-183.

Parker N (1958) 'Observations on Huntington's chorea based on a Queensland survey'. *Medical Journal of Australia* 1:351-359.

Parker N (1985) 'Hereditary whispering dysphonia'. *Journal of Neurology, Neurosurgery and Psychiatry* 48:218-224.

Parry D (1892) 'A case of hydatid of the brain'. *Australasian Medical Gazette* 11:315.

Paton RT (1894) 'On beri beri in New South Wales'. *Australasian Medical Gazette* 13:363-365.

Patrick R (1985) 'Fraud or medical genius'. In: *Horsewhip the doctor*. St Lucia: University of Queensland Press pp 194-204.

Pender MP (2012) 'CD8+ T-cell deficiency, Epstein-Barr virus infection, vitamin D deficiency, and steps to autoimmunity: a unifying hypothesis'. *Autoimmune Diseases*. 012:189096.

Penfold WJ, Butler HM, Wood IJ (1932) 'The aetiology of erythroedema (Swift's disease. pink disease, erythroedema polyneuritis, juvenile acrodynia, trophodermatoneurose), with special reference to blood culture'. *Medical Journal of Australia* 2:131-136.

Phillips G (1931) 'On the apparent diminution in skeletal muscle tonus following removal of the lumbar sympathetic trunk'. *Medical Journal of Australia* 1:628-632.

Phillips G (1937) 'Protein in the cerebro-spinal fluid: clinical significance and quantitative determination'. *Medical Journal of Australia* 2:179-181.

Phillips G (1939) 'Recent work in the study of epilepsy'. *Medical Journal of Australia* 1:922-924.

Phillips G (1951) 'Obituary. Geoffrey Trahair'. *Medical Journal of Australia* 1:100-101.

Pockley E (1915) 'Leber's disease (hereditary optic atrophy)'. *Medical Journal of Australia* 1:189-191.

Pockley FA (1891) 'Notes on a case of ophthalmoplegia acuta and double optic neuritis'. *Australasian Medical Gazette* 10:273-275.

Pridmore SA (1990) 'The large Huntington's disease family of Tasmania'. *Medical Journal of Australia* 153:593-595.

Prior GPU (1937) 'Syphilis and neuro-syphilis treated by electropyrexia'. *Medical Journal of Australia* 1:895-910.

Prior GUP, Jones SE (1916) 'Calcium and epilepsy: a preliminary report'. *Medical Journal of Australia* 1:199-203.

Read SJ, Pettigrew L, Schimmel L, *et al.* (1998) 'White matter medullary infarcts: acute subcortical infarction in the centrum ovale'. *Cerebrovascular Disease* 8:289-295.

Reeves E (1861) 'Clinical illustrations of acute softening of the corpus striata'. *Australian Medical Journal* 6:155-167.

Reid WL (1940) 'The use of histamine in the treatment of neuro-vascular headache'. *Medical Journal of Australia* 2:307-310.

Reid WL (1948) 'Studies on the tremor-rigidity syndrome: 1. Surgical treatment of human subjects'. *Medical Journal of Australia* 2:481-492.

Rennie GE (1895) 'Death after head injuries'. *Australasian Medical Gazette* 14:374-378.

Rennie GE (1897) 'Some recent work on the cerebellum and its connections'. *Australasian Medical Gazette* 16:575-578.

Rennie GE (1902) 'Three cases of meralgia paraesthetica'. *Australasian Medical Gazette* 21:446-448.

Rennie GE (1903) 'The physiology of voluntary movements'. *Australasian Medical Gazette* 22:135-141.

Rennie GE (1905a) 'Epilepsy: is it incurable?' Proceedings of the Seventh Session, Australasian Medical Congress:48-53.

Rennie GE (1905b) 'Some points in the treatment of chronic nerve disease'. *Australasian Medical Gazette* 24:359-363.

Rennie GE (1915) 'The influence of occupation on the localization of syphilitic nervous disease'. *Medical Journal of Australia* 1:375-377.

Rennie GE (1919) 'Exophthalmic goitre combined with myasthenia gravis'. *Medical Journal of Australia* 2:416-417.

Rennie GE (1921) 'The symptomatology of complete transverse lesions of the spinal cord'. *Medical Journal of Australia* 1:185-189.

Reye RDK, Morgan G, Baral J (1963) 'Encephalopathy and fatty degeneration of the viscera. A disease entity in childhood'. *Lancet* ii:749-752.

Reynolds JR (1861) *Epilepsy: its symptoms, treatment, and relation to other chronic convulsive diseases.* London: Churchill.

Rischbieth RH (1994) 'Neurology in South Australia'. In: Morris J, ed. *Neurology in Australia.* Sydney: Australian Association of Neurologists: p 90-93.

Robertson DG (2023) *E Graeme Robertson: physician, photographer, preserver.* Victoria, British Columbia: Tellwell Talent.

Robertson EG (1935) 'A clinical study of micturition'. *Medical Journal of Australia* 2:890-895.

Robertson EG (1936) 'Intracranial aneurysms'. *Medical Journal of Australia* 2:381-389.

Robertson EG (1938) 'Spinal arachnoiditis'. *Medical Journal of Australia* 1:1043-1047.

Robertson EG (1940) 'An examination of the olfactory bulbs in fatal cases of poliomyelitis during the Victorian epidemic of 1937–1938'. *Medical Journal of Australia* 1:156-162.

Robertson EG (1941) *Encephalography*. Melbourne: Macmillan.

Robertson EG (1946a) *Further studies in encephalography*. Melbourne: Macmillan.

Robertson EG (1946b) 'Toxoplasmic encephalomyelitis, with the report of two cases'. *Medical Journal of Australia* 2:449-452.

Robertson EG (1947) 'Some physical aspects of encephalography'. *Brain* 70:1-16.

Robertson EG (1949a) 'Developmental defects of the cisterna magna and dura mater'. *Journal of Neurology, Neurosurgery and Psychiatry* 12:39-51.

Robertson EG (1949b) 'Cerebral lesions due to intracranial aneurysms'. *Brain* 72:150-185.

Robertson EG (1952) 'Murray Valley encephalitis: pathological aspects'. *Medical Journal of Australia* 1:107-110.

Robertson EG (1954) 'Photogenic epilepsy: self-precipitated attacks'. *Brain* 77:232-251.

Robertson EG (1955) 'James Parkinson and his essay on the shaking palsy'. Royal Melbourne Hospital Clinical Reports 25:1-14.

Robertson EG (1957) *Pneumoencephalography*. 1st ed. Oxford: Blackwell.

Robertson EG (1959) 'A perspective of epilepsy'. *Postgraduate Medicine* 25:31-44.

Robertson EG (1967) *Pneumoencephalography*. 2nd ed. Springfield: Charles C Thomas.

Robertson EG (1968) 'John White, Surgeon-General to the colony'. *Archives of Neurology and Psychiatry* 5:1-18.

Robertson EG (1974) 'Investigation of intracranial tumours by pneumoencephalography'. In: Vinken PJ, Bruyn GW, eds. *Handbook of clinical neurology. Volume 16*. Amsterdam: North Holland: pp 530-621.

Robertson EG (1984) *Decorative cast iron in Australia*. Melbourne: Currey O'Neil.

Robertson EG, McLorinan H (1952) 'Murray Valley encephalitis: clinical aspects'. *Medical Journal of Australia* 1:103-107.

Robertson J (1860) 'Report on a case where a large tumour was discovered in the brain at the post-mortem examination'. *Australian Medical Journal* 5:37-42.

Robertson J (1881) 'Notes on two cases of hemiplegia'. *Australian Medical Journal* New Series 3:296-310.

Robinson HE (1939) 'Successful treatment of pneumococcal meningitis with "Soluseptasine" and "M&B693"'. *Medical Journal of Australia* 1:433-434.

Rocaz C (1933) *Pink disease (infantile acrodynia)*. London: Hopkinson. (translated Wood, IJ)

Romberg MH (1853) *A manual of the nervous diseases of man*. London: New Sydenham Society. Translated Sieveking, EH.

Ross-Lee L, Heazlewood V, Tyrer JH, Eadie MJ (1982) 'Aspirin treatment of migraine attacks: plasma drug level data'. *Cephalalgia* 2:9-14.

Royle ND (1924a) 'A new operative procedure in the treatment of spastic paralysis and its experimental basis'. *Medical Journal of Australia* 11:77-86.

Royle ND (1924b) 'The operation of sympathetic ramisection'. *Medical Journal of Australia* 11:587-590.

Royle ND (1927) 'The treatment of congenital spastic paraplegia by sympathetic ramisection'. *Medical Journal of Australia* 1:632-642.

Royle ND (1928) 'The sympathetic innervation of skeletal muscle'. *Medical Journal of Australia* 2:257-258.

Royle ND (1930) 'The treatment of blindness associated with retinitis pigmentosa: a preliminary note'. *Medical Journal of Australia* 2:364-365.

Royle ND (1932) 'The treatment of blindness associated with retinitis pigmentosa'. *Medical Journal of Australia* 1:111-116.

Royle ND (1933) 'The surgical treatment of disseminated sclerosis'. *Medical Journal of Australia* 1:586-588.

Royle ND (1935) 'A new treatment for anterior poliomyelitis and its experimental basis'. *Medical Journal of Australia* 1:486-488.

Royle ND (1937) 'The surgical treatment of spastic paralysis'. *Medical Journal of Australia* 1:979-982.

Rudall JT (1859) 'Case of cysticercus in the brain, with remarks'. *Australian Medical Journal* 4:161-166.

Russell KF, Bradley KC (1973) 'Obituary: Leonard Bell Cox'. *Medical Journal of Australia* 126:37-38.

Ryan G (1993) 'Professor Emeritus Sir Sydney Sunderland'. *Medical Journal of Australia* 159:828-829.

Sadka M (1980) Stroke disability, whose responsibility? Canberra. Australian Council for Rehabilitation of the Disabled.

Sadka M (1988) 'Moss, Gerald Carew'. In: McDonald GL, ed. *Roll of the Royal Australasian College of Physicians. Volume 1*. Sydney: Royal Australasian College of Physicians: pp 217-218.

Sawers WC, Thomson E (1935) 'Torulosis, with a report of a case of meningitis due to torula histolytica'. *Medical Journal of Australia* 2:581-593.

Schwieger AC (1994) 'Cox, Leonard Bell'. In: Wiseman JC, Mulhearn RJ, eds. *Roll of the Royal Australasian College of Physicians. Volume 2*. Sydney: Royal Australasian College of Physicians: pp 67-69.

Selby G (1956) 'Parietal lobe syndromes'. *Australasian Annals of Medicine* 5:89-100.

Selby G (1972) 'Subacute myelo-optic neuropathy in Australia'. *Lancet* i:123-125.

Selby G (1974) 'Obituary: Brian Turner'. *Archives of Neurology and Psychiatry* 11:248.

Selby G (1983) *Migraine and its variants*. Sydney: Adis.

Selby G (1988) 'Susman, Eric Leo'. In: McDonald GL, ed. *Roll of the Royal Australasian College of Physicians. Volume 1*. Sydney: Royal Australasian College of Physicians: pp 284-285.

Selby G, Lance JW (1960) 'Observations on 500 cases of migraine and allied vascular headache'. *Journal of Neurology, Neurosurgery and Psychiatry* 23:23-32.

Sewell SV (1920) 'Discussion'. *Medical Journal of Australia* 2:42-43.

Sewell SV (1926) 'Disseminated sclerosis'. *Medical Journal of Australia* 2:161.

Sewell SV (1937) 'Listerian oration'. *Medical Journal of Australia* 2:1019-1027.

Shallard B, Latham O (1945) 'A case of acute haemorrhagic leucoencephalitis'. *Medical Journal of Australia* 1:145-148.

Shields A (1889) 'Leprosy in Australia'. *Australian Medical Journal* New Series 11:274-282.

Simpson DA, Jamieson KG, Morson SM (1974) 'The foundations of neurosurgery in Australian and New Zealand'. *Australian and New Zealand Journal of Surgery* 44:215-227.

Sippe C (1938) 'Migraine from the allergic viewpoint: results of treatment in 105 cases'. *Medical Journal of Australia* 1:893-895.

Sippe C, Bostock J (1932) 'Some observations on bromide therapy and intoxication'. *Medical Journal of Australia* 1:85-90.

Smith ET (1920) 'A case of encephalitis lethargica'. *Medical Journal of Australia* 1:553-554.

Smith P (1873) 'On the treatment of epilepsy by large doses of bromide of potassium'. *Australian Medical Journal* 18:258-267.

Smith W (1871) 'On paralysis with apparent hypertrophy of the muscles'. *Australian Medical Journal* 16:161-171.

Southby R (1949) 'Pink disease, with a clinical approach to possible aetiology'. *Medical Journal of Australia* 2:801-807.

Spark EJS (1897) 'Notes on three cases of Friedreich's ataxy'. *Australasian Medical Gazette* 16:408-409.

Springthorpe JW (1886) 'Notes on twenty-one cases of epilepsy'. *Australian Medical Journal* New Series 8:101-112.

Springthorpe JW (1887) 'Treatment of epilepsy by removal of peripheral irritants'. *Australian Medical Journal* New Series 9:177-180.

Springthorpe JW (1888) 'Notes on fifty cases of epilepsy'. *Australian Medical Journal* New Series 10:3-6.

Stawell RH (1915) 'Huntington's chorea'. *Medical Journal of Australia* 1:245.

Stawell RR (1895) 'Two cases of Friedreich's disease'. *Australian Medical Journal* New Series 17:452-460.

Stawell RR (1919) 'Encephalitis lethargica'. *Medical Journal of Australia* 2:97.

Stawell RR (1920) 'Encephalitis lethargica'. *Medical Journal of Australia* 2:387.

Stawell RR (1923) 'Epidemic encephalitis'. *Medical Journal of Australia* 2:594-595.

Stewart-Wynne E, Jamrozik K, Ward G (1987) 'The Perth community stroke study: attack rates for stroke and TIA in Western Australia'. *Clinical and Experimental Neurology* 24:39-44.

Stoller A (1966) 'Obituary: Jacob Mackiewicz'. *Medical Journal of Australia* 2:1120.

Stoller A, Emmerson R (1969) 'General paresis in Victoria, Australia: historical study'. *Medical Journal of Australia* 2:607-611.

Sunderland S (1978) *Nerves and nerve injuries.* 2nd ed. Edinburgh: Churchill-Livingstone.

Sunderland S (1991) *Nerve injuries and their repair: a critical appraisal.* Edinburgh: Churchill-Livingstone.

Sunderland S (1994) 'The Cox-Trumble contribution to Australian neurology'. In: Morris J, ed. *Neurology in Australia.* Sydney: Australian Association of Neurologists: pp 99-111.

Susman E (1949) 'The treatment of neurosyphilis'. *Medical Journal of Australia* 2:829-831.

Susman E, Maddox K (1940) 'Guillain-Barre syndrome'. *Medical Journal of Australia* 1:158-162.

Sutherland JM (1981) *Fundamentals of neurology.* New York. Adis Press.

Sutherland JM (1989) *A far off sunlit place.* Brisbane. Ampion Press.

Sutherland JM, Eadie MJ (1980) *The epilepsies. Modern diagnosis and treatment.* 3rd ed. Edinburgh: Churchill-Livingstone.

Sutherland JM, Tyrer JH, Eadie MJ, Casey JH, Kurland LT (1966) 'The prevalence of multiple sclerosis in Queensland, Australia'. *Acta Neurologica Scandinavica* 42 (Suppl 19):57-67.

Swift H (1914) 'Erythroedema'. Transactions of the Australasian Medical Congress 10th Session:547-552.

Swift H (1917) 'A case of progressive lenticular degeneration'. *Medical Journal of Australia* 2:310.

Swift H (1923) 'Erythroedema'. *Medical Journal of Australia* 2:159-160.

Swift H, Bull LB (1917) 'Notes on a case of systemic blastomycosis – blastomycotic cerebrospinal meningitis'. *Medical Journal of Australia* 2:265.

Syme GA (1895) 'Case of tumour of the dura mater, pressing on the brain, successfully removed by operation'. *Australian Medical Journal* New Series 17:60-67.

Taylor RJ (1938) 'Muscular atrophies and dystrophies in childhood'. *Medical Journal of Australia* 2:889-892.

Tchiriew S (1879) Archives de Physiologie Normale et Pathologique 11: 89. Cited by Cobb S (1925) 'Review on the tonus of skeletal muscle'. *Physiological Reviews* 5: 518-550

Thompson JA (1898) 'On the history and prevalence of lepra in Australia'. *Intercolonial Medical Journal of Australasia* 3:65-77.

Thomson JRM (1898) 'Notes on two cases of peripheral neuritis following febrile diseases'. *Intercolonial Medical Journal of Australasia* 3:539-545.

Tiegs OW, Coates AE (1928) 'The sympathetic innervation of skeletal muscle'. *Medical Journal of Australia* 1:140-143.

Tissot SA (1840) *Traite des nerves et de leurs maladies.* Reprint of 1st (1778) edition. Paris.

Trahair G (1950) 'Some modern trends in electroencephalography'. *Medical Journal of Australia* 1:146-148.

Trahair G, Garven AK (1948) 'Electroencephalography: the localization of cerebral lesions'. *Medical Journal of Australia* 1:458-461.

Trumpy DE (1922) 'Epidemic encephalitis'. *Medical Journal of Australia* 2:282.

Turner AJ (1897) 'Lead-poisoning among Queensland children'. *Australasian Medical Gazette* 16:475-479.

Turner AJ (1908) 'Lead-poisoning in childhood'. Transactions of the Australasian Medical Congress 8th Session:3-9.

Turner EK (1946) 'Purulent meningitis in infancy and childhood: a twelve months' survey of the results of treatment with penicillin'. *Medical Journal of Australia* 1:14-18.

Tyrer JH (1993) *History of the Brisbane Hospital. A pilgrim's progress.* Brisbane: Boolarong Publications.

Tyrer JH, Sutherland JM (1961) 'The primary spino-cerebellar atrophies and their associated defects, with a study of the foot deformity'. *Brain* 84:289-300.

Tyrer JH, Sutherland JM, Eadie MJ (1981) *Exercises in neurological diagnosis.* 3rd ed. Edinburgh: Churchill-Livingstone.

Vajda FJE (2021) *We are our memories.* London. Austin McCawley.

Vajda FJE, Eadie MJ (2005) 'Maternal valproate dosage and foetal malformations'. *Acta Neurologica Scandinavica* 112: 137-143.

Vajda FJE, Hitchcock A, Graham J, Lander CM, Eadie MJ (2008)' Seizure control in antiepileptic drug treated pregnancy'. *Epilepsia* 49: 172-176.

Verco JC (1912) 'Paramyoclonus multiplex epilepticus of Unverricht'. *Australasian Medical Gazette* 31:77-80.

Vickers W (1921) 'The treatment of acute anterior poliomyelitis'. *Medical Journal of Australia* 1:396-397.

Vinken PJ, Bruyn GW eds (1975) *Handbook of clinical neurology. Volume 21.* Amsterdam: North Holland Publishing Co.

Von Bonin G (1970) 'Walter Campbell (1868-1937)'. In: Haymaker W, Schiller F, eds. *The founders of neurology.* 2nd ed. Springfield: Thomas: pp 102-104.

Wallace DC (1972) 'Huntington's chorea in Queensland. A not uncommon disease'. *Medical Journal of Australia* 1:299-307.

Wallace JAL, Latham O (1914) 'A case of sudden dementia from massive cerebral glioma of unusual nature'. *Medical Journal of Australia* 2:516-519.

Walshe FMR, Robertson EG (1933) 'Observations upon the form and nature of the 'grasping' movements and tonic innervation seen in certain cases of lesion of the frontal lobe'. *Brain* 56:40-70.

Watson JF (1911) *The history of the Sydney Hospital from 1811 to 1911.* Sydney: Government Printer.

Wehner V (2004) *A Melbourne doctor and his generation. Leonard Bell Cox, 1894-1976.* Melbourne. Leddicott Press.

Whitcomb WP (1862) 'Case III – epilepsy treated by trepanning – death'. *Australian Medical Journal* 7:41-42.

White AER (1949) 'Obituary: Sidney Valentine Sewell'. *Medical Journal of Australia* 1:666-669.

Wilcox RA, Winkler S, Lohmann K, Klein C (2011) 'Whispering dysphonia in an Australian family (DYT4): a clinical and genetic reappraisal'. *Movement Disorders* 26: 2404-2408.

Wilkinson HJ (1927) 'The Argyll-Robertson pupil: a contribution towards its understanding'. *Medical Journal of Australia* 1:267-272.

Wilkinson HJ (1929) 'The innervation of striated muscle'. *Medical Journal of Australia* 2:768-793.

Wilkinson JF (1920) 'Encephalitis lethargica'. *Medical Journal of Australia* 2:205-206.

Williams (1881) 'Intracranial aneurism'. *Australian Medical Journal* New Series 3:310.

Williams H, Macdonald WB, Callow V (1951) 'Pink disease: its relation to adrenal function and the value of salt and desoxycorticosterone in treatment'. *Medical Journal of Australia* 1:363-365.

Williams S (1937) 'Sydenham's chorea: its course and relationship to rheumatic fever'. *Medical Journal of Australia* 2:590-593.

Willis T (1683) *De anima brutorum.* (Two discourses concerning the soul of brutes). London: Dring, Harper and Leigh (Translated by Pordage, S).

Willis T (1684) 'Pathology of the brain and nervous stock: on convulsive diseases'. In: Pordage S, ed. *The remaining medical works of that famous and renowned* physician Dr Thomas Willis of Christ Church in Oxford, and Sidley Professor of Natural Philosophy in that Famous University. London: Dring, Harper, Leigh & Martyn: pp 1-89.

Wilson SAK (1918) 'Epidemic encephalitis'. *Lancet* 2:91.

Wilson SAK (1928) *Modern problems in neurology*. London: Edward Arnold.

Wolfenden WH (1994) 'Noad, Sir Kenneth Beeson'. In: Wiseman JC, Mulhearn RJ, eds. *Roll of the Royal Australasian College of Physicians. Volume 2*. Sydney: Royal Australasian College of Physicians: pp 241-244.

Wolff HG (1963) *Headache and other head pain*. 2nd ed. New York: Oxford University Press.

You R, McNeill JJ, O'Malley HM, Davis SM, Donnan GA (1995) 'Risk factors for lacunar infarction syndromes'. *Neurology* 45:1483-1487.

Young JA, Sefton AJ, Webb N eds (1984) *Centenary book of the University of Sydney Faculty of Medicine*. Sydney: Sydney University Press.

Youngman NV (1942) 'Some aspects of epilepsy'. *Medical Journal of Australia* 1:433-438.

Youngman NV (1945) 'Can epilepsy be cured? The results of treatment'. *Medical Journal of Australia* 2:332-335.

Appendix I

Minutes of the Inaugural Meeting of the Australian Association of Neurologists

MINUTES OF THE INAUGURAL BUSINESS MEETING OF THE ORIGINATING MEMBERS, HELD IN THE ANATOMY DEPARTMENT OF THE UNIVERSITY OF MELBOURNE AT 10AM, ON WEDNESDAY, 25 OCTOBER, 1950

PRESENT

Dr. Leonard B. Cox, M.D., F.R.A.C.P., M.R.C.P. (Edin.) of Melbourne, Dr. K.B. Noad M.B., Ch.M. (Syd.) F.R.A.C.P., M.R.C.P. (London), of Sydney, Dr. E. Graeme Robertson, M.D., F.R.A.C.P., F.R.C.P., of Melbourne, Dr. E. Susman; M.B., Ch.M. (Syd.), F.R.A.C.P., M.R.C P (London), of Sydney, Dr. J.J. Billings, M.D., M.R.A.C.P., M.R.C.P. (London), of Melbourne.

By unanimous agreement of those present as originating members, Professor S. Sunderland, D.Sc., M.D., B.S., F.R.A.C.P. of Melbourne and Dr J.A. Game, M.D., of Melbourne were admitted as originating members and joined the meeting.

APOLOGIES

Apologies were received from Dr. Gerald Moss, M.B., B.S., M.R.C.P. (London) of Perth.

The meeting was opened by Dr. Cox, who suggested that the order of business should be the election of officers and consideration of a constitution.

ELECTION OF OFFICE BEARERS

Thereupon Dr. Graeme Robertson proposed, and Dr. K. Noad seconded that Dr. Leonard B. Cox be elected President of the Association. This was agreed unanimously and Dr. Cox formally accepted his appointment. He thanked those present for the trust they had placed in him by electing him as their first President, and gave his assurance that he would help in any way he could to make the Association a success.

Dr. Cox then suggested from the Chair that the posts of Honorary Secretary and Honorary Treasurer be combined for the present, and called for nominations. Having been proposed by Dr. Graeme Robertson and seconded by Dr. K. Noad, Dr. John Game was appointed.

DRAFT CONSTITUTION

The President then submitted for the consideration of the meeting a draft constitution which he had prepared. He suggested that the essential provisions should be considered and decided by the meeting. The draft would then be circulated for the detailed consideration of members before submission to a legal firm. Finally, the permanent copies of the Constitution would be signed by the Originating Members and the Association registered.

The Chairman then called for discussion of the separate clauses of the draft constitution.

Clause I – Name. 'The Australian Association of Neurologists.'

Dr. E. Susman asked the President whether the alternative of 'The Association of Australian Neurologists' should be considered. Dr. Graeme Robertson mentioned the possibility of members who may not be Australians, and the former title was then unanimously adopted.

The remaining clauses of the draft, clauses II to XVIII, were accepted without discussion.

Dr. Graeme Robertson then moved that it be recorded in the proceedings of the Association that the Originating Members greatly appreciated Dr. Cox's work in forming the Association and preparing the Constitution. This was seconded by Dr. Noad and unanimously approved.

APPOINTMENT OF COUNCIL

The President said an *Ad Hoc Council* had been formed by Dr. Cox, Dr. Robertson, Dr. Noad and Dr. Susman.

Professor Sunderland moved that the *Ad Hoc Council*, including the elected Secretary and Treasurer, become the first Council. Dr. Billings seconded this.

Dr. Graeme Robertson proposed an amendment that Dr. Game be added to the Council as an elected member, apart from his exofficio membership as Hon. Secretary and Treasurer, thus conferring the right to vote in Council.

Professor Sunderland and Dr. Billings wished their motion to be resubmitted accordingly.

This was adopted by the meeting.

DINNERS

The President proposed that the cost of social functions should be shared by participating members. This would ensure an equitable distribution of costs when the Association met in any State with a small membership.

FINANCE

Dr. Cox announced an anonymous gift of £5.

Dr. Graeme Robertson proposed that initially the subscription be £1.1.0 per member per annum. Dr. Susman seconded this and proposed that the Associate

Members' fees be also £1.1.0.

Dr. Robertson agreed to incorporate this in the motion, which was adopted by the meeting.

MEMBERSHIP

Dr. Susman asked the President whether the terms of membership of the Association as defined in the draft constitution might be considered too exclusive of General Physicians who had some interest in neurology.

The President expressed the view that in order to attain the objects of the Association the existing provisions of the draft constitution allowed sufficient discretion in the appointment of members. He hoped, however, that the Scientific Meetings of the Association would be open to all who may be interested, and that guests would be invited to give papers and take part in the scientific discussions of the Association.

Dr. Robertson endorsed these views and added that he thought a high standard of membership should obtain.

It was agreed that the existing provisions of the draft constitution allowed sufficient discretion in these matters.

In the absence of any further business the President declared the meeting closed at about 10.55 a.m.

Confirmed this 10th day of April 1951.

Leonard B Cox
President.

Appendix II

Programmes of the Early Scientific Meetings of the Australian Association of Neurologists

[the original spellings are reproduced]

INAUGURAL SCIENTIFIC MEETING OF THE ASSOCIATION HELD IN THE ANATOMY SCHOOL, UNIVERSITY OF MELBOURNE, on 25 OCTOBER 1950

The following papers were presented:

The Capacity of Muscles to Function Efficiently following Reinnervation After Prolonged Denervation, Professor S. Sunderland

The Deformation of Nerves, Dr. K. Bradley

Psychogenic Impotence, Dr. E. Susman

Brief Attacks of Muscular Weakness of Endocrine Origin, Dr. E. Graeme Robertson

Cavitation of the Brainstem and Basal Ganglia (Syringoencephalia), Dr. Leonard B. Cox

The Differential Filling of Arteriovenous Malformations by Arteriography of the Internal Carotid of the Same and Opposite Sides, and of the External Carotid and The Blood Supply of the Brain after Carotid Ligation Demonstrated by Angiography, Dr. John A. Game, Dr. H. Luke

SCIENTIFIC MEETING OF THE ASSOCIATION HELD IN THE MAITLAND LECTURE THEATRE OF SYDNEY HOSPITAL, on TUESDAY, 10 APRIL 1951

The following papers were presented:

Peripheral Neuritis and Bronchial Carcinoma, Mr. Gilbert Phillips

HallevordenSpatz Disease and its Relation to Wilson's Disease, Dr. Leonard B. Cox

Lesions of Nerves in Typhus and their Pathology, Dr. K.B. Noad

What a Cerebellar Section might reveal, Dr. Oliver Latham

Some unusual Subdural Haematomas, Dr. John A. Game

Examination of Twins Joined at the Vertex, Dr. E. Graeme Robertson

SCIENTIFIC MEETING OF THE ASSOCIATION HELD AT THE ANATOMY SCHOo(L), UNIVERSITY OF MELBOURNE, ON MONDAY, 16 MARCH1953

The following papers were presented:

A Short Review of the Work of a New Neurological Diagnostic Centre in Sydney, Dr. E. Susman

Case Reports: (1) Leprosy , (2) Unilateral Proptosis, Dr. John Billings

Report of the First Thousand Electroencephalograms at the Alfred Hospital, Dr. John A. Game

The Heart in Friedreich's Ataxia: Short Case, Dr. K. Noad

Injury in the Congenitally Diseased Spinal Cord, Dr. Leonard B. Cox

The Parietal Lobe, Dr. McDonald Critchley

Self Induced Photic Epilepsy, Dr. E. Graeme Robertson

SCIENTIFIC MEETING OF THE ASSOCIATION HELD AT THE SYDNEY GENERAL HOSPITAL, SYDNEY ON THE 12 OCTOBER, 1954

The following papers were presented:

Migraine – A Clinical Study of 250 cases, Dr. G. Selby

The Clinical Importance of the Brain Stem and Thalamic Reticular Formation, Dr. L. Rail

A Clinical Survey of Optic Atrophy, Dr. J. Billings

Permanent Paralysis in Myasthenia, Dr. K. Noad

Myasthenia Gravis and Pulmonary Lesions, Dr. L. Cox

A Case of Thyrotoxicosis, Exophthalmic Opthalmoplegia and Myasthenia Gravis, Dr. J. Game

The Use of Encephalography in Suprasellar Tumours, Dr. E. Graeme Robertson

SCIENTIFIC MEETING OF THE ASSOCIATION HELD AT THE ANATOMY SCHO0L UNIVERSITY OF MELBOURNE, ON SATURDAY, 15 OCTOBER 1955

The following papers were presented:

An unusual case of Spinal Cord Disease, Dr. J. Game & Dr. Ross Anderson

Carcinomatous Neuropathy, Dr. J.J. Billings

Internal Carotid Thrombosis, Dr. George Selby & Dr. Brian Turner

Cystic pineal glands, and long suprapineal recess, Dr. E. Graeme Robertson

Infection of Tumours of the Pituitary Region, Dr. Leonard B. Cox

Some aspects of Status Epilepticus, Dr. Leonard Rail

SCIENTIFIC MEETING OF THE ASSOCIATION HELD AT THE SYDNEY GENERAL HOSPITAL, SYDNEY ON THE 17 OCTOBER 1957

The following papers were presented:

Speech Development and Hemispherectomy, Dr. L.S. Basser

A Group of Cases of Cerebral Embolism, Dr. John Billings

Ulnar Symptoms in Cortical Lesions, Dr. John Gordon

A film Depicting some wellknown Neurologists, Dr. E. Graeme Robertson

Trigeminal Nerve Lesions, Sir Geoffrey Jefferson

SCIENTIFIC MEETING OF THE ASSOCIATION HELD IN THE MAITLAND LECTURE HALL, SYDNEY HOSPITAL, on WEDNESDAY 4 JUNE and FRIDAY 6 JUNE 1958

A Symposium on the subject of the management of CerebroVascular Disease included the following papers:

Experiences with LongTerm Anticoagulant Therapy in C.V.D., Dr. G. Selby

Two Cases of Internal Carotid Artery Syndrome, Dr. J.J. Billings

Basilar Artery Syndrome, Dr. W. Burke

Treatment of Recurrent Attacks Suggestive of Localised Cerebral Ischaemia by Cervical Sympathectomy, Dr. Graeme Robertson

Some Aspects of Collateral Cerebral Circulation, Dr. John A. Game

Friday 6th June, 1958.

The following papers were presented:

Familial Polyneuritis with Four Generations of Pes Cavus, Dr. J.W. Lance

Sensory Neuropathy, Dr. L.S. Basser

Necrotic Myelitis, Dr. J.L. Allsop & Dr. Brian Turner

Episodic Behaviour Disorders in Childhood, Dr. E. Davis

A Case of Kinnier Wilson's Disease, Dr. John A. Game

Severe Torula Meningitis, Dr. G. Selby

SCIENTIFIC MEETING OF THE ASSOCIATION HELD IN THE MEDICAL SCHOOL, FROME ROAD, ADELAIDE, on TUESDAY 26 MAY 1959

The following papers were presented:

Failure of Initial Investigations to Disclose Cerebral Tumour later proven, Dr. George Selby

The Radiological Demonstration of the Full Length of the Carotid and Vertebral Arteries, Dr. H.A. Luke

Steroid Therapy of Encephalomyelitis. (Cancelled due to illness), Dr. W. Burke

Neurological Manifestations of Methyl Bromide Poisoning, Dr. P.J. Landy

Cerebellar Atrophy Associated with Alcoholism, Dr. Brian Turner

SubAcute Inclusion Encephalitis, Dr. J.V. Gordon

Late Infantile Metachromic Leucoencephalopathy, Dr. Leon Basser & Dr. Brian Turner

A Case of Megalencephaly with Hyaline PanNeuropathy, Dr. R. McD. Anderson

Some Atypical Manifestations of Acoustic Nerve Tumour, Dr. Anthony Fisher

Upward Deviation of the Eyes, Dr. Arthur Schwieger

SCIENTIFIC PROGRAMME FOR THE PLENARY SESSION OF THE ROYAL AUSTRALASIAN COLLEGE OF PHYSICIANS' MEETING held in the ACADEMY CONFERENCE CHAMBER, CANBERRA on SATURDAY 17 OCTOBER 1959

CEREBROVASCULAR DISEASE

Introduction, Dr. L.B. Cox

Pathology, Dr. R. McD. Anderson

Difficulties in Diagnosis, Dr. K.B. Noad

Cerebral Ischaemic Attacks, Dr. John Billings

Management, Dr. W. Burke

Concluding Remarks, Dr. E. Graeme Robertson

SCIENTIFIC MEETING 0F THE ASS0CIATION HELD AT THE WOOD-JONES LECTURE THEATRE, ANATOMY SCHOOL, UNIVERSITY OF MELBOURNE on 24 MAY 1960

Anticonvulsants in the Treatment of Facial Pain, Dr. R.H.S. Rischbieth

The Neurophysiology of Kuru, Dr. L.R. Rail

On Cerebellar Localisation Using Positive Contrast, Dr. A. Fisher

Olivoponto Cerebellar Degeneration with Extrapyramidal Involvement, Dr. B. Turner

Familial Myoclonic Epilepsy and its Association with Cerebellar Disorder, Dr. J.W. Lance & Dr. K.B.Noad

Some Observations on Parkinsonism. (Thoughts and Questions About the Pathological Anatomy and Physiology of Certain Aspects of the Various Forms of Parkinsonism), Dr. G. Selby

The Symptomatology of Multiple Sclerosis Based on the Review of 555 Patients, Dr. J.M. Sutherland

Experimental Encephalomyelilis, Dr. R. Anderson & Dr. G. Szego

Recent experiences in the investigation and treatment of Temporal Lobe Epilepsy, particularly in relation to Surgery, Dr. Eric Davis

AUSTRALIAN ASSOCIATION OF NEUROLOGISTS SCIENTIFIC PROGRAMME

Thursday 31 May 1962

Dystonic Seizures: Striatal or Extrapyramidal Epilepsy, Dr. J. Lance

Some Aspects of Disseminated Sclerosis in Queensland, Dr. P. Landy

Progressive Multifocal Leukoencephalopathy – A Clinical and Pathological Study, Dr. M. Sadka

Acute Toxic Encephalopathy, Dr. R. Anderson

The Present Status of Immunization Against Poliomyelitis, Dr. J. Billings

The Stiff Man Syndrome, Dr J Allsop

Temporal Lobe Epilepsy: A Critical Review of Some Thirty Cases Submitted to Temporal Lobectomy, Dr E Davis

Visual Mechanisms and the Electroencephalogram, Dr. Ross Davis

Film: The Neurological Examination of the Newborn

Friday 1 June 1962

The Falling Attacks of Myoclonus, Dr J. Lance

The Suprapineal Arachnoid Body, Dr G.C T Kenny

Some Recent Laboratory Aids to Neurological Diagnosis Dr. B. Turner

Clinical Features of Obstruction of the Proximal Part of the Major Extracranial Arteries, Dr. G. Selby

Bypassing Vertebral Artery Occlusion by Extracranial Anastomotic Channels, Dr. J.A. Game

Observations on the Prognostic Signs Following Relief of Spinal Cord Compression, Dr. A. Fisher

Deep Sensibility, Prof. A. Mclntyre

Psychomimetics and Synaptic Transmission, Dr. D. Curtis

The Problems of Subdural Gas After Pneumoencephalography, Dr. E. Graeme Robertson

Film: The Neurological Examination of the One-Year-Old

PLENARY SESSION WITH THE ROYAL AUSTRALASIAN C0LLEGE OF PHYSICIANS held at the UNION THEATRE, UNIVERSITY OF SYDNEY, on THURSDAY 6 JUNE 1963

Evaluation of Investigation of the Nervous System, Introduction, Dr. E. Graeme Robertson

Evaluation of Pneumoencephalography. Dr. E. Graeme Robertson

The Scope and Limitations of E.E.G. Examinations in Clinical Diagnosis, Dr. Leonard Rail

The Value of Angiography in the Investigation of Cerebral Disease, Dr. George Selby

Motor and Sensory Nerve Conduction Studies as Applied to the Hand, Dr. Peter Ebeling

Laboratory Investigations of Mental Retardation, Dr. Brian Turner

SCIENTIFIC MEETING HELD IN THE MAITLAND THEATRE SYDNEY HOSPITAL on SATURDAY 8 JUNE, 1963

Discussion of the Reasons for Doing Lumbar Puncture, Dr. John A. Game

Activation of the E.E.G., Dr. George Preswick

Positron Scanning in the Diagnosis of Intracranial Lesions, Dr. Paul Farrar

An Evaluation of the Echogram in Neurological Diagnosis, Mr. Robin Lowe

By Invitation:

Cortical Biopsy in Childhood, Dr. Peter Ebeling & Dr. Ross Anderson

Total Cerebral Angiography, *and* Anterior Mediastinography in the Demonstration of the Thymus), Dr. W.S.C. Hare

By Invitation:

Experience with Cortical Biopsy, Dr. Mervyn Eadie

The Hyperkalaemic Type of Periodic Paralysis, Dr. John Allsop

Necrosis of the Brain in Newborn Babies, Dr. H.F. Bettinger

By Invitation:

Serotonin and the Nervous System: A Review, Dr. J.W. Lance

Experimental Demyelination, Dr. George Szego

Experiences with Myasthenia Gravis, Dr. Arthur Schweiger

Reading Epilepsy, Dr. John V. Gordon

Study of Vascular Malformation of the Brain, Dr. Anthony Fisher

Each paper was 20 minutes long and was followed by 10 minutes' discussion.

Appendix III

The Original Constitution of
the Australian Association of Neurologists

CONSTITUTION

OF

THE AUSTRALIAN ASSOCIATION OF NEUROLOGISTS

NAME

1   The name of the Association shall be 'The Australian Association of Neurologists'.

OBJECTS

2   The objects of the Association are –

(a) to bring together physician neurologists and scientific workers in the field of the nervous system and its diseases for their mutual benefit and for the better understanding of the nervous system and its diseases.

(b) to hold scientific meetings in which all matters pertaining to the nervous system and its diseases may be discussed.

(c) to provide special facilities for members of the Association.

(d) to assist as may from time to time be considered advisable in the publication of matter pertaining to the nervous system and its diseases.

(e) generally to utilise the funds and credit of the Association in any manner which in the opinion of the Council is conducive or incidental to the encouragement of the study or appreciation of the nervous system and its diseases.

ASSOCIATION PROPERTY

3   (a) the property of the association shall be vested in three trustees who shall be appointed and may be removed by the council. the council shall also have the right to fill any vacancy occurring by resignation, death, unwillingness to act or other reasons. the following powers shall be deemed to be vested in the trustees, and may be exercised by them, subject to the direction of the council, as hereinafter mentioned:

(i)   To invest money and adopt such measures as may appear to them necessary in the interests of the Association, subject to the approval of the Council.

(ii)   To purchase or otherwise acquire any land or property of any tenure which the Council may deem desirable for, or partly for, the purposes of the Association, at such price, on such terms and upon such conditions as the Council shall think fit, and to use the Association's moneys and funds for such purposes and to hold such property on behalf of the Association and the members thereof.

(iii) To sell and procure the selling of any property of the Association, real or personal, for such consideration, on such terms and upon such conditions as the Council shall think fit.

(iv) To let any part or parts of such lastmentioned property which the Council may think is or are not required for the purposes of the Association at such rent, for such term and upon such conditions as the Council shall think fit.

(v) To borrow and arrange for borrowing, either with or without giving security, such sum or sums of money as the Association shall be of the opinion may be required by it upon such terms and at such rate or rates of interest as the Council shall think proper, and for such purpose to give (if thought fit by the Council) such security or securities over any property, real or personal, held by or on behalf of the Association as the Council shall think fit, and adopt such other measures as may appear to them necessary in the interest of the Association, subject to the approval of the Council. All securities shall be taken and investments made in the names of the trustees the property the subject matter of the trust to be nevertheless subject to the disposition of the Council.

(vi) The powers aforesaid shall only be exercised by the Trustees in accordance with the directions of the Council and the authority in writing of a majority of those assembled at a duly constituted meeting of the Council and signed by the President of the day, and attested by the Honorary Secretary, shall be binding upon and a justification to the trustees as to any purchase, sale, investment, or disposal as aforesaid, or any exercise of such powers or any of them.

(b) (i) The income and property of the Association whencesoever derived shall be applied solely towards the promotion of the objects of the Society and no portion thereof shall be paid or transferred directly or indirectly by way of dividend bonus or otherwise howsoever by way of profit to the persons who at any time are or have been members of the Association or to any of them or to any person claiming through any of them. Provided that nothing herein shall prevent the payment in good faith of remuneration to any officers or servants of the Association or to any member thereof or other person in return for services actually rendered to the Association or for goods supplied in the ordinary way of business nor prevent the payment of interest on money borrowed or the payment of rent for premises let to the Association. If the Association is dissolved and there remains after the satisfaction of its liabilities any property whatsoever the same shall not be paid to or distributed among the members of the Association but shall be given or transferred to some body whose aims are conducive to the appreciation or study of the nervous system and its diseases selected by the Council and having objects which prohibit the distribution of its or their income amongst its or their members.

MEMBERSHIP

4 The members of the association shall be:

(a) The signatories to this constitution and any other persons who in addition to such signatories are hereinafter named as members of the council.

(b) Every person who may be admitted by the council to membership of the association as hereinafter provided.

5 Members shall be divided into the following classes, namely:

Ordinary Members.
Associate Members.
Honorary Members.
Provisional Members.

6 Candidates for membership shall be nominated by any ordinary member.

7 All nominations for membership shall be placed before the Council which may elect the applicant for membership or refrain from so doing. An applicant shall not become a member of the Association unless and until elected, and the decision of the Council on nomination for membership and as to the class of membership for which the applicant is eligible shall be conclusive.

8 In judging which applicants for ordinary or associate membership shall be elected the Council shall take into consideration its knowledge of the qualifications of the applicant in the practice of neurology, his general medical and other scientific qualifications and his contribution to the knowledge of the nervous system and its diseases.

9 The Council may elect any person to honorary membership.

10 The Council may elect as provisional members those who practice neurology and who do not hold senior neurological appointments at approved hospitals although this will not of necessity preclude them from ordinary membership, and who in the opinion of the Council may not adhere to the practice of neurology, or who for other reasons should not in the opinion of the Council be appointed as ordinary members. It shall be the practice of the Council to appoint a provisional member for a period of three years after which his appointment shall be reconsidered in the light of his known professional skill and such other qualities as may seem relevant to the Council.

TERMINATION OF MEMBERSHIP

11 Membership may be terminated:

(a) by written resignation

(b) by death

(c) by resolution of the Council pursuant to Rule 4 for nonpayment of subscription.

(d) by resolution of the Council pursuant to Rule 11.

12 The Council may by resolution suspend the membership of any member for such period as the Council thinks fit or may expel any member for any conduct which in the opinion of the Council is detrimental to the interests of the Association PROVIDED ALWAYS that no resolution for suspension or expulsion shall be passed unless the Council has given the member concerned an opportunity of showing cause against his proposed suspension or expulsion.

FEES AND CONTRIBUTIONS

13 The annual subscription shall be such sums respectively as are from time to time fixed by the Council of the Association but shall not be less than

(a) for Ordinary Members $1.1.0 per annum
(b) for Associate Members $1.1.0 per annum
(c) for Provisional Members $1.1.0 per annum

14 The annual subscription shall be paid in advance in the month of October in each year and shall be for the fiscal year 1st October to 30th September.

15 If any subscription is not paid within three calendar months after notification of election or after 31st October in any year membership may at any time thereafter be terminated by resolution of the Council.

16 The members shall be expected to assist the Association by their honorary work especially in technical and professional spheres.

17 Contributions or donations may be accepted from, members to supplement their annual subscriptions which are to be regarded as minima.

VOTES OF MEMBERS

18 Each Ordinary Member shall have one vote.

19 Votes may be given either personally or by proxy or by Attorney.

20 The instrument appointing a proxy shall be in writing under the hand of the appointer or of his Attorney duly authorised in writing. No person shall be appointed a proxy who is not an ordinary member of the Association. The instrument appointing a proxy and the Power of Attorney (if any) under which it is signed, or a notarially certified copy thereof, shall be deposited at the office not less than fortyeight hours before the person named in such instrument purports to vote in respect thereof but no instrument appointing a proxy shall be valid after the expiration of twelve months from the date of its execution.

21 A vote given in accordance with the terms of an instrument of proxy shall be valid notwithstanding the previous death of the principal, or revocation of the proxy, provided no intimation in writing of the death or revocation shall have been received at the office or by the Chairman of the meeting before the vote is given.

22   Every instrument of proxy, whether for a specified meeting or otherwise shall as nearly as circumstances will admit, be in the form or to the effect following

I _____ of _____ being an ordinary member of the Australian Association of Neurologists hereby appoint_____of_____ or failing him _____ of _____ as my proxy to vote for me and on my behalf at the (ordinary or extraordinary as the case may be) general meeting of the Association to be held on the ___ day of _____ and at any adjournment thereof. As witness my hand this ___ day of _____ 195 .

or in such other form as the Council may from time to time prescribe or accept. Any instrument of proxy deposited at the office in which the name of the appointee is not filled in shall be deemed to be given in favour of the Chairman of the Meeting to which it relates.

PRIVILEGES OF MEMBERS

24   The members shall be entitled to admission to all meetings and functions held by the Association.

25   The members shall be entitled to other privileges such as will be determined by the Council from time to time.

GENERAL MEETING

26   A general meeting shall be held once in each year commencing in the year 1951 unless in the Judgment of the Council such is not practicable.

27   The annual general meeting shall be called the Ordinary General Meeting. All other general meetings shall be called Extraordinary General Meetings.

28   The Ordinary General Meetings shall where considered practicable by the Council be held at the time of a scientific session of the Association.

29   The Council may whenever it thinks fit convene an Extraordinary General Meeting and shall convene an Extraordinary General Meeting on the requisition of at least ten per centum of the ordinary members.

30   Twenty-eight days' notice at the least specifying the place day and hour of any general meeting and in the case of special business the general nature of such business shall be given to members but the accidental omission to give notice to any member shall not invalidate the proceedings at such meeting.

PROCEEDINGS AT GENERAL MEETINGS

31 The business of an Ordinary General Meeting shall be:

(a) to receive and consider the report of the Council.

(b) to receive and consider the statement of accounts and the Auditor's report.

(c) to elect officers and other members of the Council.

(d) to transact any other business which ought under the Constitution or the Rules to be transacted at an ordinary General Meeting.

All other business transacted at an ordinary General Meeting and all business transacted at an Extraordinary General Meeting shall be special business⊠

32 No member shall be at liberty to introduce any special business unless he has given not less twenty-one days' previous notice in writing to the Council or unless he has the approval of the Council.

33 The quorum for a general meeting shall be thirty per cent. of the ordinary members of the Association present in person or by proxy.

34 The president shall be entitled to take the chair at every general meeting or if at any general meeting he shall not be present within fifteen minutes after the time appointed for the holding such meeting or is unwilling to act the Council may choose a chairman and in default of their doing so the ordinary members present shall choose one of the Councillors to be Chairman and if no Councillor present be willing to take the chair shall choose some one of their number to be Chairman.

35 Every question submitted to a meeting shall be decided, in the first instance, by a show of hands, and in the case. of an equality of votes the chairman shall, both on a show of hands and on a poll, have a casting vote in addition to the vote or votes to which he may be entitled as a member.

36 At any General Meeting, unless a poll is demanded by the Chairman or by at least five ordinary members present at the meeting, a declaration by the Chairman that a resolution has been carried, or carried by a particular majority, or lost, or not carried by a particular majority and an entry to that effect in the book of proceedings of the Association, shall be conclusive evidence of the fact without proof of the number or proportion of the votes recorded in favour of or against such resolution.

37 If a poll is demanded as aforesaid, it shall be taken in such manner and at such time and place as the chairman of the meeting directs and either at once, or after an interval or adjournment, and the result of the poll shall be deemed to be the resolution of the meeting at which the poll was demanded. The demand of a poll may be withdrawn. In case of any dispute as to the admission or rejection of a vote, the chairman shall determine the same, and such determination made in good faith shall be final and conclusive.

38 Associate members, Honorary members and Provisional members shall be entitled to notice of general meetings and to attend and speak thereat but shall not be entitled to vote.

POSTAL BALLOT

39 Whenever the Council thinks fit it may submit any question to the vote of all ordinary members by means of a postal ballot in such form and returnable in such manner as the Council decides. A resolution approved by a majority or specific majority of such members voting by such ballot shall have the same force and effect as such a resolution would have if carried by such majority or specific majority at a duly constituted general meeting competent to pass such resolution.

COUNCIL AND MANAGEMENT

40 The affairs of the Association shall be managed by a Council which may exercise all powers and do all things which are not by the constitution or Rules of the Association required to be exercised or done by a general meeting.

41 The Council shall consist of the President, Honorary Treasurer, Honorary Secretary and three other ordinary members. The offices of Honorary Treasurer and Honorary Secretary may be held by one person in which case there shall be four other ordinary members. No Associate or Honorary member or Provisional member may be a member of the Council.

42 The Council shall define the duties of the President, Honorary Treasurer and Honorary Secretary, who shall in all respects be subject to the control of the Council.

43 The first Council shall be

Dr. Leonard Bell Cox (President)

Dr. John Aylward Game (Honorary Treasurer and Secretary)

Dr. Kenneth Beeson Noad

Dr. Edward Graeme Robertson

Dr. Eric Leo Susman

and they shall hold office until the Ordinary General Meeting to be held in the year 1952.

44 The election of officers and other members of the Council shall take place in the following manner:

(a) Any two ordinary members shall be at liberty to nominate an ordinary member as a candidate for office or otherwise to serve on the Council. The name of each member so nominated shall be sent in writing to the Honorary Secretary twentyone days at least before the annual general meeting, accompanied by a letter from the candidate consenting to serve if elected.

(b) Notices of the names of the nominated members shall be sent to the members fourteen days at least before the ordinary general meeting. Balloting lists shall be prepared containing the names of the candidates only and each ordinary member present at the annual general meeting shall be entitled to vote for any number of such candidates not exceeding the number of vacancies. In case there shall not be a sufficient number of candidates nominated the Council shall fill up the remaining vacancies. If two or more obtain an equal number of votes, the Council shall select by lot from such candidates the candidate or candidates who are to be members of the Council.

45   At the Ordinary General Meeting in 1952 and thereafter at every succeeding ordinary general meeting onehalf of the Councillors or if their number is not a multiple of two then the number nearest to, but not exceeding one half shall retire from office and shall be eligible for reelection. The Councillors or Councillor to retire in every year shall be determined as follows:

(a) At the ordinary general meeting in 1952 by lot.

(b) And thereafter at every succeeding ordinary general meeting the Councillors or Councillor to retire shall be those who have been longest in office and for this purpose the length of time a Councillor has been in office shall be computed from his last election. In the event of it being necessary to decide as between two or more Councillors who were elected on the same day which of them should retire the question shall (in default of agreement between them) be determined by lot.

46   Any casual vacancy on the Council shall be filled up by the Council, and any member so chosen shall retire at the following annual meeting, but shall be eligible as a candidate for election on the Council at such annual meeting. The service of any member on the Council chosen to fill a casual vacancy shall not be reckoned in calculating the seniority of such member if subsequently elected to serve on the Council.

47   The Council may from time to time make, alter and repeal bye laws for the furtherance of the objects of the Association and generally for the good conduct of the affairs of the Association. Such bye laws shall, providing they are not inconsistent with the rules of the Association for the time being, be binding on all members and be construed as part of the rules of Association until they are rescinded or varied by the Association in general meeting.

48   The Council may meet together for the despatch of business adjourn and otherwise regulate its meetings and proceedings as it thinks fit and may from time to time determine the quorum necessary for the transaction of business. Until otherwise determined three Councillors shall be a quorum.

49   A member of the Council may at any time and the Honorary Secretary upon the request of a member of the Council shall convene a meeting of the Council.

50   The President shall be entitled to take the chair at every meeting of the Council or if at any such meeting he shall not be present within fifteen minutes after the time

appointed for holding such meeting or is unwilling to act the Council may choose a Chairman from one of its members.

51 Questions arising at any meeting of the Council shall be decided by a majority of votes. In case of an equality of votes the Chairman of the Meeting of the Council shall have a second or casting vote.

EXECUTIVE COMMITTEE

52 The Council shall have the power at any time to appoint an Executive Committee consisting of Honorary Treasurer and Honorary Secretary and any member or members of the Association.

53 The Executive Committee shall appoint one of its members to be Chairman.

54 The Executive Committee shall subject to any directions from time to time given by the Council exercise all the powers of the Council.

55 The proceedings of the Executive Committee shall be in accordance with the proceedings of the Council and the number of members to be a quorum shall be determined by the Council.

SPECIAL COMMITTEES

56 The Council may from time to time appoint and delegate any of its powers to special committees upon and subject to such conditions as the Council thinks proper in relation to such matters as the Council determines.

57 Any person whether a member of the Association or not shall be eligible for appointment to a special committee.

58 Cheques and other negotiable instruments shall be drawn made signed and endorsed in such manner as the Council or Executive Committee from time to time directs.

ALTERATION OF CONSTITUTION

59 The Council may from time to time alter or amend this Constitution by a resolution passed by a majority of not less than two thirds of the ordinary members of the Council present and voting at the meeting at which such resolution is proposed, but no such resolution shall be proposed at any meeting of the Council unless not less than twentyeight days' notice of such resolution has been given to each member of the Council.

NOTICES

60 Any notice to members may be given by advertisement published in an authorised Medical Journal circulating in Australia or by posting the same by prepaid letter addressed to members at their respective addresses appearing in the Association's records.

Appendix IV

Amendments to the Constitution Made in 1961

ARTICLES 4–10A ALTERED TO READ

4   THE members of the Association shall be

(a)   The signatories to this Constitution and any other persons (male or female) who in addition to such signatories are hereinafter named as members of the Council.

(b)   Every person (male or female) who may be admitted by the Council to membership of the Association as hereinafter provided.

For the purposes of interpretation in this Constitution the masculine shall include the feminine.

5   MEMBERS shall be divided into the following classes, namely

Ordinary Members

Associate Members

Honorary Members

Provisional Members

6   CANDIDATES for membership shall be nominated by any two members, one as proposer and one as seconder. The proposer and seconder shall request a member of Council to act as sponsor. The sponsor shall present the nomination for membership at the Council Meeting at which it is considered. The proposer or seconder shall act as guarantor to the sponsor for the identity of the candidate and for the substantiation of the candidate's qualifications for membership as hereinafter prescribed. The proposer and seconder shall provide the sponsor with the candidates' curriculum vitae, including his present occupation and appointments and the relative amount of time devoted to the various occupations and appointments.

The sponsor shall submit the application together with qualifications and curriculum vitae and guarantee to the Honorary Secretary twentyeight days at least before the next Council Meeting so as to enable inclusion of. the nomination in the agenda for the Council Meeting and circulation of details of the candidate to other Council members if so desired. The proposer and seconder may if they wish suggest the suitable category of membership for the candidate.

7   Council may elect the applicant for membership, or refrain from so doing. An applicant shall not become a member of the Association unless and until elected, and the decision of the Council on Nomination for membership and as to the class of membership for which the applicant is eligible shall be conclusive.

8   AFTER the Nineteenth day of May 1961 the Council may elect to Ordinary Membership any candidate who

(a)

(i) Is either a graduate of a Faculty of Medicine already existing in one of the Universities in Australia in the year 1960 or in a Faculty of Medicine established after that date in any University in Australia and which in the opinion of the Council establishes a standard of the Faculties of Medicine in those Universities already established in Australia.

(ii) Who holds the Degree of Doctor of Medicine in one of the abovementioned Universities and/or is a Fellow or Member of the Royal College of Physicians of London or of the Royal Australasian College of Physicians or any other British Royal College of Physicians approved by the Council.

(iii) Who has been engaged preferably as a house physician in a period of training of at least one year in the clinical practice of neurology including clinical responsibility for in-patients in either a special hospital or institute for the treatment of patients suffering from disease of the nervous system or in a clinic or department for the treatment of such patients in a hospital recognised by one of the abovementioned Universities as a teaching hospital of the University:

and

(iv) Who has been occupied in the practice of clinical neurology as a primary occupation for a period of at least three years and has the purpose and intention to continue that occupation as a career.

OR

(b)

Is a graduate of any Faculty in any one of the Universities mentioned in (a) who in the opinion of Council has achieved eminence and distinction as a result of his scientific contributions to the knowledge of the nervous system and its diseases and who is engaged predominantly in the scientific study of the nervous system.
Notwithstanding the possession of these qualifications by any candidate the Council shall retain the option of accepting or rejecting the candidate for membership.

9   The Council may elect to Associate Membership any candidate who is a graduate of the Faculty of Medicine in any of the Universities mentioned in Article 8 and who is not engaged in clinical practice as a primary occupation but who in the course of his work is especially engaged with problems relating to the nervous system and who in the opinion of the Council is by virtue of his proficiency, scientific qualification, or

contributions to knowledge, worthy of Associate Membership and is likely to make valuable contributions to the objects of the Association.

10   The Council may elect to provisional membership any candidate who is a graduate of any of the Universities mentioned in Article 8 (a) (i), (ii) and (iii) of this Constitution but who has not yet attained the other qualifications of Article 8.

It shall be the practice of the Council to appoint a provisional member for a period of three years after which his appointment shall be reconsidered by the Council who may retain the member in the category of provisional membership for a further period or appoint him to the category of Ordinary Membership providing he has fulfilled all the requirements of Article 8 or terminate his provisional membership on the grounds that the member has not or is not likely to adhere to the practice of clinical neurology as a primary occupation or for other reasons is considered unsuitable by the Council.

[At this time Articles 43, 44, 45 and 46 were also modified, but these deal only with the organisation of the composition of future Councils, specifying the pattern of retirement and replacement of Council members.]

Appendix V

First Editions of Medical Books Written or Edited by Australian Neurologists (whose names appear in bold type).

Year	Edited	Authors	Edns	Title	Publisher
1905		**Campbell AW**		*Histological studies on the localisation of cerebral function*	Cambridge University Press
1941		**Robertson EG**		*Encephalography*	Macmillam
1946		**Cox LB**, Tolhurst JC		*Human torulosis; a clinical, pathological and microbiological study, with a report of thirteen cases*	Melbourne University Press
1946		**Robertson EG**		*Further studies in encephalography*	Macmillan
1950	Ed.	King ESJ, Lowe TE, **Cox LB**		*Studies in pathology: presented to Peter MacCallum*	Melbourne University Press
1957		**Robertson EG**	2	*Pneumoencephalography*	Blackwell
1969		**Lance JW**, with **Goadsby PJ** in later editions	9	*Mechanism and management of headache*	Butterworth Heinemann
1969		**Sutherland JM**, Tait H, with **Eadie MJ** in 2nd edition	3	*The epilepsies: modern treatment and diagnosis*	Churchill-Livingstone
1972	Ed.	**Lance JW** *et al.*		*A symposium on `migraine and hypertension`*	University of NSW
1973	Ed.	**Kakulas BA**		*Clinical studies in myology*	Excerpta Medica
1973	Ed.	**Kakulas BA**		*Basic research in myology*	Elsevier
1974		**McLeod JG**, Sainsbury MJ, Joseph D		*Acupuncture: a report to the National Health and Medical Research Council*	Australian Government Publishing
1975		**Burke DC**		*Handbook of spinal cord medicine*	Macmillan
1975		**Lance JW**	2	*Headache: understanding, alleviation*	Scribner
1975		**Lance JW**	2	*Headache: its cause and treatment*	Butterworths
1975		**Lance JW**, with **McLeod LG** in later editions		*A physiological approach to clinical neurology*	Butterworth Heinemann
1976		**Tyrer JH, Eadie MJ**		*The astute physician*	Elsevier
1976		**Tyrer JH, Eadie MJ**		*Queensland University aphasia and language test*	Australian Council for Education Research

1976		**Tyrer JH, Sutherland JM,** with **Eadie MJ** in later editions	3	*Exercises in neurological diagnosis*	Churchill Livingstone
1978		**Sunderland S**		*Nerves and nerve injuries*	Livingstone
1979		**Eadie MJ**		*The Duke of Marlborough's headaches*	University of Queensland Press
1979		**Eadie MJ, Tyrer JH**	3	*Anticonvulsant therapy: pharmacological basis and practice*	Churchill Livingstone
1979		**Eadie MJ Tyrer JH**		*Neurological clinical pharmacology*	Adis Press
1979		**Lance JW**		*The prevention of migraine*	Compass Publishing
1980		**Balla J I**		*Pathways in neurological diagnosis*	Year Book Medical Publishers
1981		**Eadie MJ, Tyrer JH,** Bochner F		*Introduction to clinical pharmacology*	Adis Press
1981		**McLeod JG**		*Neurology notes*	Sydney Medical Students Society
1982	Ed.	**Broe GA**, Tate RL		*Brain impairment: Proceedings of the fifth brain impairment conference*	University of Sydney Medical Society
1982		**Eadie MJ, Tyrer JH**		*Biochemical neurology*	MTP Press
1982		**Kakulas BA**	2	*Man marsupials and muscle*	Univ of W A Press
1983		**Buchanan N**		*Childhood epilepsy*	Pitman
1983		Evans LE, **Eadie MJ,** Hollister L, **Tyrer JH**		*Drug use in psychiatry*	Elsevier
1984	Ed.	**Donnan GA, Vajda FJE**		*Problem areas in acute stroke management: proceedings of a workshop held at the Austin Hospital Melbourne, Australia*	Austin Hospital Neurology Dept
1984		**McLeod JG, Lance JW**, with **Davies L** in later editions	3	*Introductory neurology*	Blackwell
1985		Adams RD, **Kakulas BA**		*Duchenne muscular dystrophy: pathological foundations of clinical myology*	Harper Collins
1985		**Balla J I**	2	*The diagnostic process: a model for clinical teachers*	Cambridge University Press
1985	Ed.	**Donnan GA, Vajda FJE**		*Grey areas in epilepsy: proceedings of a workshop held at the Austin Hospital Melbourne, Australia*	Austin Hospital Neurology Dept
1985		**Eadie MJ, Tyrer JH**		*The biochemistry of migraine*	MTP Press

1985		Kakulas BA, Adams RD		*Diseases of muscle: pathological foundations of myology*	Harper & Row
1986		Bourne DWA, Triggs EJ, Eadie MJ		*Pharmacokinetics for the non-mathematical*	MTP Press
1986	Ed.	Dimitrijevic MR, Kakulas BA, Vrbova G		*Progressive neuromuscular diseases*	Karger
1986	Ed.	Ouvrier RA		*Controversies in childhood epilepsy*	Australian Association of Neurologists
1987		Buchanan N		*Epilepsy and you*	Williams & Wilkins
1987	Ed.	Lance JW		*Recent trends in the management of migraine*	Cantor
1987		Donnan GA, Berkovic SF, Vajda FJE		*Driving and epilepsy*	Austin Hospital Neurology Dept
1987	Ed.	Donnan GA, Vajda FJE		*Perspectives in stroke; proceedings of a workshop held at the Austin Hospital Melbourne, Australia*	Austin Hospital
1988		Bladin PF, Donnan GA, Vajda FJE		*Driving and epilepsy*	Epilepsy Society of Australia
1988		Donnan GA, Berkovic SF, Vajda FJE		*Stroke*	Austin Hospital Neurology Department
1988	Ed.	Lance JW		*Mind, movement and migraine: a 25 year review: Department of Neurology, the Prince Henry and Prince of Wales Hospitals, Sydney (1962-1987)*	Butterworths
1988	Ed.	Mastaglia FL		*Inflammatory diseases of muscle*	Blackwell
1989	Ed.	Balla JI, Gibson M, Chang AM		*Learning in medical school*	Hong Kong University Press
1989	Ed.	Bladin PF, Berkovic SF, Vajda FJE, Donnan GA		*Epilepsy Australia: blueprint for the 90s*	
1990	Ed.	Kakulas BA, Mastaglia FL	2	*Pathogenesis and therapy of Duchenne and Becket muscular dystrophy*	Raven Press
1991	Ed.	Procopis PG, Kewley, GD		*Current paediatric practice*	MacKeith Press
1991		Sunderland S		*Nerve injuries and their repair*	Churchill Livingstone
1991	Ed.	Vajda FJE, Berkovic SF, Donnan GA		*Epilepsy update*	Austin Hospital Neurology Dept

1991	Ed.	**Vajda FJE**, **Donnan GA**	*Grey areas in epilepsy: proceedings of a workshop held at the Austin Hospital Melbourne, Australia*	Austin Hospital Neurology Dept
1991	Ed.	**Vajda FJE**, **Donnan GA**	*Refractory epilepsy*	Austin Hospital Neurology Dept
1991		**Vajda FJE**, **Donnan GA**	*Deprenyl: current status, clinical and pharmacological aspects*	Austin Hospital Neurology Dept
1991	Ed.	**Vajda FJE**, **Donnan GA**, **Berkovic SF**	*Focus on epilepsy*	Austin Hospital
1992	Ed.	**Donnan G A**, Fabrini GCA, **Vajda FJE**	*Stroke for the 90's*	Austin Hospital
1992	Ed.	**Eadie MJ**	*Drug therapy in neurology*	Churchill-Livingstone
1992	Ed.	**Kakulas BA**, Howell M, Roses A	*Duchenne muscular dystrophy: animal models and genetic manipulation*	Raven Press
1992	Ed.	**Mastaglia FL**, Walton JN	*Skeletal muscle pathology*	Churchill Livingstone
1993		**Donnan GA**, Burton C	*After a stroke*	North Atlantic books
1993		**Lance JW** 5	*Migraine and other headaches: a practical guide to understanding, preventing and treating headaches*	Simon & Schuster
1993	Ed.	**Mastaglia F**, Byres C	*Inflammatory myopathies*	Bailliere Tindall
1993	Ed.	Thilmann AF, **Burke DJ**, Tymer WZ	*Spasticity: mechanisms and management*	Springer
1994		**Hankey GJ**, Warlow CP	*Transient ischaemic attacks of the brain and eye*	Saunders
1994		**Hodges J** 3	*Cognitive assessment for clinicians*	Oxford University Press
1994		**McLeod JG**	*Inflammatory neuropathies*	Elsevier
1994		**Morris J**	*Neurology in Australia*	Austn. Assocn Neurologists
1994		**Morris J**	*A directory of neurology in Australia*	Austn. Assocn Neurologists
1994		**Morris JGL** 2	*The neurology short case*	Hodder
1995		**Beran RG**	*Cost of epilepsy*	Ciba-Geigy
1995		**Beran RG** 4	*Learning about epilepsy*	MacLennan & Petty
1995		**Buchanan N**	*Pseudo-epileptic seizures*	MacLennan & Petty
1995	Ed.	**Donnan GA**, Nonving B et al.	*Lacunar and other subcortical infarctions*	Oxford University Press

1995	Ed.	Enoka RM, **Gandevia SC** *et al.*	*3*	*Fatigue: neural and muscular mechanisms*	Plenum Press
1995	Ed.	**Gandevia SC**, Proske U, Stuart DG		*Sensorimotor control of movement and posture*	Springer
1995		**Pender MP, McCombe PA**		*Autoimmune neurological disease*	Cambridge University Press
1996		Baloh RW, **Halmagyi GM**		*Disorders of the vestibular system*	Oxford University Press
1996		**Beran RG**	4	*Epilepsy and law*	Yozmot
1996		Pachlatko C, **Beran RG** *et al.*		*Economic evaluation of epilepsy management*	Libbey
1997		**Beran RG**		*Epilepsy: facts about fits*	MacLennan & Petty
1997		**Blessing WW**		*The lower brainstem and bodily homeostasis*	Oxford University Press
1997		**Davis S, Donnan GA**		*Interventional therapy in acute stroke*	Blackwell
1997		**Goadsby PJ**, Olesen J		*Increasing the options for effective migraine management*	Lippincott-Raven
1997	Ed.	**Goadsby PJ**, Silberstein SD	2	*Headache*	Butterworth Heinemann
1998		**Beran RG**		*Facts about fits*	MacLennan and Petty
1998		Silberstein SD, Lipton RB, **Goadsby PJ**	2	*Headache in clinical practice*	CRC Press
1999		**Beran RG**		*Epilepsy and driving*	Yozmot
1999	Ed.	**Berkovic SF**, Genton P, Hirsch E *et al.*		*Genetics of the focal epilepsies*	Libbey
1999	Ed.	**Eadie MJ, Vajda FJE**		*Antiepileptic drugs: pharmacology and therapeutics*	Springer
1999		**Ouvrier RA, McLeod JG, Pollard JD**	*2*	*Peripheral neuropathy in childhood*	MacKeith
2000		**Beran RG**		*Epilepsy: duty of care*	Yozmot
2000		**Eadie MJ**		*The Flowering of a Waratah*	Libbey
2000		**Eadie MJ**		*Wanderings in a borderland*	Black Swan Press
2000	Ed.	Henry TR, Duncan JS, **Berkovic SF**		*Functional imaging in the epilepsies*	Lippincott Williams & Wilkins
2001		**Bladin P**		*A century of prejudice and progress: a paradigm of epilepsy in a developing society*	Epilepsy Australia
2001		**Eadie MJ, Bladin PF**		*A disease once sacred*	Libbey
2001		Fenner F, **Curtis D**		*The John Curtin School of Medical Research: the first fifty years*	Brolga Press

2001		**Goadsby PJ**, Mathew NT, Wheeler SD		*Migraine prevention?: the role of AEDs*	Health Learning Systems
2001		**North K**, with Gutmann DH		*Neurofibromatosis type 1 in childhood*	MacKeith Press
2002	Eds	Asbury AK, Mackhann GM, **McDonald WI**, **Goadsby PJ**		*Diseases of the nervous system: Clinical neuroscience and therapeutic principles*	Cambridge University Press
2002	Ed.	**Beran RG**		*Epilepsy: a question of ethics*	Yozmot
2002		**Buchanan N**		*Understanding epilepsy: what it is and how it can affect your life*	Simon & Schuster
2002		Chappell B, Crawford P, **Eadie M**		*Epilepsy at your fingertips*	McGraw Hill Australia
2002	Ed.	**Donnan GA** *et al.*	2	*Subcortical stroke*	Oxford University Press
2002		**Goadsby PJ**, Dowson AJ, Miles A *et al.*		*The effective management of headache*	Aescapulean Medical Press
2002		**Hankey GJ**	*3*	*Stroke: your questions answered*	Churchill Livingstone
2002		**Hankey GJ**, Wardlaw JM	6	*Clinical neurology*	
2003	Ed.	Davis S., Fisher M, Warach S		*Magnetic resonance imaging in stroke*	Cambridge University Press
2003	Ed.	Olesen J, **Goadsby PJ**		*Cluster headache and related conditions*	Oxford University Press
2004		**Beran RG**		*Epilepsy and the law of therapeutics*	Yozmot
2004		Wehner V, **Eadie MJ**, Wehner MS (contributions)		*A Melbourne doctor and his generation*	Leddicott Press
2005	Ed.	**Goadsby PJ**, Silberstein S, Dodick DW		*Chronic daily headache for clinicians*	Decker
2005		Maddocks I, **Brew B**, **Waddy H**, **Williams I**		*Palliative neurology*	Cambridge University Press
2005	Ed.	Saver JL, **Hankey GJ**	2	*Stroke prevention and treatment: an evidence based approach*	Cambridge University Press
2007	Ed.	**Donnan GA**, Baron J-C, **Davis SM** *et al.*		*The ischemic penumbra*	CRC Press
2007		**Kiernan M**		*The motor neuron disease handbook*	Australian Medical Publishing Co
2007	Ed.	**Mastaglia FL**, Hilton-Jones D	4	*Handbook of clinical neurology – myopathies*	Elsevier
2007		Schapira AHV, **Byrne E** *et al.*		*Neurology and clinical neuroscience*	Mosby

2008		**Goadsby PJ**, Kernick D		*Headache: a practical manual*	Oxford University Press
2010		**Gates P**		*Clinical neurology – a primer*	Churchill-Livingstone
2010		**Goadsby PJ**, etc		*The changing face of chronic migraine: who to treat, how to treat?*	BMA Publishing
2011		**Beran RG**	*3*	*Neurology for general practitioners*	Churchill Livingstone
2011	Ed.	Dimitrijevic MR, **Kakulas BA**, McKay WB, Vrbova G	*5*	*Restorative neurology of the spinal cord*	Oxford University Press
2011		Varsavsky A. Mareels I, **Cook M**		*Epileptic seizures and the EEG: measurement, models, detection and prediction*	York Press
2012		**Eadie MJ**		*Headache through the centuries*	Oxford University Press
2012		**Morris JGL**, Jankovic J		*Neurological clinical examination*	Blackwell
2012		Pierrot-Desseillingy E, **Burke D**	*2*	*The circuitry of the human spinal cord*	Excerpta Medica
2012		Scott A, **Eadie M**, Lees A		*William Richard Gower, 1845-1915: exploring the Victorian brain: a biography*	Oxford University Press
2013	Ed.	**Beran RG**	5	*Legal and forensic medicine with 34 tables*	Springer
2013		Gorelick PB, Testai FD, **Hankey GJ**, Wardlaw JM	10	*Hankey's clinical neurology*	CRC Press
2014	Ed.	Chambliss J, **Cook M**, Healy J		*Epilepsy: perception, imagination and change*	Medical History Museum, Uni Melbourne
2015		**Eadie MJ**, **Vajda FJE**		*Antiepileptic drugs and pregnancy*	Springer
2015		Turner MR, **Kiernan M**		*Landmark papers in neurology*	Churchill Livingstone
2018	Ed.	**Brew B**		*Handbook of Clinical Neurology Vol 152*	Elsevier
2019	Ed.	**Hankey GJ**, Macleod PB, Gorekick CC *et al.*	*4*	*Warlow's stroke: practical management*	Wiley Blackwell

Appendix VI

Memberships of the Council, Australian Association of Neurologists

1950–1957
President: L B Cox *Secretary:* J A Game *Treasurer:* J A Game *Council Members:* K B Noad, E G Robertson, E Susman

1957–1959
President: E G Robertson *Secretary:* J A Game *Treasurer:* J J Billings *Council Members:* L B Cox, K B Noad, E Susman

1959–1961
President: E G Robertson *Secretary:* J A Game *Treasurer:* J J Billings *Council Members:* L B Cox, L R Rail, G Selby

1961–1963
President: E G Robertson *Secretary:* J A Game *Treasurer:* J J Billings *Council Members:* L R Rail, G Selby, G C Moss

1963–1965
President: E G Robertson *Secretary:* J A Game *Treasurer:* W J G Burke *Council Members:* L R Rail, G Selby, G C Moss

1965–1967
President: J A Game *Secretary:* P Ebeling *Treasurer:* W J G Burke *Council Members:* L R Rail, G Selby, G C Moss

1967–1968
President: J A Game *Secretary:* – *Treasurer:* W J G Burke *Council Members:* L R Rail, G Selby, G C Moss

1968–1969
President: J A Game *Secretary:* – *Treasurer:* W J G Burke *Council Members:* G Selby, G C Moss, J L Allsop

1969
President: J A Game *Secretary:* J B Morley *Treasurer:* W J G Burke *Council Members:* G Selby, G C Moss, J L Allsop

1969–1970

President: J A Game *Secretary:* J B Morley *Treasurer:* W J G Burke *Council Members:* G C Moss, J L Allsop, J M Sutherland

1970–1971

President: J A Game *Secretary:* J B Morley *Treasurer:* W J G Burke *Council Members:* J L Allsop, J M Sutherland, A C Schwieger

1971–1972

President: J A Game *Secretary:* J B Morley *Treasurer:* J L Allsop *Council Members:* J M Sutherland, A C Schwieger, G Selby

1972–1973

President: J A Game *Secretary:* J B Morley *Treasurer:* J l Allsop *Council Members:* J M Sutherland, A C Schwieger, G Selby, B A Kakulas

1973–1974

President: J A Game *Secretary:* J B Morley *Treasurer:* J W Lance *Council Members:* J M Sutherland, A C Schwieger, G Selby, B A Kakulas

1974–1975

President: G Selby *Secretary:* P M Williamson *Treasurer:* J V Gordon *Council Members:* M J Eadie, B A Kakulas, J W Lance, J G McLeod

1975–1977

President: G Selby *Secretary:* P M Williamson *Treasurer:* J V Gordon *Council Members:* D R Curtis, M J Eadie, B A Kakulas, J W Lance, J G McLeod

1977–1978

President: G Selby *Secretary:* P M Williamson *Treasurer:* B S Gilligan *Council Members:* D R Curtis, M J Eadie, B A Kakulas, J W Lance, J G McLeod

1978–1980

President: J W Lance *Secretary:* M Anthony *Treasurer:* B S Gilligan *Council Members:* D R Curtis, M J Eadie, J G McLeod, J P Rice

1980–1981

President: J W Lance *Secretary:* M Anthony *Treasurer:* B S Gilligan *Council Members:* D R Curtis, A G Fisher, J P Rice, J H C Walsh

1981–1983

President: J G McLeod *Secretary:* M Anthony *Treasurer:* B S Gilligan *Council Members:* D B Appleton, A G Fisher, J P Rice, J H C Walsh

1983–1984

President: J G McLeod *Secretary:* M Anthony *Treasurer:* J O King *Council Members:* D B Appleton, A G Fisher, J P Rice, J H C Walsh

1985–1987

President: B S Gilligan *Secretary:* R J Stark *Treasurer:* J O King *Council Members:* D B Appleton, D Burke, A G Fisher, R Rischbieth

1987–1990

President: J P Rice *Secretary:* C Kneebone *Treasurer:* J O King *Council Members:* D Burke, F Mastaglia, R Rischbieth

1990–1992

President: J King *Secretary:* C Kilpartick *Treasurer:* G Donnan *Council Members:* C Kneebone, F Mastaglia, J Morris

1992–1993

President: J King *Secretary:* C Kilpartick *Treasurer:* G Donnan *Council Members:* R Burns, W Carroll, S Davis, J Morris

1993–1996

President: J Morris *Secretary:* I Lorenz *Treasurer:* B Cant. *Council Members:* R Burns, W Carroll, S Davis, R Joffe

1996–1998

President: R Burns *Secretary:* J Willoughby *Treasurer:* B Cant, R Stark. *Council Members:* E Byrne, W Carroll, M Pender, C Storey

1998-2001

President: W Carroll *President Elect*: G Donnan (in 2001) *Secretary:* A Kermode *Treasurer:* R Stark *Council Members:* D Burke, M Horne, C Kilpatrick, C Storey

2001-2003:

President: G Donnan, *President Elect*: D Burke, *Secretary*: R Macdonell, *Treasurer*: R Stark, *Council Members:* H Dewey, P McCombe, M. Pender, E Storey, C Sue, P Thompson

2004-2005:

President: G Donnan, *President Elect*: D Burke, *Secretary*: R Macdonell, *Treasurer*: R Stark, *Council Members:* H Dewey, G Hankey, G Herkes, M Kiernan, P McCombe, M. Pender, E Storey, C Sue, P Thompson

2005–2006:

President: D Burke *Secretary:* M Kiernan *Treasurer:* G Herkes *Council Members:*
H Dewey, G Hankey. R Macdonnell, J Rodrigues, E Storey, C Sue, P Thompson
[P McCombe, J Morris, E Pepper]

2007:

President: D Burke *President Elect:* S Davis *Secretary:* M Kiernan *Treasurer:*
G Herkes *Council Members:* R Frith (NZ), G Hankey. R Macdonnell, J Rodrigues,
E Storey, C Sue, P Thompson [P McCombe, J Morris, N Crump]

2008:

President: S Davis *Secretary:* P Hand *Treasurer:* G Herkes *Council Members:*
R Frith (NZ), M Kiernan, J Rodrigues, E Storey, C Sue, P Thompson, [P McCombe,
K Parratt]

2009:

President: S Davis *Secretary:* P Hand *Treasurer:* G Herkes *Council Members:*
A Barber (NZ), R Frith (NZ), M Kielly, P McCombe, J Rodrigues, B Yan, [E Storey,
R Macdonnell, M Kiernan. D Field]

2010:

President: S Davis *President Elect* R Frith *Secretary:* P Hand *Treasurer:* G Herkes
Council Members: A Barber (NZ), M Kielly, P McCombe, J Rodrigues, B Yan,
[D Field, M Kiernan, R Macdonnell, E Storey, R Webster]

2011:

President: R Frith *President Elect:* R Macdonnell *Secretary:* A Barber *Treasurer:*
M Kiley *Council Members:* J Burrow, H Dewey, R Henderson, L Kiers, C Lueck,
M Nolan, K Parratt, R Stell, B Yan, [P Hand, C Mitchell, R Webster]

2012:

President: R Frith *President Elect:* R Macdonnell *Secretary:* A Barber *Treasurer:*
M Kiley *Council Members:* J Burrow, H Dewey, R Henderson, L Kiers, C Lueck,
M Nolan, K Parratt, R Stell, B Yan, [P Hand, C Mitchell, R Webster]

2013:

President: R Frith *President Elect:* R Macdonnell *Secretary:* A Barber *Treasurer:*
M Kiley *Council Members:* J Burrow, H Dewey, R Henderson, L Kiers, C Lueck,
M Nolan, K Parratt, R Stell, B Yan, [P Hand, C Mitchell, R Webster]

2014:

President: R Macdonnell *Secretary:* H Dewey *Treasurer:* M Kiley *Council Members:* A Barber, J Burrow, R Henderson, L Kiers, C Lueck, K Parratt, R Stell, B Yan, [T Dharmadasa, J Freemen, R Gerraty, P Hand,]

2015:

President: R Macdonnell *President Elect:* M Kiernan *Secretary:* H Dewey *Treasurer:* M Kiley *Council Members:* J Burrow, R Henderson, T Kimber, A Lee, C Lueck. K Ng, K Parratt, A Ranta, R Stell, [J Freeman, R Gerraty, P Hand, K Spira]

2016:

President: R Macdonnell *Secretary:* H Dewey *Treasurer:* M Kiley *Council Members:* A Barber, J Burrow, R Henderson, L Kiers, C Lueck. K Parratt, R Stell, B Yan, [T Dharmaadasa, J Freeman, R Gerraty, P Hand]

2017:

President: M Kiernan *Secretary:* S Vusic *Treasurer:* L Kiers *Council Members:* T Kimber, A Lee, C Lueck. K Ng, K Parratt, A Ranta, R Stell, M Tan, [A Barber, J Freeman, R Gerraty, A Ma]

2018:

President: M Kiernan *Secretary:* S Vusic *Treasurer:* L Kiers *Council Members:* T Kimber, A Lee, C Lueck. K Ng, K Parratt, A Ranta, R Stell, M Tan, [A Barber, J Freeman, R Gerraty, A Ma]

2019:

President: P McCombe *Secretary:* R Henderson *Treasurer:* L Kiers *Council Members:* T Kimber, T Kleinig, K Ng, J O'Sullivan, M Parsons, A Ranta, M Tan, B Taylor, A Van Der Walt, [R Gerraty, B Giarola, M Kiley, M Slee]

2020:

President: P McCombe *Secretary:* R Henderson *Treasurer:* L Kiers *Council Members:* T Kimber, T Kleinig, K Ng, J O'Sullivan, M Parsons, A Ranta, M Tan, B Taylor, A Van Der Walt, [R Gerraty, B Giarola, M Kiley, M Slee]

2021:

President: P McCombe *Secretary:* R Henderson *Treasurer:* L Kiers *Council Members:* T Kimber, T Kleinig, K Ng, J O'Sullivan, M Parsons, A Ranta, M Tan, B Taylor, A Van Der Walt, S Vusic, [C Belder, R Gerraty, K Parratt, M Kiley]

2022:

President: A Barber ***Secretary:*** N Child ***Treasurer:*** P Hand ***Council Members:*** L Giles, T Kleinig, D Mason. M Needham, J O'Sullivan, M Parsons, B Taylor, A Van Der Walt, A Wong, B Yan [R Gerraty. K Parratt, J Ravindran, J Tilling]

Appendix VII

Dates and Venues of Annual Scientific or Associated Ordinary Meetings of the Australian Association of Neurologists

Date	City	Venue
25 October 1950	Melbourne	Anatomy Dept, University of Melbourne
10 April 1951	Sydney	Sydney Hospital
16 March 1953	Melbourne	Anatomy Dept, University of Melbourne
12 October 1954	Sydney	Sydney Hospital
15 October 1955	Melbourne	Anatomy Dept, University of Melbourne
18 October 1957	Sydney	Sydney Hospital
4 & 6 June 1958	Sydney	Sydney Hospital
26 May 1959	Adelaide	Adelaide Medical School
17 October 1959	Canberra	Academy of Sciences
24 May 1960	Melbourne	Anatomy Dept, University of Melbourne
31 May & 1 June 1962	Canberra	John Curtain School of Medical Research
6 & 8 June 1963	Sydney	University of Sydney & Sydney Hospital
27–28 October 1964	Canberra	John Curtain School of Medical Research
11 May 1965	Melbourne	Royal Australasian College of Surgeons Building
16–17 May 1966	Adelaide	University of Adelaide
27–28 May 1968	Sydney	University of Sydney
26–27 May 1969	Brisbane	Physiology Building, University of Queensland
14–15 May 1970	Canberra	Australian National University
26 November 1971	Perth	University of West Australia
10–11 May 1972	Canberra	John Curtain School of Medical Research

24–25 May 1973	Adelaide	Hotel Australia
1-3 May 1974	Canberra	John Curtain School of Medical Research
16–18 April 1975	Sydney	Sydney Hospital
19–21 February 1976	Auckland	University of Auckland
23–25 March 1977	Melbourne	Royal Australasian College of Surgeons Building
16–18 May 1978	Hobart	University of Tasmania
16 May 1979	Brisbane	University of Queensland
23 May 1980	Canberra	Canberra Rex Hotel
26 May 1981	Adelaide	Gateway Inn
22 April 1982	Sydney	Sebel Town House
3 May 1983	Perth	University of West Australia
8 May 1984	Melbourne	Hilton Hotel
14 May 1985	Singapore	Meriden Hotel
5 May 1986	Hobart	Wrest Point Hotel
28 April 1987	Broadbeach, Qld	Conrad International Hotel
11 May 1988	Sydney	Menzies Hotel
2 May 1989	Adelaide	Adelaide Convention Centre
1 May 1990	Fremantle	Fremantle Hospital
7 May 1991	Hong Kong	Sheraton Hotel
2 June 1992	Melbourne	World Congress Centre
6 July 1993	Cairns	International Hotel
24 May 1994	Canberra	Hyatt Hotel
25 May 1995	Auckland	Sheraton Hotel
23 May 1996	Broome	Cable Beach Resort
1 May 1997	Sydney	Hilton Hotel
21 May 1998	Brisbane	Sheraton Hotel
25 May 1999	Hobart	Wrest Point Hotel
18 May 2000	Melbourne	Hilton on the Park Hotel
17 May 2001	Adelaide	Convention Centre
21 June 2002	Vancouver, Canada	Convention Centre
15 May 2003	Sydney	Convention Centre
10–14 May 2004	Perth	Burwood Convention Centre

2005	Sydney	Convention Centre – World Congress
1-5-May 2006	Canberra	Convention Centre
21–25 May 2007	Alice Springs & Uluaru	Convention Centre & Sails
19–23 May 2008	Brisbane	Convention Centre
20 May 2009	Christchurch	Convention Centre
17–21 May 2010	Melbourne	Melbourne Cricket Ground
16–19 May 2011	Hobart	Grand Chancellor Hotel
4-8 June 2012	Melbourne	Convention Centre (Asian & Oceanian Association Meeting)
6-9 May 2013	Sydney	Hilton Hotel
18–22 May 2014	Adelaide	Convention Centre
12–15 May 2015	Auckland	Convention Centre
24–27 May 2016	Perth	Convention Centre
9–12 May 2017	Gold Coast	Convention Centre
29 May–1 June 2018	Darwin	Convention Centre
21–24 May 2019	Sydney	Convention Centre
2020	Cancelled	
2021	Zoom meeting	

Appendix VIII

Contents of the Journals Published by the Australian Association of Neurologists from 1963 to 1994

*An * following the name of an author indicates that he or she was not a member of the Australian Association of Neurologists. [This identifying symbol was not applied consistently in the original versions of the meeting programs.]*

PROCEEDINGS of the AUSTRALIAN ASSOCIATION of NEUROLOGISTS

Volume 1 - 1963

Contents

Immunization against poliomyelitis in Australia, J Billings

By-passing vertebral artery occlusion by extracranial anastomotic channels, J A Game

Progressive multifocal leuko-encephalopathy, G Selby

The stiff man syndrome, J L Allsop

Some aspects of disseminated sclerosis in Queensland, P J Landy

A review of the features and treatment of temporal lobe epilepsy, with special reference to surgery, E Davis

Observations on the prognostic signs following relief of spinal cord compression, A Fisher

Acute encephalopathy in childhood, R McD Anderson

Deep sensibility, A K McIntyre

Cytogenic studies in mental retardation, B Turner

Psychomimetics – a neuropharmacological study, D R Curtis

Dystonic seizures: striatal or extrapyramidal epilepsy, J W Lance

The falling attacks of myoclonus, J W Lance

Visual mechanisms and the electroencephalogram, R Davis

Further observations of the suprapineal arachnoid body, G C T Kenny

The problem of subdural gas after pneumoencephalography, E G Robertson

Volume 2 - 1964

Contents

The insigne of the Australian Association of Neurologists

A comparative evaluation of pneumoencephalography in the diagnosis of cerebral neoplasms with and without increased intracranial pressure, E. Graeme Robertson

The scope and limitations of the electroencephalograph, L Rail

The value of angiography in the investigation of cerebral disease, G Selby

Laboratory investigation of mental retardation, B Turner

Discussion of the reasons for doing lumbar puncture, J A Game

The place of positronscanning in the diagnosis of intracranial tumours, P A Farrer

Activation of the electroencephalogram, G Preswick

Cortical biopsy in childhood, P Ebeling & R McD Anderson

Experience with cortical biopsy, M Eadie

Total cerebral arteriography, W S C Hare

Anterior mediastinography in the demonstration of the thymus, W S C Hare

Some experiences with cerebral vascular malformation, A Fisher

Hyperkalemic periodic paralysis, J Allsop

Some experiences with myasthenia gravis, A Schwieger

Reading epilepsy, J V Gordon

Serotonin and the nervous system: a review, J W Lance

Cerebral necrosis in newborn babies, H F Bettinger*

Experimental demyelination, G Szego

A contribution to the study of the extrapyramidal system: cerebellorubral pathway in the cat, R Davis

Volume 3 - 1965

Contents

The nature of dystonia, D. Denny Brown

Inhibitory systems in the cerebellar cortex, J C Eccles, R Llinás & K Sasaki

The nature of the representation of the visual fields in the lateral geniculate nucleus, P O Bishop

Tactile sensory pathways from the face, I Darian Smith

Agenesis of the corpus callosum-physiopathological and clinical aspects, M A Jeeves*

An auditory feedback system, involving the organ of hearing, Jürgen Fex*

The neuromuscular junction with special reference to myasthenia gravis, J I Hubbard

The myasthenic syndromes and their reactions, G Preswick

Perception of vibration, A K McIntyre

The mechanism of reflex irradiation, J W Lance

The effects of barbiturate anaesthesia and a muscle relaxant on an extrapyramidal centre: red nucleus, R Davis

Trigeminal neuralgia – a therapeutic trial of Tegretol, W J G Burke & G Selby

Are anticoagulants of value in disease of the extracranial and intracranial arteries?, P J Landy

Observations upon a predominantly sensory hereditary neuropathy, D C Wallace*

Subacute spongiform encephalopathy, R H Rischbieth

Cerebellar degeneration associated with chronic alcoholism, B Turner & J Allsop

Dietary Deficiency and experimental allergic encephalomyelitis, G Szego

The innervation of the mammalian pineal body, G C T Kenny

Aneurysms of superficial cerebral arteries, R McD Anderson

On chiasmal arachnoiditis with reference to the pneumographic diagnosis, A Fisher

The value of pneumoencephalography in pediatrics, E G Robertson

Volume 4 - 1966
Contents

Posttraumatic epilepsy, A Earl Walker*

Symposium on Muscle

Some historical and clinical notes, J A Game

Duchenne-type dystrophy: selective aspects of diagnosis and management, G Preswick

McArdle's disease: three cases in an Australian family, J F Hammelt, P Bale, L S Basser & F C Neale

Autoimmune aspects of myasthenia gravis, S Whittingham & I R Mackay*

Type and incidence of lesions found in a human necropsy survey of skeletal muscle, B A Kakulas & F L Mastaglia

The reflex effects of muscle vibration, J W Lance

Fine control of human muscular movement, D J Dewhurst*

Theme: Neurology and General Medicine

The association between diffuse sclerosis and Addison's disease, M J Eadie

Hypoglycaemia resulting from insulin secreting tumours of the pancreas, J M Sutherland, J H Tyrer & M J Eadie

The neurological manifestations of subacute bacterial endocarditis, J LAllsop

Free Papers

Studies in migraine, J W Lance

The early diagnosis of acoustic neurilemmoma, W H Wolfenden

Ultrasound in neurological diagnosis, E Davis

Four cases of subacute necrotizing encephalomyelopathy in childhood (Leigh's syndrome), R McD Anderson

Some aspects of the neuronneuroglia relationship, C P WendellSmith

The origin of brain macrophages in the rat, R McD Anderson, S Arumugam & G B Ryan

Some aspects of the development of knowledge of the pineal body, G C T Kenny

Immunological studies in experimental allergic encephalomyelitis and in multiple sclerosis with special reference to pathogenesis and diagnosis, G Lamoureux*

Viruslike particles in proximity to myelin in a case of progressive multifocal leukoencephalopathy, J M Papadimitriou, B A Kakulas & M Sadka

Volume 5 - 1968

Contents

Part One

Symposium I: The application of recent neurophysiology and neurochemistry to clinical neurology

Symposium II: Mental effects and disorders of behaviour in children

Mental defects and disorders of behaviour in children, Y Fukuyama, l Matsui &
    M Higurashi*

The contribution of constitutional chromosomal abnormalities to mental deficiency,
    A G Baikie, O M Garson & S M Weste*

The pseudoHurler syndrome, B Turner

Phenylketonuria, D B Pitt

Clinical and neuropathological observations in phenylketonuria, B A Kakulas,
    G I L Hamilton & F L Mastaglia

Temporal lobe epilepsy in childhood, R B Aird & D L Crowther*

Intellectual impairment and behaviour disorder in 500 epileptic patients, Tsupei
    Hung*

Intelligence in cerebral palsy, P E Bharucha, S Patel, E P Bharucha &
    P K MullaFiroze*

Congenital minor anomalies in mentally retarded children, M Arima, K Komiya,
    K Ono & K Hisada*

Neurological abnormalities in primary hyperammonaemia, I J Hopkins,
    J F Connelly, B Hocking & T G Maddison

The neuropathology of the 1718 trisomy syndrome, B A Kakulas, H R Trowell,
    G I Cullity, K A Hockey & P L Masters

Prevention of Wilson's disease in asymptomatic patients, M A Rima, K Komiya,
    A Fujisawa & K Matsuoka*

Electron microscopic findings in subacute sclerosing leucoencephalitis,
    J M Papadimitriou, S S Gubbay, J S Lekias & B A Kakulas

Part Two

Symposium III:Neurological cause of blindness

Modes of reaction to central blindness, M Critchley

Metamorphosia of macular origin, D M O'Day

Neural mechanisms concerned in the development of amblyopia ex anopsia,
    J D Pettigrew, T Nikara & P O Bishop

Cranial arteritis, W H Smith & J Billings

The sella turcica in spacetaking lesions, K Thumnoon, U Chaikittisil & J Edmeads*

The evaluation of presellar expanding lesions causing blindness, A Fisher

Optic neuritis, W J Burke

The diagnosis of visual failure in clinical practice, J J Billings

Benign amaurosis fugax of uncertain cause, M J Eadie

Difficulties in pneumographic demonstration of suprasellar lesions, E G Robertson

Symposium IV: Clinical and physiological lessons from stereotactic procedures

Clinical evaluation of thalamic surgery in cerebral palsy, H Narabayashi*

Clinical and physiological data obtained in stereotaxic surgery of the hypothalamus,
    K. Sano, M. Ogashiwa & H. Sekino*

Stereotaxic amygdalotomy, V Balasubramaniam, B Ramamurthi*

Successful operations in Parkinson's disease: observations on pathological findings, M C Smith*

The adverse effect of akinesia on the success of stereotactic surgery in Parkinson's disease, R S Schwab*

Cerebral atrophy in parkinsonism, G Selby

Cryosurgical thalamotomy, R G Robinson

Analysis of cogwheel rigidity, H Narabayashi*

Stereotaxic capsulotomy for epilepsy, S Kalyanaraman & B Ramanurthi*

A study of the fibre connections in the human substantia nigra, S Masuda*

Symposium V: Neurological diseases of regional interest

Kuru, R W Hornabrook

The central nervous system in kuru, R McD Anderson

A transmission model for kuru, J D Mathews

Recent studies of amyotrophic lateral sclerosis and

Parkinsonism-dementia on Guam, J A Brody & K Chen

Motor neuron disease in the Kii peninsula, Japan, Y Yase, N Matsumoto, F Yoshimasu, Y Handa & T Kumamoto*

Clinical features of demyelinating disease in Japan, Y Kuroiwa*

Multiple sclerosis in Australia, M McCall, T Le Gay Brereton, A Dawson, K S Millingen, J M Sutherland, J H Tyrer, M J Eadie & E D Acheson

Acute necrotizing inclusion encephalitis in Taiwan, WS Lin*

Cerebral paragonimiasis, J Y Shim & C S Park*

Neurological sequelae of antirabic inoculation, A Vejjajiva*

Neurological diseases in Korea, H K Lee & C S Park*

Neurological pattern in Singapore, A L Gwee*

A clinical study of cerebrovascular diseases in Djakarta, L ToenKiong & M Mardono*

Carbon monoxide poisoning in Korea, M W Kim & C S Park*

Absorption studies in neurological disorders, B D Pimparker, E.P.Bharucha & V P Mondlkar*

Symposium VI: Malignancy and the nervous system

Peripheral neuropathy and carcinoma, R A Henson & H Urich*

Aspects of chronic polyneuropathy associated with myeloma, J B Morley & A C Schwieger

Some comments on surgical and nonsurgical adjuncts to the treatment of intracranial tumours, E B Boldrey*

Brain perfusion for tumour: the effect of nitrogen mustard on brain adenosine triphosphate, B Woodhall & A P Sanders*

A malignancy involving the cranial nerves with a possible geographic distribution, M Mardono, S Supeno & S Markham*

Myelopathy following radiotherapy of nasopharyngeal carcinoma, T Hung*

Clinical study on metastatic meningeal carcinomatosis, K Takeuchi & Y Yahagi*

Neurologic manifestations in metastatic choriocarcinoma, T E Tupasi, E A de Veyra Jr, Central nervous system infiltration in acute childhood leukaemia, J A Corrie, J H Colebach, M S Rice & H Ekert

Part Three

Free Papers

Further observations on Tourette's syndrome, K B Corbin, J R Feild, N P Goldstein & D W Klass*

Neurological diagnosis of ruptured cervical discs, R M Stuck*

Specific neural stimulation for inhibition of pain, W H Sweet*

The posttraumatic syndrome in closed head injuries accident neurosis, P J Landy

Cerebrospinal pressure mechanisms and their clinical applications, R Gye & J Pennybacker*

Preliminary experience with ^{99m}Tc cerebral scanning, J B Morley

Displacement of the superior cerebellar artery in the diagnosis of the cerebello-pontine angle tumour, M Sato, K Yoda & M Tsuru*

Electroencephalography of cerebral paragonimiasis, C S Park*

Complications of tuberculous meningitis, C Suwanwela*

Computer analysis of cortical evoked potentials – application to agnostic syndrome study, Y Kuroiwa, M Kato & H Umezaki*

Staining tissues of central nervous system with lac dye, R Wanissorn*

Regional inhibition of brain monoamine oxidase measured by microscopic photometry, M J Eadie, J H Tyrer & J R Kukums

Treatment of congenital atlantoaxial disclocation, G Sinh & S K Pandya*

Haematomyelia during pregnancy: pathogenic discussion, B Q Huong, L D Hue & N Q Khanh (With the cooperation of N L Vien, N H Can, Lichtenberger & D H Anh)*

The function of the perineurium and its relation to the flow phenomenon within the endoneurial spaces, R Mellick & J B Cavanagh

Cranial polyneuritis–a distinct clinical entity, G S Ratnavale

Femoral neuropathy with abdominal pain, M Kase & E Hiyamuta*

The natural history of human muscle diseases studied by means of serial biopsy, F L Mastaglia & B A Kakulas

The detection of female carriers of pseudohypertrophic muscular dystrophy, BA Kakulas, J O Knight, S S Gubbay & F L Mastaglia

Muscle lesions associated with bony injuries, N C Anastas & B A Kakulas

Nervous system involvement in progressive muscular dystrophy, K Nakao, S Kito, T Muro, M Tomonaga & T Mozai*

The myocardinal lesions in the Rottnest quokka with nutritional myopathy, B A Kakulas, C G Owen, J M Papadimitriou & D T Durack

Retrobulbar neuritis in the state of South Australia, R H C Rischbieth

Febrile convulsions: a clinical and encephalographic study, M P Bhagat, N M Katie & A D Desai*

Hereditary kinaesthetic reflex epilepsy, Y Fukuyama & R Okada*

Application of electroencephalographic monitoring and intracarotid therapy in reiterative focal motor seizures, P F Bladin

A particular form of muscular inhibition in epilepsy: the related epileptic silent period (R.E.S.P.), C A Tassinari, H Regis & H Gastaut*

Gliomas and epilepsy, J B Morley

Spinal vascular malformations and their treatment, R N Chatterlee & R N Roy

An angiographic analysis of the cheirooral syndrome, G W Bruyn & J C Gathier*

Vascular changes in tuberculous meningitis – an arteriographic study in 33 patients, N H Wadia & B S Singhal*

Vascular disease with cerebral effects in young identical twins, J D Bergin

The effect of serotonin on cranial vessels and its significance in migraine, J W Lance & M Anthony

Migraine and methysergide – an appraisal, G W Bruyn & J C Gathier*

Application of the averaged photopalpebral reflex in clinical neurology, K. lnanaga*

Volume 6 - 1969
Contents

Admiral Lord Nelson's neurological illnesses, W Gooddy*

Introduction to the problems of dementia, W Gooddy*

Dementia in the adult due to occult hydrocephalus, K Lethlean & R Gye

Progressive dementia in childhood due to cerebral lipidosis, B S Gilligan

On meningioma presenting with dementia, A Fisher

Post-traumatic dementia, N Parker*

The major and minor hemispheres of the human brain, W Gooddy*

Outside time and inside time, W Gooddy*

Classification and treatment of myoclonus, J W Lance

Electrophysiological observations in a patient with segmental myoclonus, M J Eadie

Paroxysmal choreo-athetosis, C A Tassinari & R D Fine

Facial myokymia, J I Balla

Postvaccinial sensory polyneuropathy with myoclonus, I T Lorentz & J G McLeod

The natural history of Duchenne muscular dystrophy – an ultrastructural study, J M Papadimitriou, F L Mastaglia & B A Kakulas

Regeneration in Duchenne muscular dystrophy; histological electronmicroscopic and histochemical study, F J Mastaglia, J M Papadimitriou & B A Kakulas

Restricted forms of muscular dystrophy: a study of 11 cases, F J Mastaglia, J M Papadimitriou & B A Kakulas

A correlative clinicopathological study of spinal cord injury, B A Kakulas & G M Bedbrook

The blood vessel permeability of peripheral nerve during primary demyelination and the effect of A.C.T.H. therapy on the permeability and on the functional disability, R Mellick

A case of cerebral cysticercosis, J B Morley & K Langlord

The additional role of the scan in the diagnosis of cerebral tumours, J B Morley & R G Sephton

Experimental allergic encephalomyelitis, experimental allergic neuritis and multiple sclerosis: an electromyographic study, T A McPherson, Z S Kiss, G Robson, R L G Kirsner & D J Dewhurst*

Volume 7 - 1970
Contents

Dr. BrownSéquard in space and time, W Gooddy*

Aspects of diphenylhydantoin metabolism, M J Eadie, J H Tyrer & W D Hooper

Investigation of an outbreak of anticonvulsant intoxication, J H Tyrer, M J Eadie & J M Sutherland

Movement induced epilepsy: three case reports and comparison with a case of hemiballismus, J B Morley

Use of the ketogenic diet in epilepsy in childhood, l J Hopkins & B C Lynch

A comparative trial of serotonin antagonists in the management of migraine, J W Lance & M Anthony

A clinical trial of an antiserotonin drug, bc105, in the prophylaxis of migraine, G Selby

Monoamine oxidase inhibitors in the control of migraine, M Anthony & J W Lance

A critical review of the treatment of migrainous neuralgia, P Mann, J M Sutherland & M J Eadie

Central synaptic transmitters, D R Curtis

The effect of germine diacetate on neuromuscular transmission, S F Jones, J. Brennan & J G McLeod

Optic neuritis and its relationship to disseminated sclerosis, P J Landy & G D Ohlrich

Cryptococcal meningitis, J L Allsop, J G McLeod & R S Gye

Alcoholic neuropathy, J C Walsh & J G McLeod

The carrier problem in progressive muscular dystrophy, J O Knight & B A Kakulas

Electrophysiological and sural nerve biopsy studies in patients with Friedreich's ataxia and Charcot-Marie-Tooth disease, J G McLeod

The mechanism of the suppression of the monosynaptic reflex by vibration, J D Gillies, J W Lance & C A Tassinari

A neurological appraisal of autistic children: results of a Western Australian survey, S S Gubbay, M Lobascher & P Kingerlee

Differing cerebral scan characteristics of different pathological lesions, J B Morley, R G Sephton, L W Steven, J T Andrews & S N Cornell

The necropsy demonstration of cerebral aneurysms by intraarterial injection, R Rodda

Volume 8 - 1971
Contents

Memory, A K McIntyre

Kuru and Creutzfeld-Jakob disease: clinical and aetiological aspects, M Alpers & L Rail

Lymphocytic studies in kuru patients, M J Simons, M G Fitzgerald & M P Alpers

Myasthenia gravis and horror autotoxicus, E Davis

Non-progressive sensory neuropathy, R E Vlietstra & M Pollock*

Histochemical and biochemical studies in pseudohyperparathyroidism, M Pollock & J G Sneyd*

Further observations on an outbreak of diphenylhydantoin intoxication, J H Tyrer, M J Eadie & W D Hooper

Whole blood histamine and plasma serotonin in cluster headache, M Anthony & J W Lance

The influence of hormonal change upon migraine in women, B W Somerville

Abnormal prothrombin times in cerebrovascular disease, J B Morley, M Korman & W G Parkin

Oxidative enzyme activity in single neurones in relation to selective vulnerability to ischaemia, M J Eadie, J H Tyrer & J R Kukums

Clinical and pathological aspects of central nervous system involvement in the haemolytic uraemic syndrome, J C Rooney, McD Anderson & I J Hopkins

The use of immunosuppressive agents in peripheral nerve homograft surgery: an experimental study, J R Pollard, J G McLeod & R S Gye

In vitro destruction of human foetal muscle cultures by peripheral blood lymphocytes from patients with polymyositis and lupus erythematosus, B A Kakulas, G H Shute & J S Lekias

Thrombosis of the internal carotid artery after closed head injury, F L Mastaglia, S Savas, B A Kakulas & J S Lekias

The vascular lesions associated with cerebellar infarcts, R Rodda

Neuropathy associated with lymphoma, J C Walsh

Ultrastructural changes in the peripheral nerves in experimental dying-back polyneuropathies, J W Prineas

Onion bulb formations in chronic polyneuropathies, J G McLeod, J W Prineas & J C Walsh

An objective assessment of a gamma aminobutyric acid derivative in the control of spasticity, D Burke, J D Gillies & J W Lance

An electromyographic analysis of the clasp-knife phenomenon, D Burke, J D Gillies & J W Lance

The supraspinal control of the tonic vibration reflex, J D Gillies, D Burke & J W Lance

Different cerebral scan characteristics of different cerebral pathologies: double isotope scanning, J B Morley & R G Sephton

Volume 9 - 1973
Contents
Polymyositis: new light on pathogenesis and treatment, J N Walton*

The nature of syringomyelia: disease or syndrome? P Hudgson & J B Foster

Chronic neuropathies of infancy and childhood, J G McLeod & J W Prineas

Infantile polymyoclonia, J I Manson

Subacute myeloopticoneuropathy (SMON) – neurotoxicity of clioquinols, G Selby

Facial thermography in cerebral vascular insufficiency and migraine, J W Lance, M Anthony & B Somerville

Amode echoencephalography (experience with 1300 midline echos), J T Holland & G Kossoff

Familial amyotrophic lateral sclerosis, W H Wolfenden, A F Calvert, E Hirst, W Evans & J G McLeod

Tuberose sclerosis in childhood, J I Manson

Hyperkalaemic periodic paralysis associated with Addison's disease, A C Schwieger

Periodic megaphagia and hypersomnian example of the Kleine-Levin syndrome in an adolescent girl, B S Gilligan

Cerebrovascular 'moyamoya' disease, D J O'Sullivan

Limb kinetic apraxia (including case report), J Vernea

Dysaesthesiadyskinesia: a syndrome of painful legs and moving toes, J W Lance & C Andrews

Spinal cord cyst: case report, V E Edwards & G Merry

A case of cauda equina tumour presenting with stupor and papilloedema, W J Burke

Geomedical aspects of neurological cryptococcosis, J M Sutherland & V E Edwards

Pathological reflexes in presenile dementia – preliminary report, J Vernea

Subacute spongiform encephalopathy – a clinical and pathological study with attention to liver involvement, P M Williamson, W H Payne, G Selby & E Davis

The treatment of selfinduced photic epilepsy, L R Rail

Spasmodic torticollis, E Davis

Results of surgical treatment of the carpal tunnel syndrome, B Mendelson & J Balla

Studies on cerebral circulation in man indicating presence of neurogenic control, J L Corbett & B H Eidelman

Bicuculline, GABA and central inhibition, D R Curtis

Reconsideration of the role of serotonin in subarachnoid haemorrhage, K M A Welch, K Hashi & J S Meyer*

The explanation of the 1968 Australian outbreak of diphenylhydantoin intoxication, F Bochner, W Hooper, J Tyrer & M Eadie

Clinical implications of certain aspects of diphenylhydantoin metabolism, F Bochner, W Hooper, JH Tyrer & M Eadie

Incidence of hypertensive intracerebral haemorrhage in Thailand: an autopsy study of sixtyseven cases, P Tangchai*

Astrocytoma in Thailand: a study of 119 cases, S Shuangshoti & R Panyathanya*

Acromegaly: assessment and selection for treatment, L Lazarus*

Radiology of the pituitary, J Bull*

Pneumographic demonstration of suprasellar tumours, E G Robertson

Cervical spondylotic myelopathy: the use of one-radiography to select certain cases for surgery, K Bleasel, T J Connelley & N G Dan*

Timing of surgery for leaking cerebral aneurysms: clinical, radiological and radioisotopic considerations, T A R. Dinning*

Computerassisted radioisotope studies with the scintillation camera in cerebrovascular disease, R J O'Reilly, P M Ronai & R E M Cooper*

Volume 10 - 1973

Contents

Central nervous system dysfunction with open heart operations, I M Williams

Carotid sinus syncope, J L Allsop

Pathologic changes in the greater splanchnic nerve of subjects with diabetic peripheral neuropathy, CY Huang & J C Walsh

A standardized test battery for the assessment of clumsy children, S S Gubbay

Ocular motor apraxia in childhood, J I Manson

Familial spastic paraplegia, R H Rischbieth

Progressive supranuclear palsy (the Steele-Richardson-Olszewski syndrome):
  clinical and electrophysiological observations in eleven cases, F L Mastaglia,
  K Grainger, F Kee, M Sadka & R Lefroy

Huntington's chorea – the rigid form (Westphal variant) treated with l-dopa: a case
  report, P A Low & J L Allsop

Central pontine myelinolysis, M G Darke & B A Kakulas

Diphenylhydantoin dosage, M J Eadie, J H Tyrer & W D Hooper

Clonazepam – a clinical study of its effectiveness as an anticonvulsant, V E Edwards
  & M J Eadie

Clonazepam in the treatment of epilepsy, C Y Huang, J G McLeod, D Sampson &
  W J Hensley

An experimental animal model for the effect of ketogenic diet on epilepsy,
  D B Appleton & D C De Vivo

The pathogenesis of trigeminal neuralgia, G Selby

Plasma free fatty acid changes in migraine, M Anthony

A serial section study for Charcot-Bouchard aneurysms in hindbrain, G Caravella,
  P F Jacobsen & B A Kakulas

The effect of humoral agents on the cranial circulation of the monkey, P J Spira,
  K M A Welch & J W Lance

A radioimmunoassay for creatine kinase, G A Nicholson & W J O'Su!livan

Experimental autonomic neuropathy, E J Post & J G McLeod

Electromyographic studies of the orbicularis oculi reflex, J Vernea & T Horvath

Activity of motor neurones during isometric contraction, H Kranz &
  R von der Heydt

Unit analysis of the F wave, J L Veale & N D Hewson

Segmental reflex changes in acute and chronic spinal cats, J Hancock, L Knowles &
  D Gillies

Obituary – Gerald Moss

Volume 11 - 1974

Contents

Subarachnoid haemorrhage in children, D B Appleton, P J Smith & W J S Earwaker

Long segment stenotic lesions of cervical arteries in cerebrovascular disease,
  P F Bladin

Cardiovascular responses to prolonged headup tilting in tetraplegic man,
  J L Corbett

Cardiovascular responses to infused noradrenaline in tetraplegic man, J L Corbett

Cortical blindness with anosognosia: subsequent simultaneous agnosia and
  persistent gross recent memory defect, J B Morley & F N Cox

Neuroophthalmic deterioration after burns, Isla M Williams

Headaches occurring during sexual intercourse, J W Lance

Landry-Guillain-Barré syndrome: a clinical and electrophysiological followup study,
  J C Walsh, J G McLeod, J W Prineas & J D Pollard

Colchicine and the peripheral nerve, R Mellick, R Kirkby, A Tail Smith &
  G Ratnavale

Demyelination in the central nervous system of the cat studied by single fibre
  isolation, G D Ohlrich & W I McDonald

Sensory function of the median nerve: preliminary studies using micro electrode
  techniques in man, D Burke, N F Shuse & A K Lethlean

Hypothesis: a biological model of schizophrenia, V I Karlov

The Aicardi syndrome, G Wise & R Ouvrier

Pituitary fossa demineralization in normal subjects, L A Cala, J Black &
  D W K Collins

Neurophysiologlcal mechanism of acupuncture analgesia, J G McLeod

Subacute sclerosing panencephalitis: a study of 25 patients, P G Procopis

Giant axonal neuropathy – a third case, R A Ouvrier, J Prineas, J C Walsh,
  R D K Reye & J G McLeod

Genetic counselling in neuromuscular diseases in Western Australia, P V Hurse &
  B A Kakulas

A new myopathy with type II muscle fibre hypoplasia, Y Matsuoka, S S Gubbay &
  B A Kakulas

A neurophysiological analysis of paramyotonia congenita, D Burke, N F Skuse &
  A K Lethlean

Neurological features in Freon freakout, J R Moon & P F Bladin

Chuckling and glugging seizures at night – Sylvian spike epilepsy, P F Bladin &
  G Papworth

Selective vulnerability of the hippocampus to hypoxia; cytophotometric studies of
  enzyme activity in single neurones, J E Penny, J R Kukums, J H Tyrer & M J Eadie

Palatal myoclonus and associated movements, F L Mastaglia, K M R Grainger &
  B A Kakulas

Preliminary observations on the clinical pharmacology of carbamazepine
  ('Tegretol'), W D Hooper, D K Dubetz, M J Eadie & J H Tyrer

Side effects of clonazepam therapy, V E Edwards

Progressive myoclonic epilepsy. The response to sodium dinpropylacetate,
  E B Tomlinson

Visual hallucinations as a symptom of right parietooccipital lesions, J W Lance,
  B Cooper & J Misbach

Hypercalcaemia and epilepsy, I T Lorentz

Partial status epilepticus with speech arrest, J J Vernea

Epilepsy and the frontal lobe, P F Bladin & J Woodward

Social problems confronting a person with epilepsy in modern society, V E Edwards

Temporal lobectomy for epilepsy – a followup, E Davis

Obituary – Brian Turner

Volume 12 - 1975
Contents

The Australian Association of Neurologists – a review of twenty-five years, J Game

Geniculate hemianopias: incongruous visual defects from partial involvement of the lateral geniculate nucleus, W F Hoyt*

Certain neuroophthalmological aspects of multiple sclerosis, J M Sutherland

A family with Charcot-Marie-Tooth disease and Leber's optic atrophy, J G McLeod, P A Low & J A Morgan

Superior oblique myokymia, K M R Grainger & S S Gubbay

The low intracranial pressure syndrome, J J Billings, E J Gilford & J K Henderson

Mechanism in cerebral lesions in trauma to high cervical portion of the vertebral artery – rotation injury, P F Bladin & J Merory

Amine turnover in migraine, M Anthony & H Hinterberger

The headaches of phaeochromocytoma, J W Lance & H Hinterberger

Sodium valproate in the management of intractable epilepsy: comparison with clonazepam, J W Lance & M Anthony

Fluctuations of plasma phenytoin levels on single dose and twice daily dose regimes, F J E Vadja, J Merory & P F Bladin

Fibre function and perception during cutaneous nerve block, R A Mackenzie, D Burke, N F Skuse & A K Lethlean

Muscular dystrophy in young girls, B A Kakulas, P E Cullity & P Maguire

Autonomic disturbances produced by lung cancer: a report of two unusual cases, J C Walsh, P A Low & J L Allsop

Enteric coated levodopa in clinical practice, E P Hicks & M W O'Halloran

Frontal agraphia (including a case report), J J Vernea & J Merory

The surgical management of extracranial cerebrovascular occlusive disease: a review of 200 consecutive surgical cases, D A Horton, R Fine & R G Hicks

Reversible cortiocospinal abnormality in the alcoholic, C Y Huang, G A Broe & P G Procopis

Interactions between anticonvulsants, C M Lander, M J Eadie & J H Tyrer

Remyelination after transient compression of the spinal cord, B M Harrison, R F Gledhill & W I McDonald

The bioavailability of carbamazepine, L M Cotter, G Smith, W D Hooper, J H Tyrer & M J Eadie

Tay Sachs disease in a child and management of a subsequent pregnancy, D B Appleton, T J Gaffney, H McGeary & N J Nicolaides

The action of thalidomide on the peripheral nervous system of the embryo, J McCredie

Ocular complications of varicella, P.G. Procopis

Congenital deficiency of horizontal gaze, P.G. Procopis

The autonomic nervous system in alcoholic and diabetic neuropathy, P A Low, J C Walsh, C Y Huang & J G McLeod

A case of spontaneously resolving 'papilloedema', G Selby & G C Hipwell

Neuromyelitis optica following infectious mononucleosis, P M Williamson

Periodic alternating nystagmus, L de Silva, B P Cooper & J G McLeod

Opsoclonus with myoclonus, J T Holland

The ocular myasthenia syndrome, W G Burke

Familial cerebellar ataxia with sexlinked recessive inheritance, P J Spira & J W Lance

Microembolism and the visual system. Part II, I M Williams, N C R Merrillees & P M Robinson

The value of the brain scan and cerebral arteriogram in the Sturge-Weber syndrome, B McCaughan, R A Ouvrier, K de Silva & A McLaughin

The chiasmal enigma, B Hughes*

Obituary – Dr Oliver Latham

Volume 13 - 1976
Contents

Obituaries:
E Graeme Robertson
Henry Miller
Bryan Cooper

Pattern visual evoked potentials in the diagnosis of multiple sclerosis and other disorders, A L Hume & B R Cant

Evoked potential studies in neurological disorders, F L Mastaglia, J L Black & D W K Collins

Computerized axial tomography for intracranial diagnosis, L A Cala

Hereditary hypertrophic neuropathy in the trembler mouse: electrophysiological studies, P A Low & J G McLeod

Computerized axial tomography findings in a group of patients with migrainous headaches, L A Cala & F L Mastaglla

Neurophysiological aspects of peripheral neuropathies, R A MacKenzie, N F Skuse & A K Lethlean

Three cases of post traumatic vascular headache treated by surgery, J T Holland

The influence of previous stereotactic thalamotomy on l-dopa therapy in Parkinson's disease, G Selby

A unique case of derangement of vitamin B12 metabolism, M Anthony & A C McLeay

Epilepsy and driving, K S Millingen

Some aspects of tuberculous meningitis in Surabaya, B Chandra*

An animal model for the study of drugs in the central nervous system, G J G Parry

The effects of phenobarbitone dose on plasma phenobarbitone levels in epileptic patients, M J Eadie, C M Lander, W D Hooper & J H Tyrer

On the visual disturbances associated with massive basal aneurysms, A Fisher & R L Cooper

Progressive facial hemiatrophy (Parry-Romberg syndrome), R H C Rischbieth

Electrophysiological and pathological studies in spinocerebellar degenerations, J G McLeod & J A Morgan

The use of clonazepam in the treatment of tic douloureux (a preliminary report), B Chandra*

Serial nerve conduction studies in patients with maturity onset diabetes mellitus, G Danta

Measurement of cerebrospinal fluid IgG in the diagnosis of multiple sclerosis, E W Willoughby

Histamine receptor blockade with cimetidine in the monkey cranial circulation, G D A Lord, E J Mylecharane, J W Duckworth & J W Lance

Performance changes during recovery from closed head injury, D Gronwall*

The continual administration of neostigmine and the neuromuscular junction, J D Gillies & J Allen

Volume 14 - 1977
Contents

Transient ischaemic attacks, J P Whisnant

Postirradiation extracranial cerebrovascular disease, P F Bladin & J Royle

Tremor in alcoholic brain disease, S Bajada & A Fisher

A case of dacrystic epilepsy, C Y Huang & G A Broe

An investigation into reading epilepsy, G Danta, P J Dowling & S R Hammond

The late form of pure familial spastic paraplegia, J Vernea & G R Symington

Motor neuron disease in Australia (State of New South Wales), J W Lance, J Enis & J W Duckworth

The carpal tunnel syndrome: a clinical and electrophysiological study in 250 patients, S.C. Loong

Ocular motor involvement in post-infective polyneuropathy, W M Carroll & F L Mastaglia

Syndrome of ophthalmoplegia, ataxia and areflexia, C E Storey, G Selby & P M Williamson

The H reflex in the forearm muscles in normal subjects and patients with mild pyramidal syndrome, J Vernea

Intestinal giardiarsis, steatorrhoea and peripheral nerve dysfunction, M L Bassett, T A Cook & G Danta

Intermittent hydrocephalus due to cysts of the septum pellucidum: a study of three cases, S S Gubbay, R Vaughan & J S Lekias

Brachiocephaliac arteritis in a young female (Takayasu's disease), B S Gilligan

A case of Creutzfeldt-Jakob disease, R A Rodda

Saccadic velocities in multiple sclerosis and myasthenia gravis, F L Mastaglia, J L Black & D W K Collins

Diagnostic significance of autoantibodies and HLA in myasthenia gravis and multiple sclerosis, R L Dawkins, F L Mastaglia & P Kay

Electrophysiological and immunological studies in optic neuritis, R Garrick, J C Walsh & J G McLeod

Relapsing allergic neuritis, J D Pollard & G Selby

Clinical electrophysiological and pathological features of three cases of cerebromacular degeneration in childhood, J l Manson, R F Carter, M E Haynes & C G Keith

Peroneal muscular atrophy with autosomal dominant inheritance, J G McLeod & P A Low

Acupuncture for chronic back pain: patients and methods, G Mendelson, H Kranz, A Kidson, S T Loh, D F Scott & T S Sehvood

Observations on vascular neuropathies, H Urich

Pharmacokinetics of drugs used for petit mal 'absence' epilepsy, M J Eadie, J H Tyrer, G A Smith & L McKauge

Factors influencing plasma carbamazepine concentrations, C M Lander, M J Eadie & J H Tyrer

Phenobarbitone dosage in the neonate: preliminary communication, R A Ouvrier &
R Goldsmith

Therapeutic problems related to tonic status epilepticus, P F Bladin, F J Vajda &
G R Symington

Plasma sodium valproate levels and clinical response in epilepsy, M Anthony,
H Hinterberger & J W Lance

Spinal and cortical evoked potentials in multiple sclerosis, R Garrick & J G McLeod

Electrophysiological and computerised tomography findings in multiple sclerosis: a
comparative study, F L Mastaglia, J L Black, L A Cala & D W K Collins

Computerised tomography findings in multiple sclerosis and Schilder's disease,
L A Cala & F L Mastaglia

Computerised tomography of the cranium in patients with epilepsy: a preliminary
report, L A Cala, F L Mastaglia & T L Woodings

Parietal lobe atrophy: a report on two patients, J C Walsh & J L Allsop

Distal chronic spinal muscular atrophy involving the hands, D J O'Sullivan &
J G McLeod

Myosins in murine muscular dystrophy, R B Fitzsimons, J F Y Hob & J G McLeod

A syndrome of myopathy and polycythaemia in a young man, B A Kakulas

Effects of neostigmine and pyridostigmine at the neuromuscular junction,
J D Gillies & J Allen

Volume 15 - 1978
Contents

The E Graeme Robertson Memorial Lecture 1978:

Graeme Robertson and the golden age of neurology, R Hooper

Central pain mechanisms, A W Duggan

A review of some aspects of the pharmacology of levodopa, J G L Morris

The pharmacology of anticonvulsant drugs, M J Eadie

A case of spinal cysticercosis, I T Lorentz

Parasitic diseases of the nervous system in Thailand, A Vejjajiva

Vertebral metastases and spinal cord compression, B A Kakulas, C G Harper,
K Shibasaki & G M Bedbrook

Wernicke-Korsakov syndrome lesions in coronial necropsies, R Rodda,
R Cummings & K S Millingen

Association of central nervous system sarcoma with familial polyposis coli,
P M Williamson & K V Smith

Preliminary observations on the pharmacokinetics of methylphenobarbitone,
M J Eadie, F Bochner, W D Hooper & J H Tyrer

Sodium valproate: dose-plasma level relationships and interdose fluctuations,
F J E Vajda, G W Mihaly, J L Miles, P M Morris & P F Bladin

A comparison of the absorption of phenobarbitone given via the oral and the
intramuscular route, J K Graham

Posterior fossa arachnoid cysts: two case reports, G H Purdie & R H C Rischbieth

The causalgia syndrome treated with regional intravenous guanethidine,
J T Holland

Detection of experimental carotid ulceration by radionucleotide labelled particles,
G A Donnan, W J McKay, D P Thomas & P F Bladin

Acupuncture analgesia for chronic low back pain, G Mendelson, M A Kidson,
S T Loh, D F Scott, T S Selwood & H Kranz

Visuomotor skill and visual perception in left and right handed children of superior
intelligence, R Mellick, I Klajic, H Grahame & B Higgins

Individual free fatty acids and migraine, M Anthony

Autonomic dysfunction in the Landry-Guillain-Barre syndrome, R R Tuck &
J G McLeod

Electromyographic study of polysynaptic responses from muscles not supplied by
the stimulated nerve: preliminary report, J. Vernea

Memory disorder in vertebrobasilar disease, G A Donnan, K W Walsh & P F Bladin

Delayed radiation-induced damage to the brachial plexus, R Burns

An evaluation of bromocriptine in the treatment of Parkinson's disease,
R A MacKenzie & J W Lance

Neurological features of polyarteritis nodosa, G L Walker

Primary empty sella syndrome and benign intracranial hypertension, S Davis,
B Tress & J King

Occipital neuralgia, S R Hammond & G Danta

Some specific neurological complications of acute lymphocytic leukaemia of
childhood, D B Appleton, A F Isles & J R Tieman

The contribution of evoked potentials in the functional assessment of the
somatosensory pathway, F L Mastaglia, J L Black, R Edis & D W K Collins

Patterns of response to levodopa in Parkinson's disease, F J E Vajda, G A Donnan &
P F Bladin

Volume 16 - 1979

Contents

The E Graeme Robertson Memorial Lecture 1979:

I. Aspects of cuprogenic disorder in Wilson's disease in India, D K Dastur &
    D K Manghani

II. Pathology and pathogenesis of chronic myelopathy in atlantoaxial dislocation,
    with operative or postoperative haematomyelia or other cord complications,
    D K Dastur

Thoracic outlet syndrome secondary to childhood poliomyelitis, N W Knuckey &
    S S Gubbay

A retrospective study of carotid endarterectomy, G D Ohlrich & J R Kukums

The stroke syndrome of long intraluminal clots with incomplete vessel obstruction,
    G A Donnan & P F Bladin

Neuromyotonia in the spinal form of Charcot-Marie-Tooth disease, J W Lance,
    D Burke & J Pollard

Contribution of single motor units to the surface electromyogram, J L Veale &
    W J Russell

Brain infarction in young men, R J Burns, P C Blumbergs & M A Sage

The application of prolonged EEG telemetry and videotape recording to the study of
    seizures and related disorders, V Vignaendra, J Walsh & S Burrows

The epoxide of carbamazepine, L McKauge, J H Tyrer & M J Eadie

The neurological aspects of atrial myxoma, R Beran & E P Hicks

Cerebellar malformations: some pathogenetic considerations, H Urich

Adrenoleucodystrophy: a study of four patients, P G Procopis & R A Ouvrier

Primary lymphoma of the central nervous system: a case report, R A Mackenzie &
    S C Braye

Hypoglycaemia secondary to pancreatic islet cell adenoma, G L Coffey,
    D J O'Sullivan & W J Burke

Idiopathic communicating hydrocephalus: the prognostic significance of ventricular
    size after shunting, K S Millingen

Factors likely to affect the development of multiple sclerosis in patients presenting
    with optic neuritis in a tropical and subtropical area, P J Landy, M Innis &
    R Boyle

Antipyrine half-life as a measure of hepatic enzyme induction: clinical applications
    in a chronic epileptic population, E Byrne, A W Harman, D B Frewin &
    J F Hallpike

Urticaria pigmentosa: change in conscious state associated with rise in plasma
   histamine levels, G A Donnan & B J Jarrott

Oscillations in performance in levodopa-treated Parkinsonians: treatment with
   bromocriptine and 'Deprenyl', C M Lander, A Lees & G Stern

Ischaemic optic neuropathy, J King

Clinical application of the patterned light visual evoked response (a two-year
   experience at the Adelaide Children's Hospital), J I Manson, P F Weston &
   R G Beran

Observations on voluntary nystagmus, A Fisher, H Davies & S Wallis

Motor fibre refractory period and motor conduction velocity range, J Vernea

Trimethadione embryopathy: case report with review of the literature,
   R H Rischbieth

Two-dimensional echo encephalography in paediatric neurology, J I Manson,
   P F Weston & R Gent

Carbamazepine in two pregnancies, E P Hicks

Lepromatous leprosy as a model of Schwann cell pathology and lysosomal activity,
   D K Daslur & G L Porwal*

The neuropathology of a case of Pick's disease, R A Rodda

Idiopathic scoliosis, Scheurmann's disease and myopathy: two case reports,
   R B Fitzsimons

Computerised tomography in the leucodystrophies, P G Procopis

Familial trigeminal and glossopharyngeal neuralgia, N W Knuckey & S S Gubbay

Lipoma of the cauda equina: case report and review of the literature,
   R H C Rischbieth

Some aspects of the clinical use of clonazepam in refractory epilepsy, C M Lander,
   G A Donnan, P F Bladin & F J E Vajda

Volume 17 - 1980
Contents

The E Graeme Robertson Memorial Lecture 1980:
Myasthenia gravis: a clinical review, W J Burke
Music and neurology, J B Morley
A W Campbell: Australia's first neurologist, M J Eadie
Innovation in electroencephalography, F YingK'un, H ChingChin & K TanHua*
Clinicoelectroencephalographic studies in multiple sclerosis, F YingK'un
Patient perspectives of epilepsy, R G Beran & T Read
The clearance of anticonvulsant drugs in pregnancy, C M Lander, I Livingstone,
   J H Tyrer & M J Eadie

The effects of anticonvulsants on memory function in epileptic patients: preliminary findings, A T Butlin, L Wolfendale & G Danta

Method of source derivation for the EEG, L S Basser

Spontaneous dissecting aneurysms of the cervical internal carotid artery, J P Rice

Barlow's syndrome and cerebral emboli: a common cause of stroke in young patients?, K M R Grainger

Carotidynia: aetiology, diagnosis and treatment, B R Chambers, G A Donnan, R J Riddell & P F Bladin

Progressive multifocal leukoencephalopathy, J O King, D H L Hart, J R Sullivan, V M Surtees & R McD Anderson

Muscle disease and viruses, L Herzberg, G B Hamell, J Papadimitriou & N Tan

Transcutaneous sympathetic stimulation: effects on autonomic nervous function, S Bajada & A Touraine

Subacute cholinergic dysautonomia in childhood, I J Hopkins, L K Shield & M Harris

A clinical and electrophysiological study of neurologically induced winging of the scapula, S R Hammond & G Danta

The anatomy of occipital neuralgia, N Bogduk

The mitochondrial myopathies: 9 case reports and a literature review, R B Fitzsimons

Immunological studies of brainspecific antigens, R D Helme & J L Stow

Experimental neurogenic pulmonary oedema after discrete lesions in the ventrolateral medulla oblongata, W W Blessing

Neuropathology of the cortical lesions of the Parkinsonian-dementia (PD) complex of Guam, N T Tan, B A Kakulas, C L Masters, J C Gibbs & D C Gajdusek

Volume 18 - 1981

Contents

The E Graeme Robertson Memorial Lecture 1981:

Stretch compression neuropathy, Sir Sydney Sunderland

Myasthenia gravis: immune mechanisms and implications, J Newsom-Davis

Disordered muscle tone and movement, J W Lance

Hypotensive central spinal cord infarction: A clinicopathological study of 3 cases of aortic disease, P C Blumbergs, D Chin & J P Rice

A comparison of Australian caucasian and aboriginal brain weights, C Harper & L Mina

Bilateral optic nerve hypoplasia , R A Ouvrier, D Lewis, G Procopis, F A Billson, M Silink & M de Silva

Acetylcholine receptor antibodies in the diagnosis and management of myasthenia gravis, G A Nicholson & L R Griffiths

Serum induced demyelination: an electrophysiological and histological study, J D Pollard, B Harrison & P Gatenby

Compression of the tibial nerve by the tendinous arch of origin of the soleus muscle, F L Mastaglia, J Venerys, B A Stokes & R Vaughan

Hypokalaemic periodic paralysis unresponsive to acetazolamide, R H Rischbieth

A case of cortical deafness, C S Kneebone & R J Burns

Metachromatic leucodystrophy in children, P G Procopis

Preservation of acquired music performance functions with a dominant hemisphere lesion: a case report, D Erdonmez & J B Morley

Changes in peripheral and central nerve conduction with aging, A Mackenzie & H Phillips II

Evaluation of therapists by patients with epilepsy, C Sutton & R G Beran

How worthwhile is plasma primidone level measurement?, M J Eadie, R Heazlewood & J H Tyrer

Stroke syndromes in young people, B R Chambers, P F Bladin, K McGrath & A J Goble

Carotid endarterectomy at Royal Brisbane Hospital and Princess Alexandra Hospital, Brisbane, G D Ohlrich & J R Kukums

Retention of urine and sacral paraesthesia in anogenital herpes simplex infection, R H Edis

Substance P in the central nervous system, R D Helme & D W White

Optic nerve decompression in benign intracranial hypertension, C J Kilpatrick, D V Kaufman, E K Galbraith & J O King

Familial occurrence of meningioma: a case report, R Pamphlett & R A Mackenzie

Senile Parkinsonism and DOPA pharmacokinetics, G A Broe, M A Evans & E J Triggs

Assessment of disability in multiple sclerosis: a new approach to epidemiological study, R G Beran, V R Jennings & T Read

Volume 19 - 1982
Contents

The E Graeme Robertson Memorial Lecture 1982:

Multiple sclerosis: 50 years on, J Sutherland

Measles encephalitis, R T Johnson, D E Griffin, R Hirsh & A Vaisberg*

Experimental demyelinating optic neuropathy, W M Carroll, A Jennings & F L Mastaglia

Immunological studies in myotonic dystrophy, G L Walker, F L Mastagia, R J M Lane & U Karagol

Substance P in the trigeminal system at postmortem: evidence for a role in pain pathways in man, R D Helme & J L Fletcher

Comparison of diagnostic tests in myasthenia gravis, G A Nicholson, J G McLeod & L R Griffiths

Hormonal influence on water permeability across the blood-brain barrier, A C Reid, G M Teasdale & J McCulloch*

Myelopathy associated with decompression sickness: a report of six cases,
 F L Mastaglia, R I McCallurn & D N Walder

The hypereosinophilic syndrome, G H Putdie, D Kotasek & R H C Rischbieth

Concentric sclerosis, G YuPu & G ShuFang*

Amoebic meningitis also occurs in NSW, P G Procopis, Z Stuart & A Kan

Encephalitis in infectious mononucleosis, D H Todman

Hypopituitarism with arachnoid cyst, R H C Rischbieth

Diffuse infiltrating astrocytoma (gliomatosis cerebri) with 22 year history,
 P C Blumbergs, D K F Chin & J F Hallpike

Oculopharyngeal dystrophy: clinicopathological study of an Australian family,
 P C Blumbergs, D Chin, D Burrow, R J Burns & J P Rice

Hemimasticatory and hemifacial spasm: a common pathophysiology?,
 P D Thompson & W M Carroll

A case of Lhermitte-Duclos disease, P McCombe & B A Warren

Developmental anomalies affecting the fourth ventricular outflow region: a report
 of four cases, G L Coffey, D J O'Sullivan & T J Connelley

Neurophysiological evidence of aging in Down's syndrome, R A Mackenzie,
 H Creasey & C Y Huang

Parenchymal brain lesions in spontaneously hypertensive strokeprone rats,
 R A Rodda, T Brain & S Jones

Embolisation of cerebral arteriovenous malformations, P G McManis, G M Selby &
 W A Sorby

Senile dementia and hydrocephalus due to carotid dolichoectasia, C Huang,
 Y W Chan & R Wang

Carotid plaques and retinal emboli: a clinical, angiographic and morphological
 study, S F Berkovic, P F Bladin, L R Ferguson, J P Royle & D P Thomas

Steady-state valproate pharmacokinetics during long-term therapy, M J Eadie,
 V Heazlewood, L McKauge & J H Tyrer

Hepatotoxicity of sodium valproate, S F Berkovic, P F Bladin, D B Jones,
 R A Smallwood & F J E Vajda

Absence status in adults, S F Berkovic & P F Bladin

Demographics of an epileptic population, R G Beran, C Sutton & T Read

Volume 20 - 1984

Contents

The E Graeme Robertson Memorial Lecture 1983:
The longterm prognosis of Parkinson's disease, G Selby

Anticonvulsant effects on the memory performance of epileptics, A T Butlin,
 G Danta & M L Cook

Experience with continuous ambulatory EEG monitoring, S F Berkovic, P F Bladin,
 M D Connelly, L A Gossat, G R Symington & F J E Vajda

Convulsive status epilepsy: is there a role for thiopentone induced narcosis?, K
   Burton & J T Holland

Anti convulsants, folic acid and memory dysfunction in epileptics, A T Butlin,
   G Danta & M L Cook

Dilatation in the carotid vascular territory of the cat in response to activation of cell
   bodies in the locus coeruleus, P J Goadsby, G A Lambert & J W Lance

An analysis of the decision-making process in the management of malignant
   gliomas, R Iansek & J I Balla

Latency of late responses in lesions of lumbosacral nerve roots, P T Yeo

Fatal migraine, G Selby & J A Fryer

Neurovascular disturbances in headache patients, P D Drummond & J W Lance

Symptomatic hydrocephalus due to an elongated and ectatic basilar artery, R H Edis
   & T M H Chakera

Dexamethasone: pharmacokinetics in neurological patients, M J Eadie,
   T R O'R Brophy, G Ohlrich & J H Tyrer

Rubral tremor: clinical features and treatment of three cases, S F Berkovic &
   P F Bladin

Segmental motor paralysis in herpes zoster, J P Rice

Progressive myoclonic epilepsy, nerve deafness and spinal muscular atrophy,
   J W Lance & W A Evans

Neurological complications of mycoplasma pneumoniae infection, M A Hely,
   P M Williamson & T R Terenty

Psychometric and cranial CT study in myotonic dystrophy, G L Walker, R Rosser,
   F L Mastaglia & J N Walton

Scapuloperoneal myopathy, D H Todman & R A Cooke

Brainstem auditory evoked responses and quantitative saccade studies in multiple
   sclerosis: a comparative evaluation, W Knezevic, F L Mastaglia, Black &
   D W K Collins

Neuropathological findings in a case of coexistent progressive supranuclear palsy
   and Alzheimer's disease, D G Milder, C F Elliott & W A Evans

Central pontine myelinolysis with widespread extrapontine lesions: a report of two
   cases, R M Kalnins, S F Berkovic & P F Bladin

The plasticity of the Purkinje cell, H Urich

F-response studies. Computer analysis and recovery cycle, F L Mastaglia,
   W M Carroll &G W Thickbroom

Vaso activity of cerebrospinal fluid from patients with brain swelling, A C Reid,
   M Stewart & G M Teasdale

Volume 21 - 1985

Contents

The E Graeme Robertson Memorial Lecture 1984:

Some disorders of the central grey matter in children: clinical and radiological
    diagnosis, J Aicardi

Adult onset rod disease: a clinicopathological reappraisal, E Byrne

Peripheral neuropathy in IgM kappa paraproteinaemia: clinical and ultrastructural
    studies in two patients, J D Pollard, J G McLeod & D Feeney

Duchenne de Boulogne and human facial expression, R A Cuthbertson

Use of total and free anticonvulsant serum levels in clinical practice, R G Beran,
    J H Lewis, J L Nolte & A P Westwood

Valproate hepatotoxicity: a review and report of two instances in adults,
    R G Dickinson, M L Basset, J Searle, J H Tyrer & M J Eadie

Adult Lennox-Gastaut syndrome: features and diagnostic problems, P F Bladin

Adult Lennox-Gastaut syndrome: patients with large focal structural lesions,
    P F Bladin

The effect of infusion of various peptide antisera on vasodilatation in the cat
    common carotid vascular territory, P J Goadsby & G J Macdonald

The prognostic significance of intraventricular haemorrhage, P Kerr, R Iansek,
    R D Helme & A Rosengarten

Ocular and ocular motor aspects of primary thalamic haemorrhage, A Fisher &
    W Knezevic

Familial myasthenia gravis: a study of three families, D Chin & S S Gubbay

Brainstem auditory evoked responses in hereditary spinocerebellar ataxias,
    W Knezevic & E G StewartWynne

Triplicate posttraumatic sciatic nerve palsy: evoked potentials in the diagnosis,
    V M Synek & A E Hardy

Neuropathological findings in a case of chronic inflammatory polyneuropathy,
    D C Milder, D H L Rail & G A Broe

Availability of drug assay results and dosage advice improves antiepileptic care in a
    specialist neurology outpatient clinic, L L Ioannides Demos, A J McLean,
    J Wodak, N Tong, U Heinzow, M Horne, P M Harrison & B S Gilligan

Clinical experience with clobazam: a new 1,5 benzodiazepine in the treatment of
    refractory epilepsy, F J E Vajda, P F Bladin & B J Parsons

Examination of the problems confronting those with epilepsy, R G Beran &
    P L Flanagan

A simple and validated tool for the clinicjan to assess psychosocial status when
    conducting anticonvulsant drug trials, P J Flanagan & R G Beran

Peripheral neuropathy with gammopathy responding to plasmapheresis, J Frayne &
    R J Stark

Peripheral autonomic surface potential: a quantitative technique for recording
    autonomic neural function in man, W Knezevic & S Bajada

Vulnerability of the dorsal root ganglion in experimental allergic encephalomyelitis,
    M P Pender & T A Sears

Experimental allergic encephalomyelitis: effect of neonatal exposure to
neuroantigen or neuroantigen immune cells on subsequent reactivity as adults,
D O Willenborg & G Danta

Spatial contrast sensitivity in patients with multiple sclerosis, R Carter & G Danta

A decision analytic approach to the role of visual evoked response and cerebrospinal
fluid abnormalities in the management of singular spinal sclerosis, R Iansek &
J l Balla

Cerebral abscess in leukaemia: an unusual presentation of a rare complication,
M C Patterson, I H Bunce & M J Eadie

Ophthalmological complications of cryptococcal meningitis, J D Blackie, G Danta,
T Sorrell & P Collignon

Cryptococcal infection of the central nervous system, P A Sandstrom

Infantile Refsum's disease: a peroxisomal storage disorder?, J I Manson, A C Pollard,
A Poulos & R F Carter

Phytanic acid oxidase deficiency in childhood, G A Wise, B J Duffy, J D Mitchell,
A C Pollard, A Poulos & J Pollard

Volume 22 - 1986
Contents

Edrophonium test in myasthenia: quantitative oculography, I M Williams,
P Dickinson &A C Sum

A case of invasive thymoma associated with myasthenia gravis, myositis and
demyelinating neuropathy, H Miller, B D Shenstone, R Joffe & S Kannangara

Chronic subdural haematomas presenting with Parkinsonian signs, R F Peppard,
E Byrne & D Nye

Global stereopsis in stroke patients, B Fenelon, K Grant, A Delahunty, R Neill,
D Dunlop, P Dunlop, B Frost & A Quayle

Extradural malignancy simulating brachial neuritis, P C Gates, P A Kempster,
D Risebin & J l Balla

Peripheral sympathetic conduction velocity calculated from surface potentials,
T J Day, D Offerman & S Bajada

Myopathy with fatiguability: myositis or myasthenia?, R Peppard, E Byrne &
X Dennet

A clinical study of convulsive syncope, P A Kempster & J I Balla

Effects of age on the axon reflex response to noxious chemical stimulation,
R D Helme & S McKernan

The use of lisuride in severe Parkinson's disease, D Chin, Y L Yu & C Y Huang

The natural history of syringomyelia, N E Anderson, E W Willoughby &
P Wrightson

Thoracic intervertebral disc protrusion with spinal cord compression, B Gilligan &
J Frayne

Substance P in human hypothalamus, R D Helme & K Thomas

The neuropathology of progressive autonomic failure of central origin (the
Shy-Drager syndrome), B A Kakulas, N Tan & V J Ojeda
Cryoglobulinaemic neuropathy – a clinical spectrum, R F Peppard, E Byrne,
R McD Anderson & B J Clarke
Nonbacterial thrombotic endocarditis and stroke, R A L Macdonell, R M Kalnins &
G A Donnan
Evaluation of an introductory course in neurology, J l Balla & H Edwards
Lumbosacral nerve plexus compression by ovarian fallopian cysts, P T Yeo &
A C Grice
Genitofemoral neuropathy, R H Rischbieth
Transfer factor as a therapy for multiple sclerosis: a followup study, J A Frith,
J G McLeod, A Basten, J D Pollard, S R Hammond, D B Williams & P A Crossie
The neurochemical and clinical effects of 1-methyl-4-phenyl 1,2,3,6
tetrahydropyridine in small animals, G A Donnan, S J Kaczmarczyk,
T Solopotias, P Rowe, R M Kalnins, F J E Vajda & F A O Mendelsohn
Normative data for somatosensory evoked potentials from upper limb nerves in
middle-aged subjects, V M Synek

Volume 23 - 1987
Contents

The E Graeme Robertson Memorial Lecture, 1985:
Neurology of the sphincters, M Swash
Crossed facilitation and post-contraction depression of abductor pollicis brevis
motor neurones, W Knezevic, F L Mastaglia, G W Thickbroom & W M Carroll
Unusual paraspinal muscle lesions in ankylosing spondylitis, B A Kakulas,
I Morrison, E T Owen & R Kitridou
The pyriformis syndrome: review and case presentation, V M Synek
Clonic perseveration, G L Morris & J Leicester
The basis for aspirin dosage in stroke prevention, R A Brandon & M J Eadie
Cerebral infarction due to presumed haemodynamic factors in ambulant
hypertensive patients, G D McLaren & G Danta
Subcortical arteriosclerotic encephalopathy: Binswanger's disease, S E Mathers,
B R Chambers, J R Merory & l Alexander
Cranial CT scan appearances that correlate with patient outcome in acute stroke,
G J Hankey, S J Davis, E G Stewart-Wynne & T M H Chakera
Clinically unsuspected cardiac disease in patients with cerebral ischaemia, P Gates,
R Peppard, P Kempster, A Harris & M Pierce
Electrically evoked skin vasodilatation: a quantitative test of nociceptor function in
man, R A Westerman, A Low, A Pratt, J S Hutchinson, J Szolcsanyi, W Magerl,
H O Handwerker & W M Kozak
Neurogenic flare responses in chronic rheumatic pain syndromes, R D Helme,
G O Littlejohn & C Weinstein

Neurogenic plasma extravasation in response to mechanical, chemical and thermal stimuli, P V Andrews & R D Helme

Magnetoencephalography: locating the source of P300 via magnetic field recording, E Gordon, G Sloggett, I Harvey, C Kraiuhin, C Rennie, C Yiannikas & R Meares

Gliomas presenting outside the central nervous system, B J Brew & R Garrick

Neoplastic angioendotheliosis, B J Brew, D J O'Sullivan, P Darveniza, G Selby, J Fryer & W Evans

Cryptococcal infections of the central nervous system: a ten year experience, J A Waterson & B S Gilligan

Clobazam in the treatment of epilepsy, C Kilpatrick, R Bury, R Fullinfaw & R Moulds

The management of epilepsy in women of childbearing age and the Australian experience of valproate in pregnancy, M A W Curran*

Intensive neuromonitoring for complex partial seizures: focal seizure pattern variability in surgical patients, P F Bladin

Tolerance to the anticonvulsant effects of clonazepam and clobazam in the amygdaloid kindled rat, F J E Vajda, S J Lewis, Q L G Harris, B Jarrott & N A Young

Evaluation of the first 18 months of a specific rehabilitation programme for those with epilepsy, R G Beran, M Major & L Veldze

Impairment of consciousness in migraine, P A Kempster, R lansek & J I Balla

Cervical spondylosis and headaches, R lansek, J Heywood, J Karnaghan & J I Balla

Whiplash headache, J Balla & J Karnaghan

Diagnostic strategies of fifth year medical student in a neurological case. The importance of the first hypothesis, M Gibson, J Kaaden & J I Balla

An analysis of cranial computerized tomography scanning in private neurological practice, G J Hankey & E G StewartWynne

Acute encephalopathy following petrol sniffing in two aboriginal patients, R H Rischbieth, N Thompson, A Hamilton Bruce, G H Purdie & J N Peters

Bilateral intracerebral haemorrhage presenting with supranuclear ophthalmoplegia, bradykinesia and rigidity, G J Hankey & E G StewartWynne

Amnesia following right thalamic haemorrhage, M M Tsoi, C Y Huang, A O M Lee & Y L Yu

Ventriculoperitoneal shunting of acute hydrocephalus in vein of Galen malformation, K K Pun, Y L Yu, C Y Huang & E Woo

Isolated unilateral hypoglossal nerve palsy due to a chondroid chordoma, K Millingen & M Prentice

Herpes zoster arteritis: pathological findings, R A Mackenzie, P Ryan, W E Karnes & H Okazaki

Otocerebral mucormycosis a case report, R A L Macdonell, G A Donnan, R M Kalnins, M J Richards & P F Baldin

Lumboperitoneal shunting as a cause of visual loss in benign intracranial
   hypertension, B J Brew, R Garrick & T J Connelley

Volume 24 - 1987

Contents

Pregnancy and multiple sclerosis. An Australian perspective, J A Frith &
   J G McLeod

Diagnostic value of cerebrospinal fluid myelin basic protein in patients with
   neurological illness, L Davies, J G McLeod, A Muir & W J Hensley

Pseudo-multiple sclerosis: a clinico-epidemiological study, G J Hankey &
   E G Stewart-Wynne

Unreported symptomatic and asymptomatic ischaemic heart disease in patients
   presenting with TIA or minor stroke detected by the London School of Hygiene
   cardiovascular questionnaire and Minnesota coding of a routine ECG, P Gates,
   S Marwood, M Jelinek & M Scott

Lacunar infarction: a 12 month study, J Reimers, C de Wytt & B Seneviratne

A case-control study of cerebrovascular disease in Western Australia, K Jamrozik,
   E Stewart-Wynne, G Ward, P Giele, J Perica & C Phatouros

The Perth community stroke study: attack rates for stroke and TIA in Western
   Australia, E StewartWynne, K Jamrozik & G Ward

Paramedian thalamic and midbrain infarction: the 'mesencephalothalamic
   syndrome', J A Waterston R J Stark & B S Gilligan

Spinal arteriovenous malformations: some diagnostic difficulties with illustrative
   cases, E Byrne, R McD Anderson, K Henderson, J Cummins, P McNeill &
   E Gilford

Lipids in cerebrovascular disease: is there an association?, L Herzberg, J R L Maserei
   & A Taylor

Selection criteria for surgery in patients with refractory epilepsy, R Mackenzie,
   J S Smith, J Matheson, C Bucovaz, M Dwyer & C Morris

Post-temporal lobectomy seizures, P F Bladin

Scalp and intracerebral P300 in surgery for temporal lobe epilepsy, A Puce &
   P F Bladin

Clinical relevance of therapeutic drug level estimation with respect to clonazepam
   and carbamazepine: preliminary report, R G Beran, J Lewis, J Nolte & E Yip

Changes in clearance of sodium valproate with changes in dose, C J Kilpatrick,
   R W Bury, R O Fullinfaw & R F W Moulds

Oxcarbazepine: preliminary clinical and pharmacokinetic studies on a new anticonvulsant, W D Hooper, R G Dickinson, P R Dunstan, S C Pendlebury &
   M J Eadie

Glossopharyngeal neuralgia, J King

Pathological changes in the vagus nerve in diabetes and chronic alcoholism,
   YP Gui, J G McLeod & J Baverstock

Volume 25 - 1988

Contents

Abnormalities of visual evoked responses in hyperprolactinaemia, P T Yeo,
    S Kamaldeen & D Walker
Somatosensory evoked potentials, electroencephalography and CT scans in the
    assessment of the neurological sequelae of decompression sickness, C Yiannikas
    & R Beran
The flight of colours test. Its value as an indicator of dysfunction of the visual
    pathways, M A Hamilton-Bruce & A B Black
A prospective study of the predictive value of electroencephalographic
    abnormalities for epileptic loss of consciousness, S Collins & R Iansek
Transition from alpha to theta pattern coma in fatal cerebral anoxia, V M Synek &
    B J L Synek
Choreoathetosis and thalamic haemorrhage, R J Freilich & B R Chambers
Neurologists' use and interpretation of antiepileptic drug monitoring in the
    treatment of epilepsy, R G Beran, E Y S Yip & J J Ashley
Further clinical and pharmacokinetic observations on the new anticonvulsant,
    oxcarbazepine, R G Dickinson, W D Hooper, S C Pendlebury, D Moses &
    M J Eadie
Necropsy study of GABA/benzodiazepine receptor binding sites in brain tissue from
    chronic alcoholic patients, J J Kril, P R Dodd, A L Gundlach, N Davies,
    W E J Watson, G A R Johnston & C G Harper

Volume 26 - 1989
Contents

Optic neuritis and its significance, W I McDonald
Epilepsy in Gowers' understanding, a century ago, M J Eadie
Effect of haemodilution on experimental cerebral ischaemia, K Yamashita,
    S Kobayashi, S Yamaguchi & T Tsunematsu*
Spinal cord lesions induced by antigalactocerebroside serum, F L Mastaglia,
    W M Carroll & A R Jennings
Sympathetic neurons modulate plasma extravasation in the rat through a
    nonadrenergic mechanism, Z Khalil & R D Helme
Concordance between different measures of small sensory and autonomic fibre
    neuropathy in diabetes mellitus, R A Westerman, C Delaney, A Ivamy Phillips,
    M Horowitz & A Roberts
Hereditary motor and sensory neuropathy type ii followed in the next two
    generations by a clinically distal motor neuropathy, G Selby
The P300 event-related potential and regional cerebral blood flow in patients with
    Alzheimer's disease C Rennie, P Landau, A Singer, E Gordon, C Kraiuhin,
    Y Zurynski, A Howson & R Meares
The relationship between reaction time and latency of the P300 event-related
    potential in normal subjects and Alzheimers disease, C Kraiubin, C Yaannikis,
    S Coyle, E Gordon, C Rennie, A Howson, R Mears

Evaluation of evoked potentials and cerebrospinal fluid analysis in the differential diagnosis of multiple sclerosis, M A Hamilton Bruce, A B Black, D J Chappelt & P R Pannail

Neurological complications of sarcoidosis, R C Y Chen & J G McLeod

Can psychometric tools be used to analyse pain in a geriatric population?, R D Helme, B Katz, S Gibson & T Corran

Validity of a revised EEG coma scale for predicting survival in anoxic encephalopathy, V M Synek

The addition of bromocriptine to long-term dopa therapy in Parkinson's disease, G Selby

Daily salivary anticonvulsant monitoring in patients with intractable epilepsy, G K Herkes & M J Eadie

Possible extension of SPECT cerebral imaging in the investigation of epilepsy using radioiodinated benzodiazepines, D J Maddalena, R G Beran, A Jenkinson & G M Snowdon

Minocyline-induced benign intracranial hypertension, C M Lander

Factors influencing the yield of cranial CT scanning in a private neurological practice, D C Reutens & E G Stewart Wynne

A review of 20 cases of spastic dysphonia, S Whyte & P Darveniza

CNS cryptococcosis: unusual aspects, J l Cochius, R J Burns & J O Willoughby

Cerebral infarction in cryptococcal meningitis, Y L Yu, E Woo, F L Chan, T Y K. Chan & G CY Chan*

Iophendylate-induced basal arachnoiditis, C K Wong, E Woo & W L Yu*

Infarction of the conus medullaris: clinical and radiographic features, G K Herkes, G Selby & W A Sorby

Cerebral deposits of carcinoid tumour, E G Butler, R J Stark, K Siu & R A Sinclair

Obstructive hydrocephalus caused by multiple sclerosis, E G Butler & B S Gilligan

Posterior cortical atrophy, R S Delamont, J Harrison, M Field & R S Boyle

Focal cerebral ischaemia induced by postural change, L Sedal & J Heywood

Orthostatic tremora: case report, D Thyagarajan & P Gates

Traumatic hypoglossal nerve palsy, R S Delamont & R S Boyle

Volume 27 - 1990

Contents

The value to the clinical neurologist of electromyography in the 1990s, E. Stolberg

The evolution of J. Hughlings Jackson's thought on epilepsy, M J Eadie

Thirteen years longitudinal study of computed tomography, visual electrophysiology and neuropsychological changes in Huntington's chorea patients and 50% at risk asymptomatic subjects, L A Cala, J L Black, D W K Collins, R M Ellison & S A Zubrick

Mitomycin C induces a delayed and prolonged demyelination and conduction block due to Schwann cell destruction, K Westland, J D Pollard & A J Sumner

Pleuropulmonary fibrosis due to bromocriptine treatment for Parkinson's disease, D H Todman, W A Oliver & R L Edwards

Commencement of a paediatric EEG video telemetry service, A Bye, P Lamont & L Healy

P300 event-related potentials in de novo Parkinson's disease, J S Graham, C Yiannikas, E Gordon, S Coyle & J G L Morris

Revised LEG coma scale in diffuse acute head injuries in adults, V M Synek

Magnetoencephalography and late component ERPs, E Gordon, C Rennie & L Collins

Physical disability after stroke in the Perth community stroke study, C Anderson, K Jamrozik & E G Stewart-Wynne

Perth community stroke study: design and preliminary results, C Anderson, E StewartWynne, K Jamrozik, P Buryill & T Chakera

Volume 28 - 1991
Contents

The E Graeme Robertson Memorial Lecture - 1991:

Vertebrobasilar embolism, L R Caplan

Superior sagittal sinus thrombosis, A Mohammed, J G McLeod & J Hallinan

The influence of age on atrial fibrillation as a risk factor for stroke, R X You, J J McNeil, S J Farish, H M O'Malley & G A Donnan

Preliminary experience with 99mTcHMPAO SPECT in cerebral ischaemia, A E Baird, G A Donnan, M Austin, M R Newton & W J McKay

Mechanisms and clinical features of internal watershed infarction, A E Baird, G A Donnan & M Saling

Regional cerebral blood flow and recognition memory in elderly normals: potential application to Alzheimer's disease, R S Schwartz, C Burke, J Sears, E Gordon, J Batchelor, G Kostalas, R Meares & C Yiannikas

Colour duplex flow imaging in carotid arterial disease: correlation with intraarterial digital angiography, D H Todman, D J Hewson B Seneviratne & P Walsh

Pattern of memory deficits in a controlled psychometric study of thalamic haemorrhage, A Au, Y L Yu, M Tsoi & C M Chang*

A clinical and pathological study of progressive supranuclear palsy, J Frasca, P C Blumbergs, P Henschke & R J Burns

Ataxia telangiectasia presenting as an extrapyramidal movement disorder and ocular motor apraxia without overt telangiectasia, A Churchyard, R Stell & F L Mastaglia

Familial spastic paraplegia: an electrophysiological study of central sensory conduction pathways, P K Panegyres, G H Purdie, M A HamiltonBruce & R H C Rischbieth

Lithium neurotoxicity, G L Sheean

The chronic fatigue syndrome: a reappraisal and unifying hypothesis, E. Byrne

Lack of neurological abnormalities in Lewis rats with experimental chronic
   serum sickness, P A McCombe & M P Pender
Sensorimotor peripheral neuropathy in rheumatoid arthritis, P A McCombe,
   A C Klestov, A E Tannenberg, J B Chalk & M P Pender
Palmar cold threshold test and median nerve electrophysiology in carpal tunnel
   compression neuropathy, R A Westerman & C A Delaney
Intravenous immunoglobulin therapy in the inflammatory neuropathies,
   A Churchyard, T Day, K Grainger & F L Mastaglia
A prospective study of acute radioculopathy after scoliosis surgery, J W Dunne,
   P L Silbert & M Wren
Bicycling induced pudendal nerve pressure neuropathy, P L Silbert, J W Dunne,
   R H Edis & E G StewartWynne
Botulinum toxin treatment of spasmodic torticollis, L Davies & I T Lorentz
The value of non-invasive spinal cord monitoring during spinal surgery and
   interventional angiography, J W Dunne & C M Field
Late-onset acid maltase deficiency in a Chinese girl, K S Wong, C Lai & H K Ng*
Inter-operator variability in quantitative electroencephalography, M A Hamilton-
   Bruce, K L Boundy & G H Purdie
The use of magnetic resonance imaging in neurological practice - a local
   experience, D Chin & P Lo*
Neuropsychological assessment in lamotrigine treated epileptic patients, G K
   Banks & R G Beran
Zeta waves: a distinctive type of intermittent delta wave studied prospectively,
   J W Dunne & P L Silbert
Intrathecal baclofen for severe spasticity: five years experience, E G Stewart-
   Wynne, P L Silbert, S Buffery, D Periman & E Tan
Noxious heat hyperalgesia test instrument, R A Westerman, R W Carr, W
   Brenton, J C Kiln, I Pano, A Rabavilas, C A Delahunty & R D G Roberts

Volume 29 - 1992

Contents

The E Graeme Robertson Memorial Lecture - 1992:
Interesting Neurological Syndromes, J W Lance
History of neurology in Australia, G Selby
XIXth Century pre-Jacksonian concepts of epileptogenesis , M J Eadie
Update on surgical treatment of epilepsies, J Engel Jr
Psychosocial aspects of epilepsy and of epilepsy surgery, P F Bladin
The influence of other anticonvulsants on the plasma concentration
   of E-2-en-valproate, D B McLaughlin, G E McKinnon & M J Eadie
Videoaudio/EEG monitoring in epilepsy: the Queen Elizabeth Hospital experience,
   S A Koblar, A B Black & G J Schapel

Salivary concentrations of antiepileptic drags, oestradiol and progesterone throughout pregnancy in epileptic women, G K Herkes & M J Eadie

Automatisms: the current legal position related to clinical practice and medico-legal interpretation, R G Beran

Video EEG analysis of nonictal events in children, A S Bye & J Nunan

P300 eventrelated potentials correlated with cerebral blood flow in nondemented patients with lacunar infarction, K Yamashita, S Kobayashi, H Koide, K Okada & T Tsunematsu*

Vigabatrin plasma enantiomer concentration and clinical effects, G Sheean, T Schramm, D S Anderson & M J Eadie

Predicting survival after stroke: experience from the Perth community stroke study, C S. Anderson, K D Jamrozik & E G Stewart-Wynne

Thrombolytic therapy in vertebrobasilar occlusion, D Thyagarajan, J Stark, J Frayne, B S Gilligan & N Sacharias

Comparison of transcranial doppler with DSA in vertebrobasilar ischaemia, L M Cher, B R Chambers & V Smidt

Confounding factors in noninvasive tests of neurovascular function in diabetes mellitus, R A Westerman, L E Lindblad, D Wajnblum, R G D Roberts & C A Delaney

Frontal signs following subcortical infarction, A J Corbett, H Bennett & S Kos

The molecular genetics of mitochondrial cytopathies: the Melbourne experience, D Thyagarajan, E Byrne, X Dennet & S Marzuki

Antiganglioside antibodies in peripheral neuropathy, P A McCombe, R Wilson & R L Prentice

Hereditary sensory radicular neuropathy: defective neurogenic inflammation, R A Westerman, A Block, A Nunn, C A Delaney, A Hahn, X Dennett & R W Carr

Reflex sympathetic dystrophy: altered axon reflex and autonomic responses, R A Westerman, I Parto, A Rabavilas, A Hahn, A Nunn, R G D Roberts & H Burry

Enigmatic trigeminal sensory neuropathy diagnosed by facial skin biopsy, P L Silbert, G R Kelsall, J M Shepherd & S S Gubbay

Late radiation associated neurological injury, A G Kerrnode, T J Day & W M Carroll

Postinfectious myelitis, encephalitis and encephalomyelitis, C M Chang, H K Ng, Y W Chan, S Y Leung, K Y Fong & Y L Yu

The cervical spine in fatal motor vehicle accidents, J Leditschke, R M D Anderson* W S C Hare

Low osmolar and nonionic xmy contrast media and cortical blindness, A G Kermode, T Chakera* F L Mastaglia

Effect of ritanserin, a highly selective 5HT2 receptor antagonist, on Parkinson's disease, J Henderson, C Yiannikas* J S Graham

334

Volume 30 - 1993

Contents

Volume 31 - 1994

Contents

Huntington's disease in Hong Kong Chinese: epidemiology and clinical picture, C M Chang, E L Yu, K Y Fong, M T H Wong, Y W Chan, T H K Ng, C M Leung & V Chan*

Isaac's syndrome: report of a case responding to valproic acid, T J O'Brien & P Gates

Routine use of lamotrigine, a new antiepileptic medication, and the value of measuring its blood levels, R G Beran, K Sheehan & M I Tilley

Rhinocerebral mucormycosis presenting as periorbital cellulitis with blindness: report of 2 cases, T J O'Brien & P McKelvie

Primary cerebral abscess due to nocardia asteroids presenting as stroke, R T F Cheung, Y L Yu & C M Chang

Alzheimer's disease and Alzheimer type of cerebral degenerations in Chinese, H K Ng

Appendix IX

E Graeme Robertson Memorial Lecturers
and their Lecture Titles

Year	Lecturer	Lecture title
1978	R Hooper	Graeme Robertson and the golden age of neurology
1979	D Dastur	Aspects of cuprogenic disorder in Wilson's disease in India
1980	W Burke	Myasthenia gravis: a clinical review
1981	S Sunderland	Stretch-compression neuropathy
1982	J M Sutherland	Multiple sclerosis fifty years on
1983	G Selby	The long-term prognosis of Parkinson's disease
1984	J Acardi	Some disorders of the central grey matter in children: clinical and radiological diagnosis
1985	H J Barnett	Vascular disease
1986	M Swash	Neurology of the sphincters
1987	R Balogh	Neuro-otology
1988	W I Mcdonald	Optic neuritis and its significance
1989	J Morgan-Hughes	The molecular biology of mitochondrial disease
1990	E Stalberg	The value to the clinical neurologist of electro-myography in the 1990s
1991	L B Caplan	Vertebro-basilar embolism
1992	J W Lance	Interesting neurology syndromes
1993	A Harding	Mitochondrial genes and neurological disease
1994	W Landau	—
1995	J B Posner	Neurological paraneoplastic syndromes: a review of diagnosis and prospects for therapy
1996	M J Eadie	Concerning a very noble lady of a most curious shape
1997	J G McLeod	Multiple sclerosis in Australia
1999	B Kakulas	Molecular genetics in the diagnosis of neuro-muscular disease
2000	F Mendelsohn	Neuroscience at the Howard Florey Institute
2001	T Brandt	The vestibular cortex: its location, function and disorders

2002 S Berkovic   Causes of epilepsies: how do genetic and acquired factors interact?

2003 R Burns   The neurology of leadership

2004 W Carroll   Demyelinating optic neuropathy: and insight into the changing practise of neurology

2005 P Doherty   Immune memories are made of this

2006 J Morris   Cases and faces

2007 C Storey   From vital spirit to vital time

2008 J Pollard   Mechanisms and management of inflammatory neuropathy

2009 R Stark   Headaches and homicides

2010 E Byrne   Crossing the crevasses, new major challenges for clinical neuroscience

2011 D Burke   The primacy of the spinal cord in the control of movement

2012 S Davis   Stroke in evolution - a tale of two strategies

2013 C Yiannikis   Evoked potentials: the relationship between structure and function

2014 F Mastaglia   Immune-mediated inflammatory myopathies

2015 R Frith   Is Australasian neurology ready for the next golden era?

2016 E Somerville   Self-induced syncope: not for the faint of heart

2017 M Halmagyi   Disorders of the vestibular system: what we have learned in the last 100 years

2018 N Anderson   The spectacular advance of the autoimmune encephalopathies

2019 R Macdonell   Achievements and challenges in multiple sclerosis

2021 C Lueck   The optic chiasm: studies in architecture and neurology

2022 S Vusic   Pathogenesis of motor neuron disease: from the motor cortex and beyond

Appendix X

Other Named Lectures and Orations of the Australian Association of Neurologists

Mervyn Eadie Lectures

Year	Lecturer	Lecture title
2001	David Burke	The properties and functions of myelinated axons
2002	John Pollard	Mechanisms and management in inflammatory demyelinating neuropathy
2003	Frank Mastaglia	Parkinson's disease – what role do genes play?
2004	Stephen Davis	Stroke in evolution – imaging and management
2006	Graeme Hankey	Stroke treatment and prevention: an evidence-based approach
2007	Neil Anderson	Limbic encephalitis, viruses and antibodies
2008	Geoffrey Donnan	Clinical neuroscience trials in Australia: is there a future?
2009	Phillip Thompson	The signs of a neurologist
2010	Garth Nicholson	Viewing diseases: seeing history and looking for preventions and cures through genes
2011	Robert Ouvrier	Charcot-Marie-Tooth disease in the 19th and 21st centuries
2012	Pamela McCombe	Something old, something new
2013	Ingrid Scheffer	Is the epilepsy exome changing clinical practice?
2014	Elsdon Storey	The neurologist and the *arbor vitae*
2015	Sam Berkovic	Precision medicine: a new pharmacology of epilepsy
2016	Matthew Kiernan	Chance and design: translations in clinical neurology
2017	Robert Henderson	Evolution, handedness and MND
2018	Victor Fung	The patient as pearl: personalised research and the treatment in Parkinson's disease
2019	Carolyn Sue	An unplanned path to discovering the importance of *chi*
2021	Mark Cook	Seizures and cycles: patterns and prediction
2022	Amy Brodtmann	Nuns and orthodoxies: charting vascular neurodegeneration

W Ian McDonald Lectures

Year	Lecturer	Lecture title
2008	A Lees	The Parkinson sphinx
2009	D Miller	Perspectives of multiple sclerosis over thirty years
2010	A Compston	Limiting and repairing the damage in multiple sclerosis
2011	M Hanna	Translational research in muscle channelopathies – genetics, disease mechanisms and treatment trials
2012	S Kuwabara	Neuromyelitis optica: concepts in evolution
2013	A Ascherio	Can we prevent multiple sclerosis
2014	M Pender	The role of Epstein-Barr virus in the pathogenesis of multiple sclerosis
2015	S Pittock	NMO spectrum disorders
2016	M Reilly	Emerging therapies in hereditary neuropathies
2017	X Montalban	Multiple sclerosis: a 30-year tale
2018	G Giovanoni	Trialling new drugs and approaches in progressive multiple sclerosis
2019	J Hillert	Patient value of multiple sclerosis research – from genes to quality of life care
2021	E Willoughby	MS redux: looking back over 48 years
2022	T Anderson	Parkinson's and NZP3 - is it worth the effort?

James Lance Orations

2019	D Burke	James W Lance: the science of neurology.
2021	I Scheffer	The promise of precision medicine for the epilepsies
2022	G Donnan	The new frontier – prehospital stroke care

Appendix XI

L B Cox Awards & ANZAN Medal Awards

L B Cox Awards

Year	Awardee	Paper title
2000	T Kilpatrick	LIF and life for academic neurology
2001	S Kolbar	Wiring the nervous system – a matter of guidance
2002	M Kiernan	Demyelinating neuropathies
2003	C Sue	Expanding the umbrella of mitochondrial disease
2004	P Batchelor	Neural regeneration after spinal cord injury
2006	L Vadlamudi	Genetics of epilepsy – the testimony of twins
2007	D Williams	The tau of PSP: untangling the diagnosis of atypical Parkinsonism
2008	M Parsons	Guiding stroke therapy with advanced brain imaging
2009	R Henderson	A tale of three cities
2010	A Krishnan	Novel clinical paradigms for neuropathy identification and treatment
2011	S Vudic	Novel insights into the physiopathological mechanisms of ALS
2013	B Campbell	Individualising ischaemic stroke management using advanced imaging
2014	S Lewis	The many (masked) faces of Parkinson's
2015	M Needham	Trying to understand inclusion body myositis: the importance of collaboration
2016	K Kumar	Use of next generation sequencing to shed light on movement disorders and mitochondrial disease
2017	M Farrar	Findings in nerve neverland: a neuromuscular adventure
2018	P Menon	ALS pathogenesis: site of disease onset and mechanisms underlying disease spread
2019	T Kalincik	Multiple sclerosis: navigating treatment choice
2020	R Ahmed	Physiological changes in neurodegererative dementias
2021	P Perucca	The genetics of focal epilepsies: from research to clinical practice
2022	D Ramanathan	Fighting friendly fire: the immunology, diagnosis and therapeutics of auto-immunity

ANZAN Medal Awards

2010	John Morris
2011	no award
2012	Richard Stark
2013	William Carroll
2014	John King
2015	Pamela McCombe
2016	Geoffrey Herkes
2017	Elsdon Storey
2018	David Burke
2019	Mervyn Eadie
2021	Richard Frith
2022	Amanda Jones

Index

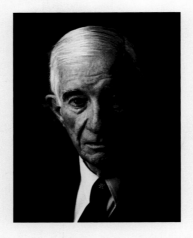

Mervyn J Eadie AO, MD, PhD, FRCP Edin, FRACP

Emeritus Professor of Clinical Neurology and Neuropharmacology, University of Queensland and Honorary Consultant Neurologist, Royal Brisbane and Women's Hospital, Brisbane. His medical interests are epilepsy and headache and their treatment, and also the history of neurology.

Books

Eadie M J (2000) *Wanderings in a Borderland – the Eadie Historical Collection.* Perth. Black Swan Press.

Eadie MJ (2012) *Headache – through the centuries.* New York. Oxford University Press.

Books co-authored

Eadie, M J & Tyrer, J H (1974) *Anticonvulsant therapy: Pharmacological basis and practice.* Churchill-Livingstone, Edinburgh and London. (Translated into Italian and Japanese.)

Sutherland, J M & Eadie, M J (1980) *The epilepsies – modern diagnosis and treatment.* Edinburgh, London, New York. Churchill-Livingstone, 3rd edition.

Eadie, M J & Tyrer, J H (1980) *Neurological Clinical Pharmacology.* New York. ADIS Press.

Eadie, M J & Tyrer, J H (1982) *Biochemical Neurology. Lancaster.* MTP. Press.

Eadie, M J & Tyrer, J H (1985) *Biochemistry of Migraine.* Lancaster, MTP. Press.

Eadie M J & Bladin P F (2001) *A Disease Once Sacred.* Sydney. John Libbey & Co.

Scott, AE, Eadie M J & Lees A (2012) *Sir William Richard Gowers 1845–1915 – exploring the Victorian brain.* Oxford. Oxford University Press.

Eadie M J & Vajda FJE (2015) *Antiepileptic Drugs and Pregnancy.* Heidelberg. Springer.